HOMŒOPATHIC PROVINGS,

CONTAINING THE VIENNA PROVINGS OF

COLOCYNTH AND THUJA-OCCIDENTALIS,

AND THE SYMPTOMS OF

AETHUSA-CYNAPIUM,
ALCOHOL-SULPHURIS,
AMPHISBÆNA-VERMICULARIS,
ANAGALLIS-ARVENSIS,
APIS-MELLIFICA,
ARISTOLOCHIA-MILHOMENS,
ARSENICUM-METALLICUM,
ARTEMISIA-VULGARIS,
ASTERIAS-RUBENS,
CINNABARIS,
TURPETHUM,
COCCUS-CACTI.

BEING THE APPENDIX TO THE

NORTH AMERICAN HOMŒOPATHIC JOURNAL.

EDITED BY

JAMES W. METCALF, M.D.

NEW-YORK:
WILLIAM RADDE, 322 BROADWAY.
PHILADELPHIA: RADEMACHER & SHEEK.—BOSTON: OTIS CLAPP.—ST. LOUIS
C. F. WESSELHOEFT.—MANCHESTER: TURNER, 97 PICCADILLY.

1853.

CONTENTS.

CONTENTS.

HOMŒOPATHIC MEDICINES.

WILLIAM RADDE,

322 BROADWAY, NEW-YORK,

Respectfully informs the Homœopathic Physicians, and the friends of the System, that he is the sole Agent for

THE LEIPZIG CENTRAL HOMŒOPATHIC PHARMACY,

and that he has always on hand a good assortment of the best Homœopathic Medicines, in complete sets, or by single vials, in

TINCTURES, DILUTIONS, AND TRITURATIONS.

Also, *Pocket Cases of Medicines; Physicians' and Families' Medicine Chests to Laurie's Domestic* (60 to 82 Remedies)—Epp's (60 Remedies)—Hering's (60 Remedies to 102).

Small Pocket Cases at $3, with Family Guide, and 27 Remedies.

Cases containing 415 vials, with Tinctures and Triturations for Physicians.

Cases with 268 Vials of Tinctures and Triturations to Jahr's New Manual, or Symptomen-Codex.

Physicians' Pocket Cases, with 60 Vials of Tinctures and Triturations.

Cases from 200 to 300 Vials, with low and high dilutions of medicated pellets.

Cases from 50 to 80 Vials of low and high dilutions, &c., &c.

Homœopathic Chocolate.

Refined Sugar of Milk, pure Globules, &c.

Arnica Tincture, the best specific remedy for bruises, sprains, wounds, &c.

Arnica Plaster, the best application for Corns.

Arnica Salve, Urtica urens tincture and salve, and Dr. Reisig's Homœopathic Pain Extractor, are the best remedies for Burns.

Canchalagua, a specific in Fever and Ague.

ALSO,

BOOKS, PAMPHLETS, AND STANDARD WORKS ON THE SYSTEM,

IN THE ENGLISH, FRENCH, SPANISH, AND GERMAN LANGUAGES.

☞ Physicians ordering medicines will please mark after each one its strength and preparation, as:

moth. tinct. for mother tincture.

1. *trit.* or 3. *trit.* for first or third trituration.

6. *in liq.* or 30. *in liq.* for six or thirtieth attenuation in liquid.

3. *in glob.* or 30. *in glob.* for third or thirtieth attenuation in globules.

Thuja Occidentalis.

The following exhausting proving of *Thuja Occidentalis* is translated from the *Oesterreichische Zeitschrift*, *Band* 2, *s*. 289 *et seqq*:—a part of it has already appeared fragmentarily in the *Homœopathic Examiner*, volume 5, page 159, &c. It is here reproduced entire, with corrections, that it may be more conveniently studied and referred to by students of the Materia Medica and the Profession.

EDS. NORTH AM. HOM. JOURNAL.

THUJA OCCIDENTALIS.

AN ESSAY.

BY CARL MAYRHOFER, M. D.

CHAPTER I.

Etymology, synonymes, description and chemical constitution of Thuja.

THE term "*arbor vitæ*," has a threefold acceptation in literature; pharmacological, botanical, and anatomical.

Van Helmont wrote a special treatise entitled "*arbor vitæ*," by which he understood a macrobiotic mixture, among the ingredients of which the wood and resin of the cedar hold the principal rank. It was supposed that life was prolonged by the continued use of this drug; that it was a prophylactic against every disease, and that it gave strength to patients; it was looked upon as a sort of elixir of life, such as are found in abundance in the older books on medicine, evidences of the mystic faith of those times, and such as are sold even now to the credulous public for their weight in gold.

Every physician knows what is meant by "arbor vitæ" anatomically. On making a deep longitudinal cut through the lobes of the cerebellum, the substance of the brain presents the appearance of a tree, called by the anatomists *arbor vitæ*, because the cerebellum was supposed to be the principal seat of life.

The subject of our essay is, however, a real tree, the western *arbor vitæ* or *Thuja occidentalis*. In the time of Francis I., king of France, this tree was imported into France from Canada. The first specimen was seen by Clusius in the royal garden of Fontainebleau, and a tolerably correct figure and description of it were furnished by him under the name of *arbor vitæ*.* The Greek name *θύα* also *θύεια* or *θύια* from *θύειν*, *suffire*, to fumigate, points to a resinous tree, and is first seen in Theophrastus Lesbius, a disciple of Aristotle; in his work, "*περι φυτων ἱστοριας*," he describes a tree resembling the cypress and called *θύον* (*δένδρον*) or *θύα* (*ἰδεα*, *species*). Roman authors latinized the word *θύα*, changing it to Thya, Thuya, Thuia, Thuja, as *θύς* gen. *θύεος*, was changed to *thus*, gen. *thuris*, and the word *κυπαρισσος* to *cupressus*. We have adopted in this essay the spelling *Thuja*, which is most frequently used and is most correct.

* Caroli Clusii Rarior. Plantar. Histor., 1601.

A

In the copious synonymes of *Thuja*, there seems to be some confusion. According to Theophrastus, the precious carvings in the temples of the ancient Greeks were made of the indestructible wood of the *ϑύα*. In his Natural History,* Pliny quotes Theophrastus, with the remark that the tree which was called by the Greeks *ϑύον* or *ϑύα* was known to Homer. Clusius says (loc. cit.): "*Ad quam arborem veteribus descriptam referenda sit* (*arbor vitæ*), *non facile quis conjiciat*," adding that it was generally believed that the arbor vitæ is the *ϑύα* of Theophrastus. Bauhinius calls the arbor vitæ *Thuja Theophrasti*, and even in our own time the belief is entertained by some that the Thuja Theophrasti is our Thuja.

We do not accede to this opinion. The native region and habitat of the Thuja of Theophrastus, according to his account, is the territory of Cyrene, in Africa, and especially the region in which the temple of Jupiter Ammon was situated, whereas our Thuja is a native of North America and Siberia, and could not, therefore, have been known to the ancients.

Our own inquiries have led us to assume that the Thuja of Theophrastus is the *Thuja articulata* of Vahl, who has shown to a certainty that it is from the *Thuja articulata* that we obtain sandarac, and not, as has been falsely believed heretofore, from a species of juniper. Shaw described the tree as a species of cypress, but in the Flora Atlantica by Desfontaines it is considered as a species of Thuja; and recently we have accurately ascertained by the French expedition to Algiers and Morocco, that sandarac (*el grassa*), of which Morocco furnishes from 600–700 hundred weight, is derived from the *Thuja articulata*, which the French botanists found throughout the territory of Algiers, and which probably likewise exists in Tunis and Tripoli, the ancient Cyrene, whence the ancients also may have derived it.

The terms "*arbor vitæ, arbor paradisea, arbre de vie, tree of life*," are derived from the French, who first cultivated it. Clusius thinks that the term *arbor vitæ* arose from the perennial verdure of the tree, *immortalis coma*, and from its strong and reputed healthy odor, and that it was afterwards adopted by all subsequent writers.† Dioscorides calls our Thuja *Cedrus major;* Bellonius, *Sabina altera;* Targione, *Cupressus arbor vitæ;* Camerarius calls it simply *Thuja*, and Mönch, *Thuja obtusa*. Linnæus finally gave it the name of *Thuja occidentalis*, in contradistinction from the Eastern Thuja, *Thuja orientalis*, which was brought to Europe from northern China.

The *Thuja occidentalis*, which is found in the West Indies, in the United States of North America and in Canada, belongs, according to

* Hist. Nat., lib. xiii, cap. xvi.

† We take this opportunity of observing that the symptoms which the provers of Thuja experienced, by no means reminded them of the golden fruits of Paradise; the consciousness, however, of something paradisaical in the sacrifice of his own health at the shrine of science and humanity, that by that means the health of others may be preserved, sustains the prover in the midst of the ingratitude of the indifferent and the contumely of opponents.—*Mayrhofer.*

the natural system of plants, to the family of the *Coniferæ Strobilaceæ*, and more particularly to the variety "cypress;" according to Linnæus' sexual system it belongs to the class *Monoecia.* The common Thuja attains a height of from thirty to forty feet; its branches spread horizontally in the shape of a fan; the twigs are broad and flat; the scales of the leaves are placed over one another in four rows like the tiles of a roof; each scale is provided with a gland in the middle of the upper surface, from which the Thuja-oil is secreted. The little cones are egg-shaped, and contain winged seeds which, like all the varieties of Thuja, Cypress and Juniper, are provided with two cotyledons; this distinguishes them from the varieties of pine which are of the class *polycotyledoneæ.* On pressing out the oil from the glands by rubbing the twigs, they emit a strong odor, and their beautiful green changes in winter by the alteration of the chlorophyll into a reddish brown which is dark in proportion to the coldness of the season.

The native regions of the Thuja are North America and Siberia. In Germany it is frequently used as an ornament in parks, and is frequently cut into all sorts of stiff shapes according to the French taste. In Upper Austria single Thujas are frequently found on farms, like the Sabina, and are called Cedars. The Thuja orientalis is distinguished from the Thuja occidentalis by its erect branches, the furrowed scales of its leaves, its unwinged seeds, and the absence of the peculiar odor.*

Constituents of the Thuja occidentalis.—Besides the ordinary constituents which are found in every plant, the Thuja contains, like most coniferæ, an ethereal oil of a strong odor, and a resin, its usual attendant.

The ethereal oil, which exists in a lesser quantity in the Thuja than might have been expected from its strong smell, is obtained by distilling

* Thuja Occidentalis. *Common arbor vitæ.* Branchlets two-edged, spreading; leaves imbricated in four rows, ovate-rhomboid, closely compressed, with a small flattened gland on the back; cones nodding, obovoid, the scales few (5–7), inferior ones truncate, gibbous at the tip; seed compressed, winged all round. *Linn. sp.* 2, *p.* 1002; *Michx. fl.* 2, *p.* 226; *Pursh. fl.* 2, *p.* 646; *Michx. Sylv.* 2, *p.* 156; *Ell. sk.* 2, *p.* 644; *Bigel. fl. Bost. p.* 361; *Beck, bot. p.* 338; *Hook, fl. Bor.-Am.* 2, *p.* 165; *Loud. Enc. tr. & shr., p.* 1068.

A tree with a narrowly conical and tapering head, [in New York] seldom more than 30–35 feet high and 6–12 inches in diameter, much branched; the ultimate divisions flattened and covered with numerous obtuse shining leaves, each furnished with a little vesicle which (as in the white Cedar) is filled with a thin aromatic turpentine. Sterile aments minute at the extremity of the branchlets, consisting of a few concave, scale-like anthers. Cones about five lines long, yellowish-brown; the scales loosely imbricated, opening to the base. Seeds conspicuously winged, emarginate, one under each scale.

Rocky banks of rivers and hill-sides, also in swamps; abundant and very conspicuous on the Hudson above Newburgh; Oriskany swamp; and various parts of the northern and western counties [of the State of New York]. *Fl.* May. The wood is light, of a reddish color and though soft, is very durable. It is not much used for lumber, as its trunk does not afford pieces of sufficient length. It is often planted about houses and in pleasure-grounds. In some parts of the country it is called White Cedar, and in New England it is often called Hackmatack.—*Torrey, Fl. State N. Y.*

the branches with water. It has been recently examined and analyzed by Schweizer with great care. It is a mixture of at least two kinds of oil containing oxygen. It does not contain any carburetted hydrogen.*

When freshly prepared it is entirely colorless, but it soon becomes yellowish. It occasions the peculiar odor of Thuja and possesses an acrid taste. It is lighter than water, is but sparingly soluble in that liquid, but dissolves readily in alcohol and ether.

The anhydrous oil, the water having been removed in two different ways by chloride of calcium, was found to contain:

Carbon	77,99	77,25.
Hydrogen	10,73	11,11.
Oxygen	11,28	11,64.

CHAPTER II.

Ante-Hahnemannian notions of the medicinal virtues of Thuja.

The medicinal powers of Thuja were first brought from the regions of faith into those of knowledge by Hahnemann: it is he who, by means of physiological provings, has given us the golden key to all the treasures of nature in her medicinal preparations.

He says†—"Before me no serious medicinal use was ever made of this plant in Europe; the remarks of Parkinson and Hermann about the virtues of Thuja are mere theoretical conjecture, after the fashion of their beloved *Therapia generalis.*

Clusius says (l. c.): "*Non dubium est, quin ad pleraque sit utilis (arbor vitæ); nemo vero illius facultates nostro ævo prodidit. Cum tamen magnam habeat partium tenuitatem, et amariuscula sit, verosimile est digerendi et abstergendi facultate proditam esse.*"

We must excuse the age of Clusius for the breakneck conclusion, that Thuja must have a dissolvent and a detergent power because it is a fine and bitter plant.

Tabernæmontanus, dutiful disciple of Galen as he is, declares as follows: "The taste and odor of Thuja show that it must be of a warm and dry nature; but we do not yet know what it is good for."

Camerarius‡ expresses himself in a similar manner: "This tree ought not to be lightly esteemed, not only on account of its strong smell, but also on account of its other virtues. A water and an oil may be prepared from it, which are said to be an excellent remedy against gouty pains, if properly used."

* The presence of oxygen distinguishes the oil of Thuja from the oil of Sabina and from turpentine, these two latter oils being free from oxygen and having an analogous composition. C^{10} H^{16}.

† Rein. Arzn. M. L., 2 Anfl. B. 5, s. 123.

‡ Hort., p. 186.

In the *Cynosura Materiæ Medicæ Pauli Herrmanni*, which was continued by *Bocclerus* (editio II., Argentorati, 1747, p. 565) the following virtues are ascribeed to Thuja: "*Folia (thujæ) resolvunt, exsiccant, flatus pellunt, et sudorem cient. Parkinsonus folia tenera et cruda cum butyro pani illito comesta ad tenaces et viscidos 'humores expectorandos nonnullis in usu esse scribit.*"

Krunitz (Encyklop. B. 66) gives the following extended version of this passage (probably from the first edition of Herrmann's Cynosura): "The leaves disperse, dry, expel flatulence, and bring out sweat. The wood is cleansing, it is good for the head, excites sweat, resists poison, and is good in infirmities of the eyes and ears, either in the shape of a powder or decoction."

Krunitz must have been staggered by the unbounded praise which Herrmann bestows upon Thuja, for he adds: "I dare not relate all the marvellous things which Herrmann tells of Thuja."

According to *Boerhaave* the water which has been distilled from the branches of Thuja is useful in swellings; according to others, a decoction of the cones is useful in fever and ague.

According to Halm, the natives of America prepare an ointment from the crushed leaves, and rub the limbs with it when they are affected with pain.

These few quotations, which might be increased, are sufficient to show, that, previous to Hahnemann, scarce anything was known of the curative virtues of Thuja, and that the supposed remedial properties above mentioned were merely hypothetical notions.

The Thuja occidentalis has never been used as an officinal drug by the physicians of the Old School, nor is it mentioned in the common works on pharmacology, not even in Vogt's pharmacodynamics.

It is therefore the original and exclusive property of the new school, a pearl of price for which we are indebted to Hahnemann.

CHAPTER III.

(1.) *Hahnemann's Proving of the* ARBOR VITÆ *on the healthy.*

The great medical reformer proved Thuja on himself and on ten of his pupils. He gives us 330 symptoms,* which he had observed partly on himself and partly on others among his immediate followers, and some of which he had gathered from the sick. He had no assistance from previous authors, as there was nothing known of the action of Thuja before his time, and he conducted its proving with zeal and perseverance. The symptoms collected by him present the characteristic features of Thuja in the clearest manner.

We give below the results of Hahnemann's proving, with the omission of the characterless, bracketed symptoms, and of those obtained

* R. A. M. L., 2 Aufl., B. 5, S. 125.

from the sick, and for greater convenience of inspection, take the liberty of changing the anatomical order, of which Hahnemann was so fond, for one founded on an anatomico-physiological basis.

General.

Sticking, tearing, and drawing in different parts of the body, particularly in the limbs; itching, as from fleabites, on the body and limbs; pricking itching over the whole body; *crawling itching over the whole body; burning of the itching spots* after having been rubbed; limbs go to sleep; cracking in the joints on stretching the limbs; aggravation of the symptoms in the afternoon and night.

Skin.

Painful sensitiveness of the skin over the whole body; *inflamed eruptions* and *tubercles* on various places; *red,* painful *tubercles* on the *temples;* white *tubercles of the size of a hazelnut* on the calf, which itch violently and for some distance around, and *burn* after being rubbed; *isolated pimples, like chickenpox, with a red areola and pus at the summit, on the thighs, elbows and forearms; pimples on the knees, like smallpox, which itch and suppurate; an itching boil on the small of the back; a red mottled spot on the dorsum of the left foot and on the left forearm; eruptions on the left buttock, which itch and burn after having been scratched.*

Sleep.

Early sleepiness; late going to sleep; restlessness before going to sleep; restless sleep; restless tossing during sleep; sleeplessness; crying out in sleep; talking in sleep; anxious dreams, with loud exclamations; weeping when asleep; dreams of the dead, voluptuous dreams.

Fever.

Chilliness, without thirst; chills only on the left side in the evening in bed; *chilliness every morning or every evening;* chills for five hours, with thrice vomiting; *violent chill* for a quarter of an hour at about three o'clock, followed *by thirst and sweat over the whole body,* except the head; chilliness, with external heat of the body; *chilliness in the back, with numbness in the fingers;* coldness of the body, with great restlessness; coldness of both legs, which are covered with cold sweat.

Dry heat at night; heat in the face, with burning and redness of the cheeks; violent ebullition of blood every evening, with throbbing and beating in every vein; redness and burning of the left cheek; heat, with sweat, towards morning; dry mouth, with thirst.

Mental and Moral.

Activity of the mind, with weakness of the body; inability to rid himself of the thoughts that occupy his mind; unfitness for thinking, with confusion in the head; slowness of thought and speech.

Anxiety; *restless moral state; vexation and depression;* tired of life; discontent; great anxiety about trifles; *anxiety and solicitude* about the future.

Head and Face.

Vertigo when seated; when lying; reeling vertigo, with tottering when walking; headache in the forehead in the morning; drawing, sticking, pressing, boring headache; *sensation in the vertex, as if a nail were driven into it with a sudden blow;* tearing in the right side of the sinciput and face to the zygoma, morning and evening; *fine prickling crawling in the head; itching of the occiput.*

Drawing in the temporal muscles, worse when chewing; prickling pain in the temples; *crawling and filliping in the zygomata; twitching in the buccinatores;* an itching, scurfy eruption on the corner of the mouth.

PERCEPTIVE FACULTIES.

Visual Organs.

Eyes.—Sticking, *pressing in the eyes;* redness and inflammation of the sclerotica, with biting and pressing in the eye as if from sand; burning pressing in the external canthus of the left eye; *pressing in the eyes, with the feeling as if they were protruded from their sockets;* single, piercing stitches in the right inner canthus; *lachrymation of the left eye;* secretion of gum in the inner canthi.

Eyelids.—A red tubercle on the edge of the lower eyelid.

Sight.—Shortsightedness; *dim sight,* with the feeling as though the eyelids were swollen; *sensation as if looking through gauze* at near objects, as well as at distant ones; darker appearance of objects around, when reading; *weak, obscure vision.*

Auditory Organs.

Hammering and tearing in the ear until midnight; forcing and constriction in the ear, and afterward a sudden, violent stitch there; pressing in the meatus.

Olfactory Organs.

Daily epistaxis; nasal mucus mixed with coagulated blood; crawling in the nose as though from a cold; feeling as of coryza, with stuffed nose; *violent, rapidly appearing coryza;* profuse running at the nose, with catarrh; coryza, with nocturnal cough; an ulcerous scab in the nose.

Gustatory Organs.

Lips.—Twitching in the upper lip; burning in the red part of the lip and in the palate.

Tongue.—Sore pain on the tip of the tongue, when touching it; raw, scratching feeling on the tongue, with a white fur; *great swelling of the tongue; a white vesicle on the root of the tongue;* a white, painful blister on the middle of the tongue.

Palate.—Burning in the palate; sore pain in the whole palate when swallowing; feeling as if the oral cavity were full of blisters or scorched; pressing like weight in the velum palati.

Jaw and Teeth.—Sticking in the underjaw: sticking, drawing or twitching toothache, especially early in the morning and in the evening; toothache, as though the nerve were touched.

Gums.—Great swelling of the gums; swollen, sore gums.

Tonsils and Salivary Glands.—Swelling of the tonsils; sticking in the throat; rough, scraped throat; *copious flow of saliva;* saliva mixed with blood.

Appetite and Taste.—Flat, sweetish taste; appetite without relish for food; slimy taste (after eating); food tastes too little salted.

Respiratory Organs.

Trachea.—Sticking in the trachea; hoarseness as though from constriction in the pharynx.

Lungs.—Difficult, embarrassed breathing with thirst and anxiety; constriction of the left breast which provokes a slight cough; night-cough; oppression of the chest as though something had swollen there; constriction, forcing him to breathe deeply.

Heart.—Visible palpitation; pain in the cardiac region; violent palpitation on going up stairs; feeling of anxiety in the scrobiculus cordis.

Thorax.—Pressing on the chest after eating; paroxysms of pressure on the chest in the region of the axilla; feeling as if the chest were inflated from within; blue coloration of the skin on the clavicles.

Digestive Organs.

Pharynx.—Inclination to swallow; pressing behind in the throat when swallowing, feeling as though the pharynx were constricted and swallowing obstructed by mucus.

Stomach.—Cramp in the stomach, becoming worse in the evening; rancid, foul eructations; inflation and eructations as if from disordered stomach; heartburn.

Abdomen.—Pressing in the scrobiculus immediately after eating; constriction in the epigastric region; tension in the abdomen; inflated hypogastrium; pressure as from fulness in the right side of the abdomen; rumbling in the abdomen; ***jerking tearing in the abdomen; movement in the abdomen, as of something alive.***

Fæces.—Diminished evacuations; ineffectual desire for stool; desire for stool with erection; ***violent pain in the rectum during stool;*** painful constriction of the anus during stool; diarrhœic stool.

Anus.—*Burning at the anus; violent burning in the furrow between the buttocks when walking; burning sticking in the rectum* when not at stool.

Urinary Organs.

Urethra.—***Burning in the urethra*** especially when urinating and also afterwards, and even without passing water; *cutting pain when urinating;* biting and itching in the (female) urethra when urinating; *flow of mucus from the female urethra;* a very violent stitch from the rectum through the urethra; ***stitches in the urethra*** from behind forwards (when not urinating), ***stitches in the urethra with stiffness of the penis;*** tearing stitches in the anterior part of the urethra; *twitching-cutting sticking in the urethra* (when not urinating); *feeling in the urethra as if moisture were oozing along it.*

Urine.—***Frequent urination; reddish urine;*** pressing when urinating with jerking ejection of the urine; frequently interrupted stream; ***after urinating, a feeling as if a few drops were still passing on;*** after urinating, a little urine continues to flow in drops.

Sexual Organs.

Male.—*Sticking and itching in the glans; burning sticking in the end of the glans* when urinating; *single stitches in the end of the glans* when not urinating; *sticking itching on the side of the glans; a roundish, flat, foul ulcer with a red border and burning pain on the corona glandis; behind the glans, red, smooth excrescences in which there is formication; on the glans a small, low vesicle* which is painful when urinating; *moisture of the glans; balanorrhœa.*

Painful stitches on the inner side of the prepuce; great swelling of the prepuce; on the external surface of the prepuce, a red, ashy, elevated spot, which passes into an ulcer with a scab, itches and burns; small pustules on the inner surface of the prepuce which are depressed in the middle, are moist and suppurating; a red excrescence on the interior of the prepuce like a condyloma.

Fine stitches in the scrotum; *itching of the scrotum; sweat on the scrotum; profuse sweat on the genitals; scratching and itching on the scrotum, with burning if the places are rubbed; a moist pimple on the scrotum; drawing in the testicle; retraction of the left testicle towards the inguinal ring;* long-continued erection; nocturnal erections.

Female.—*Biting and itching in the female organs; sore pain in the female parts, especially during urination; swelling of both labia which burn* when walking and on being touched; *biting and burning in the vagina* when sitting and walking; pressing and constriction in the genital organs; constrictive pain in the genital organs and perinæum.

Glands.

Swelling of the salivary glands, with increased flow of saliva; swelling of the tonsils; swelling of glands in the left cheek; pain in the swollen glands of the neck; *drawing pain in the groin* when standing and walking; drawing from the inguinal glands outwards through the thigh into the knee; stitches from the groin through the thigh when sitting down; painless *swelling* in the groin.

Spinal Column.

Nape.—Pain in the left side of the neck, as if from an uncomfortable bed or position in lying; swelling and blue coloration of the cervical veins; alternate contraction and relaxation in the cervical muscles and in the nape.

Back.—Drawing pain in the back when sitting; *pressing in small spots on the back* when sitting; boring in a small spot in the back; sore pain in the back; tearing in the left scapula; crushing pain below the shoulder-blade; *twitching over the upper part of the body.*

Small of the back.—Tension; drawing; crushing pain after standing up, more violent when standing and turning the trunk, less painful when walking.

Extremities.

Upper.—Beating and throbbing in the shoulder-joint; cracking of the shoulder-joint when bending the arm backwards; formicating-itching on the upper arm, and a fine stitch afterwards in a small spot; feeling of heaviness from the middle of the left upper arm to the fingers; raging pain in both arms from three, A. M., until six; *involuntary twitching of the arm;* drawing in the arm of several hours' duration, feeling as though it were in the bones; digging-drawing pain in the whole arm as if in the periosteum with the sensation, on deep pressure, as if the flesh were loose from the bone; pain in the humerus on pressure; painful difficulty of movement in both arms; beating and throbbing in the elbow-joint, and in the evening drawing in the arms down to the fingers; tearing in the left wrist; pain as of dislocation in the right wrist; fine sticking in the fingers; fine prickling pain in the first joints of the fingers; fine sticking in the ends of the three left middle fingers; redness and swelling of the balls of both indices; the anterior joints of the three left middle fingers become red and swollen with fine sticking down to the ends; sweat on the hands.

Lower.—Tension from the hip-joint to the groin and in the posterior part of the thigh to the popliteal space; sticking in the most upper part of the thigh; the leg and thigh go to sleep when sitting; *sweat of the thigh near the genitals;* crushing pain over the middle of both thighs when walking; cracking in the elbow, knee and ankle-joints when stretching the limbs; paroxysms of weariness in the thighs; single stitches in the knees when rising up and beginning to walk; heaviness and stiffness of the leg when walking; drawing pain jerking downwards in the right leg as if from weariness; pressing in the tibia; inflammation, redness and swelling of the dorsum of the foot and of the toes which are painful and tensive when treading on or moving them; *involuntary upward twitching of the foot* as the pain increases; pain in the heel as though it were asleep; a sharp stitch in the tendo Achillis (after 2 h.); drawing in all the toes; drawing in the great toe; tearing stitches on both sides in the nails of the great toes; shining redness and swelling of the toes which itch and burn after being rubbed; sweat on the toes and feet proceeding upwards over the legs and thighs to the head and thence to the scrobiculus, with nausea.

The contributions of the pupils of Hahnemann follow in the alphabetical order of their names:

(2.) Franz.

Cloudiness of the head; pressing in the left parietal bone (after 2 h.); drawing in the left parietal bone (after 4 h.); *sensation as if a nail were driven into the right parietal bone (disappearing on touching it)*; pressing drawing in the left temple; occipital headache; *black points before the eyes*, which move about among each other, and are present even when the eyes are closed; itching in the face; cramp pain in the ear (after 4½ h.); rancid smell in the throat; *pressing* in the right groin (after 4 h.); formicating sticking in the right side of the chest (after 3 h.); painful sticking in the right shoulder (after 5 h.); aching in the small of the back when bowing; painful sticking in the right shoulder, opposite the clavicle (after 5 h.); pain, as of excoriation, on the forearm and inner side of the thigh; sensation in the knee as if it were cut into with a sharp knife; cutting pain in the left ankle when walking; drawing in the right great toe; warmth over the whole body, with cold fingers, especially on the left hand, without thirst (evening, after 3½ h.); *creeping chilliness, with icy cold hand,' after gentle heat* (evening); heat, with thirst, without chilliness, with pleasant state of mind.

Dr. Franz seems to have had but little sensibility to the action of Thuja, or to have experimented with too small doses; for, in the foregoing picture, the image of the drug is but faintly distinguishable.

(3.) Gross.

A spot is painful on the occiput, when lying on his left side, the hairs on which are sensitive to the touch; hawking up of bloody mucus from the throat; want of appetite; flatulence, with inflated abdomen (after a meal); weakness and weariness, with nausea, which compel him to lie down; frequent passage of pappy stools; evacuation of hard fæces in balls, which are streaked with blood * (after 14 h.); *frequent passing of copious clear urine, watery;* red urine, which deposits a lateritious sediment on standing; epistaxis; blowing of blood from the nose; intermitting stitches in the chest; warm perspiration on the covered parts of the body, which disappears on awaking.

An unimportant proving.

(4.) Frederick Hahnemann.

Headache on awaking; toothache; nausea, with several turns of vomiting of sourish fluids and food (after 3 h.); after vomiting, a chill, with heaviness in the limbs; *copious flow of urine;* tearing in the occiput; sticking tearing in the little finger.†

Who, from these insignificant *vitæ symptomata,* could recognize the effects of the *vitæ arbor?*

(5.) Haynel.

Drawing-tearing headache; corroding gnawing (*obscure expression —Mayrhofer*) in the skin of the occiput for half an hour (after 13 h.); feeling of dryness in the eyes; sneezing; tension over the right ala nasi; frequent epistaxis; swelling and hardness of the left ala nasi; *itching of the upper lip; cutting* pain in the vesical region before and during urination, and when not urinating (after 12 h.); *burning stitches at the orifice of the urethra,* when not urinating (after 9 h.); *cutting pain in the urethra* when walking (after 10 h.); drawing-tearing in the right upper jaw in the evening; sticking in the right deltoid when walking in the open air; interrupted, burning stitches in the popliteal space; a lasting stitch in the left knee and external malleolus of the right foot when at rest (after 28 h.); continuous burning in the left popliteal space, as if an eruption were breaking out (after 25 h.); lasting stitches in the right patella, with twitching of the skin (after $7\frac{1}{2}$ h.); fine, rapidly succeeding stitches in the hollow of the right sole; coldness in the back.

Thuja speaks out clearly from this proving.

(6.) Hartmann.

Giddiness as if from turning around in a circle (after $\frac{3}{4}$ h.); heaviness in the head (after $1\frac{1}{2}$ h.); momentary pressing in the head, now here, now there (after 2 h.); jerking stitch through the whole head (after

* A symptom of the prover's hæmorrhoids?—*Mayrhofer.*

† This prover communicates the following remarkable symptom of a female prover: "Walking is wonderfully easy to her; it seems as though her body were borne along by wings; she ran several miles in an uncommonly short time, and with unusual good feeling."

Was this a dream or a reality? a mystification, a tarantula-dance, or an effect of Thuja?—*Mayrhofer.*

1 h.); *jerking pressing on both frontal eminences* (after 4 h.); constrictive pressing on the left frontal eminence, which seems to depress the upper eyelid (after 1½ h.); pressing in both temples; itching tearing in the occiput (after 1 h.); a violent stitch in the left inner canthus (after 1¼ h.); pressing over the right eye; humming in the left ear (after 3 h.); pinching pain in the right ear; a gradually increasing stitch under the tongue, as if a needle had been stuck in there (after 4 h.); jumping stitches in the right side of the fauces, running rapidly into the ear (after 6½ h.); violent tearing in the left upper jaw (after 2 h.); *stiffness of the nape* and of the left side of the neck (after 2½ h.); pinching in the stomach; painful throbbing in the scrobiculus; *frequent copious urination* (after 4½ h.); *violent stitches in the glans, with desire to urinate;* the urine is discharged by drops; the sticking during urination is sometimes violent and sometimes absent, and the tenesmus continues as long as the sticking (after 7¼ h.); pressing in the middle of the chest, not interfering with the respiration, when sitting (after ¼ h.); jerking stitch in the sacrum, disappearing when rubbed (after 3¼ h.); occasionally a tearing stitch in the right, and sticking tearing in the left forearm;* feeling of heat in all the fingers of the left hand, while the right is as cold as ice (after 2½ h.); restless sleep, with dreams; heat in the face, with icy cold hands, and body moderately warm (after 2 h.); *chill over the whole body,* without perceptible coldness to the touch.

The subjective side of the Thuja-sickness is here clearly discerned; it also produced fever, but no permanent products of its power.

(7.) Hempel.

Drawing between the mouth and the nose; sore pain in the right posterior molars; tension in the abdomen; constipation for several days; pollution with the feeling in the urethra, as though it were too narrow; discharge of prostatic juice (without semen? M.); *twitching pain of the penis* on walking; crushing pain in the upper and lower extremities; deceptive feeling, as if he could not stand another attack, and was in danger of falling to pieces.

These few symptoms seem to be the meagre results of a short and timid proving.

(8.) Langhammer.

Embarrassed head when sitting and walking; pressive headache in the forehead (after ½ h.); dull pain in the whole body (after 1 h.); lancinations along the forehead (after 5½ h.); *tearing pain in the left superciliary arch, disappearing on touching it* (after 11 h.); swelling of the upper lid; reddening of the left sclerotica (after 74 h.); great dilatation of the pupils; distension of the veins of the temples

* Vague symptoms lead the prover into obscure expressions, while those which are sharply defined leave him no choice in the description. "*Doloresipsi loquuntur.*"—*Mayrhofer.*

and hands (after 18 h.); *itching and boring in the left zygoma diminished by touching it* (after ½ h.); boring pain in the left under-jaw (after 1½ h.); fine stitches in the left under-jaw; feeling of dryness in the lips and palate, without thirst (after 11 h.); itching *eruption of pimples between the eyebrows, with pus at the points; pimples over the whole face* (after 17 h.); *itching pimples on the knee* (after 5 h.); eructations of food; bitter taste of the saliva; violent thirst, without heat; nausea and vomiturition, with sweat over the whole body, without thirst; pinching and gnawing in the belly; discharge of flatulence; several loose stools; *frequent urgency to urinate and discharge of urine; nocturnal pollutions; crushing pains in the testicles* when sitting, aggravated by walking (after 2 h.); dry coryza, which becomes fluent in the open air, and which comes on sometimes in the morning, sometimes in the evening; cough in the morning on rising; sticking in the loins when sitting and walking (after 10 h.); pains in the back in the evening in bed; paralytic pain in the middle of the muscles of the left forearm, recurring both in rest and motion (after 1¼ h.); *transient sticking and drawing pains in various parts of the limbs, disappearing on handling the parts;* voluptuous itching on the dorsum of the right foot and under the toes; great weariness in all the limbs; drowsiness, without being able to go to sleep; restless sleep, with perspiration; *continued heat in the face and on the body, with cold fingers, without thirst; deadness of the ends of the fingers, which are icy-cold while the body is hot, and no thirst* (after ¼ h.); *frequent general shuddering* (after 2¼ h.); congestion of blood to the head with sweat on the face, and thirst after partaking of cold drink (after 11¾ h.); dissipation of mind, unsteadiness and inclination first to this and then to that matter; serene temper and desire to talk (after 12, 15, 16, h.).

Langhammer unquestionably produced the best proving of all of the pupils of Hahnemann. It gives evidence that it is the result of an energetic and persevering experiment in a constitution susceptible to the effects of Thuja, by means of which both the objective and subjective symptoms were brought to light.

(9.) Teuthorn.

Headache; sticking in the temples and over the left eye; contraction of the pupils for five days; (? *Mayrhofer*); trembling of surrounding objects while writing; white fur on the tongue after eating; bitter taste of bread.

No marks of life in this abortive production.

(10.) Wagner.

Occipital headache for six hours, heaviness of the head with peevishness and indisposition to talk (after 3 h.); drawing in the right side of the neck, when at rest (after 3 h.); pressive sticking pain in the right meatus auditorius (after 5 h.); ringing and roaring in the ears (after

1 h.); pressing in the region of the left kidney (after ½ h.); burning heat in the lumbar region (after 1 h.); beating and sticking in the right groin (after 1 h.); *frequent burning stitches through the penis into the testicles, disappearing on motion,* returning during rest (after 24 h.); burning stitches in the glans; *repeated stitches in the left testicle* (after 7 h.); *tickling and itching between the prepuce and the glans;* pressing sticking in the left side of the chest, equally perceptible when inspiring and expiring; sticking between the shoulder-blades, in the back and small of the back, when sitting; great lassitude of the body with disinclination to walk (after 11 h.); terrific dreams at night, heat and an emission.

Thuja appears here subjectively but not objectively.

(11.) Wislicenus.

Stupefaction of the head (after 6 h.); *tension of the skin of the nape on moving the head* (after 16 h.); boring in the right inner canthus (after 3 h.); squeezing in the right external meatus auditorius (after 4 h.); *stiffness in the masticatory muscles of the left side, which are painful when opening the mouth* (after 4 h.); sticking and twitching in the gum of the inferior posterior molars (after 34 h.); *a streak of small red pimples on both sides of the neck* (after 26 h.); red pustules on the hip which bleed when scratched off (after 36 h.); pressing in the hypogastrium as if from flatulence; ineffectual urging to stool; stool difficult to evacuate; loose evacuation; *single lancinations in the perinæum, disappearing on drawing in the anus* (after 8 h.); tension in the left ribs (after 1 h.); boring pressure over the scrobiculus cordis (after 40 h.); drawing in the small of the back, in coccyx and thighs when sitting (after 4 h.); sudden cramp pain in the small of the back on attempting to change feet after standing a long while (after 6 h.); paralytic feeling in the arms (after 8 h.); sticking in the middle finger, aggravated by bending it (after 16 h.); pain in the left thigh when walking as though it would break down (after 10 h.); cramp pain above the left knee when sitting: intermittent pinching in the calves (after 4 h.); fine stitches on the right external malleolus and crawling twitching in the soles of the feet; *stiffness* and heaviness in all the limbs; occasional shuddering over the back; *cold shivering* with frequent yawning (after 3 h.); *disquieting dreams;* thirst without heat, in the morning; weak pulse, below 60 (after 4 h.); peevishness and morose humor.

There are but few clear developments of the action of the drug in this proving.

CHAPTER IV.

Results of our own Provings of Thuja on the healthy organism.

Thuja was proved by twenty-six persons, among whom eighteen were males, five females, and three children. All the provings were instituted with the tinctures and the attenuations of Thuja, except one with the oil and the triturated twigs.

A.

Dr. Böhm instituted two provings.

(12.) *First proving, with the first trituration of the dried twigs* (1 : 99).

1844, Nov. 12th. Böhm took five grains of the first trituration an hour before breakfast (bread and milk); in the forenoon he experienced slight vertigo and dull pain at the root of the nose, with a feeling of warmth as if a cold would set in; in the evening he experienced several times fleeting stitches in the heel and in the ball of the right foot, a sensation which he had never before experienced.

13th. No medicine.

14th. In the morning, B. took ten grains of the first trituration. In the forenoon he experienced an increased feeling of warmth over the forehead and a pressing in the right temple from without inward; bleeding at the nose in the evening.

15th. In the morning, took ten grains. Experienced drowsiness in the afternoon and evening; restless sleep at night, and *frequent urination.*

16th and 17th. Took no medicine.

18th. In the morning, took again ten grains of the first trituration. Aching in the forehead, with obstruction of the nose, from which a quantity of blood was blown in the evening; *painful stitches in the glans.*

19th. No medicine.

20th. Took ten grains in the morning. Great flow *of saliva into the mouth*, frequent sneezing, bleeding at the nose, and remarkable drowsiness after dinner.

24th. Took again ten grains of the first trituration in the morning. Unusual dryness in both nasal cavities, *frequent urination, with urging at first, as though there was always water to come away*, afterwards without urging; fleeting stitches in the heel and big toe of the left foot.

Took no medicine for seven days.

Dec. 1st. Twenty grains of the first trituration. Dryness of the palate; slight *swelling* of the tonsils, painful, and inducing frequent deglutition; small white *vesicles* on the tongue, *resembling miliary rash.*

4th. Took another twenty grains. The above-mentioned vesicles on the tongue, which had almost vanished, re-appeared with burning, especially after eating warm food. This was accompanied with painful compression in the region of both malleoli of the left foot, and slight *burning* during urination, the urine being redder than usual.

8th. Another twenty grains. They produced frequent eructations, as of rancid grease; *desire to urinate;* great drowsiness in the evening.

12th. Another twenty grains in the morning. They occasioned rancid eructations, *violent bleeding at the nose* almost every time he blew it, and frequent urination, with *burning in the fossa navicularis.*

(13.) *Second proving, with the tincture.*

After an interval of more than two months and a half, Dr. B. instituted a second proving with the tincture of Thuja. He diluted ten drops of the tincture with six ounces of distilled water, of which he took two table-spoonfuls on the morning of the 3d of March, 1845, before breakfast. After the lapse of two hours he experienced frequent eructations; frequent *urging to urinate* in the daytime. Next day: obstruction of the nose, *which began to bleed* as soon as he attempted to expel air through it.

March 5th. In the morning, B. took four tablespoonfuls of the abovementioned dilution. Headache in the forehead with warmth, *frequent urination with urging,* slight *burning* under the sternum, painful pressure at the root of the nose. These symptoms disappeared gradually within three days.

10th. Eight spoonfuls of the same dilution. Result: continued rancid eructations; oppression of the chest; frequent hawking and hacking; continued *burning* along the whole length of the sternum; *frequent urination followed by long-continued urging.*

15th. B. took, as a final experiment, ten drops of the undiluted tincture on sugar. The effects were rancid eructations (for eight hours); fluent coryza, disturbing the night's rest; weight on the chest; painful stitches in the big toe of the left foot; *frequent urination with urging.* All these symptoms increased on the day following, subsequently decreased, and disappeared entirely in a few days.

It is to be regretted that B., whose organism seemed to possess a great susceptibility to the effects of Thuja, did not pursue his experiments with more perseverance.

B.

Doctor Fröhlich proved the Thuja on himself, and on one girl and two rabbits.

I.

FRÖHLICH'S PROVINGS OF THE THUJA ON HIMSELF.

F. instituted six separate provings with Thuja.

(14.) *First proving, with the juice of the chewed branches of Thuja.*

1844, Dec. 20th. F. began his proving by chewing a few fresh twigs, and swallowing the juice. He experienced no change in his feelings.

21st. In the morning he repeated the experiment, and experienced, in the afternoon, protrusion of the hæmorrhoidal vessels, with sticking in those vessels when walking; in the evening, ten hours after swallowing the juice, he felt a tearing in the left knee-joint, extending to the middle of the calf, commencing while sitting and lasting only a short while.

22d. In the morning the experiment was made a third time. Soon after he felt a continuous, digging and burning pain in two upper hollow molars of the right side; in the evening, ten hours after swallowing the juice, he experienced short but frequently returning paroxysms of a lancinating pain from the left acetabulum down to the calf, deep in the bone (while walking in the street). The toothache was removed by a dose of *Merc-sol.* 3.

No chewing on the 23d, lest the toothache should occur again. The toothache returned, nevertheless, whenever he entered a warm room from the street and remained there a little while. He tried the nitrate of silver 6. with but temporary relief; and the troublesome toothache, for which cold water was the only palliative when the pain was very violent, disappeared gradually in some days.

(15.) *Second proving, with the third dilution.*

The symptoms of the former proving having entirely ceased for several days, on the 2d of Jan., F. took three drops of Thuja 3. in a tablespoonful of water, before breakfast. No result.

Jan. 5th. In the morning, six drops of the same preparation. *A painful stitch through the centre of the left eye, commencing in the centre of the brain;* a few stitches in the external tuberosity of the left thigh when walking; the above-mentioned toothache again made its appearance, but only under similar circumstances.

12th. Twelve drops in a glass of water. After walking in the open air for half an hour, he entered a warm room, where the above-described toothache again made its appearance, but soon abated, and disappeared on using cold water. This symptom returned as often as F. entered a closed apartment, even though not heated, and remained in it for a while. The toothache was immediately diminished by inhaling the air at an open window for a few moments. On the same day the following symptoms were observed: drawing *tension in the nape of the neck* (more on the left side), recurring several times; feeling of weakness in the chest; frequent emission of flatulence which had not much smell; drawing, and *fleeting deep stitches* in various parts of the body.*

* These fleeting stitches resemble slight electric shocks.—*Mayrhofer.*

No medicine was taken from the 8th to the 19th; the toothache recurred during all this time under the circumstances indicated above, although several remedies, such as *merc-sol.*, *camph.*, *sabina* and *nux* were taken to remove it.

(16.) *Third proving, with the tincture.*

Jan. 22d. After the toothache had entirely subsided, F. took twenty drops of the tincture in a glass of water. That same forenoon the toothache returned ten minutes after having entered a room without fire; after dinner he experienced a piercing stitch in the left hypochondria, and a continuing squeezing-sticking pain in the concha of the left ear.

23d. In the morning, thirty drops. At noon he was unable to distinguish by the taste what sort of soup he was eating (it was dark). Nor was he able to discern the vegetables by the taste, and black coffee tasted like warm water, without aroma.

24th. Forty drops: stitches in the region of the liver when sitting.

25th. The same dose produced a slight colicky pain in the small intestines and a few stitches in the right thumb.

26th. Another forty drops: painful stitches in the inner side of the left knee-joint when standing.

27th. Sixty drops. In the forenoon he experienced a few deep stitches in the left hypochondria.

28th. Eighty drops. In the forenoon: pinching pain in the stomach, and a feeling of fulness and of being bruised in the chest under the sternum; which last symptom he had observed for several days past.

No Thuja was taken from the 29th of January to the 3d of February. During this period the following symptoms were observed: single deep stitches in the right and left hypochondria; gnawing-stinging pain in the stomach (coming on in bed and going off after rising); drawing-sticking pain in the head of the left femur; dulness of the senses of taste and smell.

Feb. 3d. F. took one hundred drops of the tincture in a tumblerful of water before breakfast. An hour after, he experienced a single stitch through the lower portion of the lungs from behind forward. This was accompanied by a bruised sensation in the chest with dulness of the head, sad mood and discouragement, being the same in the open air and in the room. Afterwards the well-known toothache made its appearance again in the usual paroxysms, and in the evening, while sitting in a crowded theatre, he experienced a drawing-sticking pain in the right forearm, extending from the elbow to the wrist-joint.

4th. He experienced a painful stitch through the occiput from above downward.

5th. The troublesome toothache came on again as often as F. entered a closed apartment from the open air, and continued until the 23d of February. During that period F. had several characteristic symptoms of Thuja, especially in the limbs, but which were not noted down because he had taken several remedies, such as *sabina*, *rhus*, and *mezereum*, against the toothache with only transitory relief.

(17.) *Fourth proving, with the eleventh dilution.*

April 4th. Before breakfast, F. took twenty drops of the 11th dilution, in three ounces of distilled water. While proving the attenuations, he avoided every kind of spirituous beverage, and partook of the plainest food.

6th. He felt vertigo with fulness in the head, and the hands became easily stiff and tired when moving them.

7th. Twelve drops of the 11th potency produced the following result: in the forenoon, while walking in the street, he felt a few deep stitches in the right groin; afterwards he felt a violent drawing tearing from the left elbow-joint as far as the two middle fingers; vertigo at home, with vanishing of the letters when reading, and a continued digging pain in two hollow upper molares of the right side, relieved by cold water, but increased by warm soup and tobacco-smoke.

8th. F. feeling *debilitated all over as by fatigue, and gloomy*, was compelled to take a little wine, after which all the above symptoms disappeared.

(18.) *Fifth proving, with the tincture again.*

April 22d. After all the symptoms of Thuja had ceased and the carious teeth had become entirely free from pain, F. took eighty drops of the tincture before breakfast, after which he swallowed a glass of water. No effects were observed either this or the next day. On the 24th and on the 26th he took one hundred drops each day. On the latter day the prover experienced considerable dulness of the head and *mistiness of sight;* on the dorsum of the right foot a small blotch was discovered with a *red areola*, which rendered walking in boots difficult.

28th. Another hundred drops. The blotch is diminishing, and nothing remains of it except a dark-red, somewhat elevated spot with a lighter areola, still impeding walking. General weariness during the day, as if he had slept none all night. These symptoms are accompanied by dulness of the head, *sad mood*, dulness of taste, *indistinct sight*, and bad, sunken appearance.

Nevertheless, on the 30th, F. took another hundred drops. In the forenoon: dulness of the head, with vanishing of objects when attempting to fix them. In the afternoon: painful *stiffness of the nape of the neck* when moving the head, bruised sensation in the chest, dulness of taste and *very gloomy mood.* The efflorescence on the dorsum of the foot began to subside.

May 2d. Another hundred drops elicited no new symptoms.

No medicine was taken on the 3d and 4th of May; during this period F. observed the following symptoms: dulness and feeling of fulness in the head, with ill-humor and drowsiness. After a siesta of three quarters of an hour: vertigo so that he could scarcely walk without holding on to something; great sensitiveness of the skin to cool air.

5th. F. took the last hundred drops. Result: sticking tearing in the right tarsal joint in the forenoon, while walking. Another *little blotch* makes its appearance in the still existing red spot on the dorsum of the right foot, impeding the walking very much.

6th. In the morning, in bed: sticking beating in the right hand extending as far as the tips of the fingers and in the anterior part of the right foot. Towards noon: pressive headache with pressure in both eyes, accompanied with gastric uneasiness and reddened urine. F. had to lie down on account of his increasing debility, and was not able to go to sleep for several hours.

7th. He felt a general debility as from fatigue; feeling of fulness in the head; a paralytic *burning sensation*, which had been felt already for some days past in all the *muscles* of the forearm, and which extended as far as the tips of the fingers, was particularly troublesome (coming on when moving the arm, going off in rest). In the afternoon and evening: feeling of coldness through the back, with debility and stiffness in all the limbs; dulness of the head; sticking pain in the left patella when going up stairs; great debility in the small of the back and feet, and a feeling of weakness in the chest.

8th. After having spent a night full of dreams, F. woke greatly improved; the head continued dull, and he was attacked with turns of vertigo after talking long; at noon he felt *chilly* all over, especially on the extremities; he was *ill-humored* and *restless*, and had canine hunger without thirst. A small quantity of wine which he took at dinner without relishing it, aggravated the headache very much, and smoking increased it to vertigo.* At eight o'clock in the evening: *aching pain*, especially in the *frontal eminences* and temples; vertigo when walking; bruised pain in the shoulder-joints and upper arms; weak feeling in the chest with pressure under the sternum and difficulty of breathing, especially while going up stairs.

9th. F. felt better in every respect, all the symptoms disappeared within a few days, except the weak feeling in the chest and the difficulty of breathing in going up stairs, which did not entirely leave him until the end of the month.

(19.) *Sixth proving, with the recent juice.*

May 21st. F. swallowed before breakfast a table-spoonful of recently expressed juice, obtained by crushing the twigs of Thuja and pouring upon them a mixture of equal quantities of distilled water and alcohol. Of this nauseous juice F. took another table-spoonful on the first and second of June, and two table-spoonfuls on the third.

* As the use of wine was beneficial previously, this aggravation seems to be rather attributable to the effects of a meal eaten with canine appetite.—*Mayrhofer.*

On the last day he experienced in the forenoon frequent paroxysms of tearing and sticking in both hands, which became so violent in the middle of the right ulna while he was writing, that he had to give it up. In the afternoon, while driving in a carriage, he experienced a very violent tearing in the left forearm, which was especially violent in the anterior tuberosity of the humerus, that region becoming very sensitive to the touch. Moreover, ***prickings in the fingers*** of the same hands. These symptoms continued while driving, and did not abate until F. got into a profuse perspiration in the evening, while in a crowded theatre. Upon moving the hand quickly and strongly he felt ***a burning pain in all the muscles*** of the forearm.

June 4th. F. again took two table-spoonfuls of the recent juice, which did not produce any new symptoms. The tearing pain in the anterior tuberosity of the left humerus continued, was increased by motion, and was heightened to a burning pain by contact, especially after the painful spot on the arm had been knocked against something though only slightly. The red spot on the dorsum of the foot impeded his walking very much. Under the sternum he experienced an oppression with a bruised sensation in the chest. These symptoms were accompanied by frequent hawking of mucus, dulness of taste, with great appetite and swelling of the hæmorrhoidal veins.

5th. The following symptoms were observed: sensitiveness of the anterior tuberosity of the left upper arm, especially when touched; in the afternoon, feeling of fulness in the head with drawing pain in the nape of the neck; feeling of weakness in the chest; painful stiffness in the left forearm extending as far as the fingers, and impeding motion: pressing sensation in the ***turgid hæmorrhoidal veins;*** sticking-burning pain in the external tuberosity of the left tibia (coming on when sitting and increased by pressure). All these symptoms disappeared gradually on the following days except the great sensitiveness in the tuberosity of the humerus, which seemed to become more and more circumscribed every day, but which only entirely disappeared in the course of a week. The last to yield was the *hæmorrhoidal congestion*, to remedy which he used several bottles of mineral water.

II.

FRÖHLICH'S PROVING OF THUJA ON AN UNMARRIED WOMAN.

(20.) *First proving, with the third dilution.*

Caroline Philipp, forty-five years old, the same person who assisted in proving Colocynth, took ten pellets, moistened with the 3d dilution of Thuja, on the 14th of November, 1844, before breakfast. Two hours after, she experienced a *drawing* from the left axilla as far as the elbow-joint; afterwards a *drawing* along the vertebral column and in the calves, with a feeling of weakness in the feet.

Nov. 13th. The prover again took ten pellets, which elicited the following symptoms: *drawing* from the right wrist-joint as far as the tips of the fingers, and from the right calf as far as the malleoli, with the sensation as if that foot were lame; afterwards a drawing from the right elbow as far as the wrist-joint; then a transient paralytic feeling in both thighs as far as the knees.

14th. After another ten pellets, she experienced a weakness in the knees and a decrease of appetite.

No medicine was taken on the 15th, 16th, and 17th; during the first two days the above symptoms were yet slightly felt.

From the 18th to the 23d, Caroline took ten pellets every day, and observed the following symptoms: *drawing sticking* in the right upper arm as far as the elbow-joint, and in the right thigh as far as the knee; *sticking* in the right forearm as far as the finger-joints; *drawing* in both scapulæ in the direction of the *nape of the neck*, in both legs from the knees to the malleoli, and at the same time in both forearms from the elbows to the wrist-joints. These symptoms generally appeared three or four hours after taking the drug, and lasted from ten to sixteen hours.

The prover discontinued the medicine until the 26th of November, when she took another ten pellets. On that day she experienced a *sticking* in the left thigh as far as the knee, *single stitches* in the left tarsal joint, and in the evening *drawing* in both thighs.

27th and 28th. She again took ten pellets each time, after which she experienced a *tearing* in the left upper arm, afterwards in the left leg; sticking in the left wrist-joint extending as far as the tip of the index finger; *drawing* in the left calf, afterwards in the right forearm from the elbow as far as the wrist-joint.

Dec. 5th, 6th, and 10th. She took ten pellets each time without experiencing any new symptoms. The same drawing and sticking was experienced in various parts of the limbs. On the inner surface of the left forearm a *red, round, itching spot* (of what size?—M.) was observed with *white vesicles* raised upon it, which burst, poured out a clear lymph, and left a yellowish crust behind.

(21.) *Second proving, with the two hundred and second dilution.*

Dec. 12th. Before breakfast, F. gave the prover ten pellets of Thuja 202, without her knowing that the preparation was different from what she had previously taken. Results: *drawing* in both hands and feet, afterwards only in the forearms as far as the wrist-joints, and *sticking* in both sides of the chest.

13th. She took another ten pellets, with the same result.

19th and 20th. She took the usual number of pellets, and observed, besides the symptoms mentioned above: *drawing in both hips* from without inward and from above downward toward the *genital parts*. After an interval of twelve days, the prover took ten pellets of Thuja

202 on each of the following days: 2d, 3d, 4th, 6th, 7th, and 9th of January, 1845. After every dose she experienced *tearing*, *drawing* or *sticking* sensations, accompanied with repeated attacks of vertigo, and *a feeling of stiffness in the feet* and back, as far *as the nape of the neck.*

The prover having taken cold, in consequence of which she was attacked with toothache and a swelling of the cheek, the experiments were concluded. F. mentions that the prover had frequently asserted with great positiveness, that she had experienced with more intensity all her former symptoms ever since the 12th of December, when she took the first dose of Thuja 202. We ought to state that the prover observed a very plain diet during the whole period of the proving.

From the results of the last two provings, Dr. Fröhlich draws the following inferences:

1. Thuja specifically affects the sero-fibrous tissues.

2. It develops its effects chiefly in the extremities, and mostly in the direction of the limb from joint to joint.

3. The symptoms of Thuja produced by the different dilutions have much more similarity to one another than is the case with other drugs.

4. By this experiment with the 202d dilution, the power of the high attenuations (*hoch-potenzen*) to produce effects on the healthy human organism is perfectly established. Dr. F. does not consider this astonishing, inasmuch as the delicately-organized prover lived very plainly, and inasmuch as he had seen decided effects from many of the other highest potencies in his ordinary practice.*

C.

Doctor William Huber, of Linz, instituted three provings upon himself with the Thuja.

(22.) *First proving, with the lower dilutions (prepared according to the decimal scale).*

One drachm of the third attenuation which H. took on the 14th of September, 1844, at 8 o'clock in the morning, produced no effect. He took a similar dose on the 13th at 5 o'clock in the morning; after an hour and a half, while lying in bed, he experienced a momentary starting in the epigastric region, in the direction of the left hypocon-

* We may here be allowed to remark that the alleged effects of high potencies on the healthy and on the sick, must be considered as exceptional cases until more copious statistics shall be at our command. We must remember that one swallow does not make a summer; of a hundred magnetic subjects scarce one or two become clairvoyant, and it may be that the same relative proportion holds as to the sensibility of sound and sick to high potencies—"*High potencies for highly-potentized nerves—Similia similibus!*"—*Mayrhofer.*

drium, as of something alive. Next day he took a third dose of the same dilution, but observed no further symptoms.

Sept. 15th. At 6 o'clock in the morning, H. took one drachm of the fifth dilution. One hour after dinner he experienced a fine, transitory stitch in the posterior surface of the left ulna near the elbow; soon after a sudden starting-bounding sensation in the right iliac region, as though from something alive; a quarter of an hour afterwards, he experienced *a painful drawing* in the outer surface of the left upper arm near the olecranon, *recurring several times at short intervals.* At 8 o'clock in the evening, H. experienced a sensation on the glans near the frænulum præputii, as if the spot had been excoriated, although no change was visible.

16th. Took a similar dose, after which: the same feeling of soreness on the glans, only when touching it; at 4 o'clock, after dinner, he experienced a few fine stitches in the *fossa navicularis* of the urethra; an hour afterwards, during the siesta, he experienced a second time a sudden bounding up in the abdomen, accompanied with starting of the whole upper part of the body, as if from fright.

17th. After a similar dose a *drawing intermittent pain in the left side of the forehead,* and at the same time symptoms of colic, accompanied by emission of flatulence.

18th. A drachm of the fourth dilution morning and evening; this caused a profuse secretion of insipid saliva in the night, and a painful *tension* in the *right side of the nape* and *in the small of the back.*

19th. The dose was repeated, causing a slight tension in the *left side of the nape,* and a pretty severe sticking crosswise where the radius and the carpus unite, from without inwards (in rest).

20th. In the morning, H. repeated the dose. After the lapse of an hour he felt as if his stomach were deranged, with pressure over the scrobiculus, which impeded respiration. At 9 o'clock he experienced a pain in the left side of the forehead when writing, which continued the whole forenoon; upon being waked from the siesta H. became quite giddy, and had great trouble in collecting his thoughts.*

21st, 22d, and 23d. H. took one drachm of the third dilution at 7 o'clock in the morning. On the first day, towards 9 o'clock in the morning, he experienced an aching in the epigastrium, towards the right hypochondrium, for half an hour (more in rest than when walking). On the morning of the second day, dulness of the head, and at 10 o'clock, painful drawing in the left thumb, lasting only a short while, but returning frequently. On the third day a sudden sensation of giddiness was experienced at 11 o'clock in the forenoon while writing. He felt as if a current of air was ascending from the occiput and penetrating towards the forepart of the head, causing vertigo and a loss of thought.

24th, 25th, and 26th. H. took one drachm of the second dilution in the morning. Result: after the first dose he experienced a *momentary*

* Was this the effect of sleep or of Thuja?—*Mayrhofer.*

tearing in the dorsum of the left hand, at noon, while writing; after the second dose several stitches were experienced periodically in the left side of the chest, apparently deep in the pectoralis major muscle. The third dose was without result. One drachm of the first dilution, taken on the 27th, 28th, and 29th of the same month, was likewise without result.

(23.) *Second proving, with the tincture.*

Five drops on the morning of the 30th September, produced no effect.

Oct. 1st. Eight drops. In the evening, while chewing a piece of bread, H. experienced an *intense sticking pain* between the left *ear and zygomatic arch*, as if the jawbone had suddenly become *dislocated*, extorting a scream. This pain was experienced every time he attempted to chew, continued the whole evening, and was still felt the next morning.

2d. In the morning, ten drops. As soon as he awoke he felt an extremely disagreeable, painful sensation in the *nape of the neck*, close to the occiput, as if he had been *lying on a hard couch*. In the course of the day this pain spread over the whole of the right side of the back as if the muscles in that part of the body were *sprained*, and was felt especially when bending the head forward and raising the right arm.*

In the evening the pain moved more into the region of the right shoulder and neck; upon chewing bread the before-mentioned pain in the muscles of mastication was again experienced.

3d. In the morning, sixteen drops. After dinner a *voluptuous itching* in the forepart of the *urethra*, while the penis was relaxed. The pain in the right posterior cervical and dorsal muscles continued the whole day, accompanied with *whizzing* and *buzzing* in the right ear. On bending the head forward he experienced a sensation as if the muscles were *too short*, and as if the pain was caused by the tension of the muscles. Had a quiet night after taking forty drops in the evening.

4th. Twenty-six drops. Shortly after taking the drug the pain in the nape of the neck, shoulder and back, was increased to such an extent that the raising of the right arm and carrying the hand behind the head caused the most exquisite pain. He was unable to bend the head forward or to turn it; in order to accomplish this he had to move the whole upper part of the body. The pain was a sort of *tumultuous digging*, as if the muscles had been *crushed*, and as if a gathering were taking place in the subcutaneous and intermuscular areolar tissue. On the same day he had two papescent fetid stools, and, in the evening, after eating a warm soup, a vaporous perspiration broke out all over the body, continuing for half an hour, and followed by a diminution of the pain in the nape of the neck; on the following

* Dr. Huber observes that he had never been affected with rheumatism of the nape of the neck.—*Mayrhofer.*

day, however, H. was not yet able to tie his cravat behind, or to hang the chain of his watch around his neck. On looking at the right shoulder in the glass, it was found to be somewhat more elevated than the left, and swollen; the taste in the mouth was insipid, with a sensation as if the stomach were disordered.

5th. Thirty drops. At 8 o'clock in the morning he had a large evacuation, which was at first hard, afterwards papescent, clayish and fetid. The disagreeable sensation in the stomach continued all day. At half past 7 in the evening, painful *tension* in the bottom of the left *orbit* for several minutes.

8th. Sixty drops. After the lapse of half an hour: several painful *stitches* in the forepart of the *urethra*, the penis being relaxed; afterwards he felt a transitory cramp pain in the right ear, and several times *fine prickings in various parts of the skin as if with needles*, which sometimes changed to a *burning;* also a *painful burning sensation between the prepuce* and *glans*, continuing from 6 to 7 seconds, and returning several times *at short intervals*, without any change in the parts perceptible to the eye. At 10 o'clock in the forenoon he experienced a painful *drawing* in the left *frontal eminence* (while walking in the open air) and an *itching of the anus*, which induced scratching. At 4¾ in the afternoon, while sitting, *a sensation in the urethra, as if a drop of viscid fluid were pressing forward.* At 5 o'clock *drawing pains* were experienced directly below the right internal malleolus (for a few seconds). On the morning of the following day, the orifice of the urethra was closed with a *slimy fluid*, consisting of a serous liquid and a lump of mucus, which could be drawn into threads by the fingers. After removing this liquid a slight *burning* was experienced on urinating.

9th. In the morning, H. took eighty drops. After the lapse of fifteen minutes the left eye began to water, the right one remaining dry; confusion of the head the whole forenoon; *whizzing* in the left ear; painful pressure in the superior and posterior angle of the left parietal bone, as if a small *convex button were pressed against that part* (going off rapidly when touching it). At 10 o'clock in the forenoon painful *drawing*, extending from the bend of the right thigh to the internal surface of the thigh for a few seconds (in rest).

After dinner a pain in the right *parietal bone*, as if *a pointed nail had been driven in;* violent vertigo when sitting and closing his eyes, as if the sofa upon which he was sitting were balancing to and fro (going off immediately when opening his eyes).

At 4½ o'clock, during the siesta, he experienced a momentary, darting pain in the gums of the right upper jaw. (The affection of the back and nape of the neck had again by degrees wholly disappeared.)

10th. One hundred drops: after the lapse of two hours transitory *jerking formication in the fossa navicularis of the urethra*, accompanied with a voluptuous feeling without erection; dulness of the head the whole forenoon, with *paroxysms* of a drawing pain in the middle of the forehead, which was especially violent *in the left frontal eminence*, and thence extended to the posterior portion of the left eyeball, and at times as far as the occiput, and at 3 o'clock in the afternoon passed into a constant digging pain. This headache was as violent in the open air as in the room, and lasted until 10 o'clock at night. Occasional sensation in the right epigastric region as of something alive moving there; frequently a painful *jerking in the penis*, accompanied by a sensation as if a viscid liquid were exuding from the urethra, which, however, was not the case. He fell asleep after midnight; on the following day, when waking at half past 6 o'clock, a dull drawing pain was experienced in the right *frontal eminence*, extending as far as the right orbit and the right nasal bone, setting in in paroxysms and ending at 8 o'clock.

The right eye was dry and in the margin of the lower lid there was a burning spot as if a stye were about to form. He felt, besides, whizzing in the left ear, and once a fleeting stitch in the left testicle.

11th. At 8 o'clock in the morning, H. took one hundred and twenty drops. After the lapse of an hour, a *jerking, voluptuous formication* was experienced in the forepart of the *urethra* (while walking in the street), his penis being relaxed. At 10 o'clock in the forenoon: painful drawing in the *right side of the forehead*, ceasing and returning several times. At half past 12: painful *drawing* in the left *posterior cervical region*, close to the occiput, alternating with a similar pain in the right *frontal eminence*. Afterwards creaking in both ears *when swallowing*, resembling the turning of a wooden screw, accompanied with sticking and a feeling of dryness in the right outer *canthus*, as if a *grain of sand* had got into it. At 2 o'clock in the afternoon he experienced frequent attacks of a painless *twitching* in the back towards the left loin like a muscular twitch.

On waking the next morning, the scrotum, perinæum, and the inner surfaces of the thighs were dripping with sweat,* and, a few minutes after, paroxysms of a drawing pain were experienced in the bottom of the right orbit, continuing a quarter of an hour.

The same phenomena continually recurring, H. concluded the provings with the tincture by taking 140 drops of it at 8 o'clock in the morning on the 12th. After the lapse of a quarter of an hour, a feeling of dryness in both eyes, with painful sticking and creaking in both ears, as when a wooden screw is turned, especially during empty deglutition. Half an hour after, a short painful *drawing* in the left side of the occiput. Two hours after, a clawing aching pain in the left *frontal eminence*, becoming fixed in a small place (for a few minutes) accompanied with rumbling in the bowels. After nine and a half hours colicky pain in the right iliac region, for a few minutes, while walking in the room; shortly after, a few shooting *stitches* in the *urethra*, and a drawing

* Dr. H. observes that this sweat of the genital organs reminded him involuntarily of the assertion of his teacher, Von Hildenbrandt: "*Amant condylomata loca uda ut fungi.*"

headache in the right forehead. These symptoms lasted with more or less intensity during the subsequent days, and a few more were felt on the 21st, such as *feeling of soreness* about the hard *palate*, as if burnt and covered with vesicles; periodical pinching in the middle of the left calf as if *a convex button were pressed upon that part*, the same sensation being experienced in the mastoid process of the right side; shooting stitches from the *neck of the bladder* towards the *urethra.*

These phenomena became gradually weaker, though some of them were yet experienced on the 30th of Nov., 1844, more than six weeks after the prover had taken his last dose of Thuja.

(24.) *Third proving, with the sixtieth dilution.*

After all the symptoms produced by the increasing doses of the tincture of Thuja had entirely disappeared, H. experimented with the 60th dilution (1 : 99), not, however, without a pre-formed conviction that the experiment would be wholly without result and was therefore much astonished at again experiencing not only many of the old symptoms, but also others, which he had never before felt.

1845, Jan. 16th. H. took ten drops of the 60th dilution at 11 o'clock in the forenoon. After a quarter of an hour a slight pressure in the pit of the stomach and in the chest, impeding respiration. Sticking tearing pain in the muscular parts of the right side of the nape of the neck, in the evening, extending as far as the scapula (continuing only a short while, but returning several times with considerable violence). Soon after, a similar pain in the left forearm, where the ulna joins the carpus. On the morning of the day following, H. experienced a sensation in the abdomen as if a child's knee were pushing against the anterior abdominal walls from within.

17th and 18th. Ten drops produced no symptoms.

19th. The same dose occasioned the following symptoms: voluptuous itching in the forepart of the urethra, the penis being relaxed, accompanied with a sensation as if a few drops would flow out; jerking in the left hypochondrium, towards the epigastrium; transitory pain in the left *frontal eminence* as if a *nail* were driven in. This pain disappeared at once on touching the part, returned, however, immediately at the superior posterior angle of the left *parietal bone*, as if a *convex button* were pressed against the part.

20th. Twelve drops at 10 o'clock in the morning; frequent *lachrymation* of the left eye (when walking in the open air); digging headache in the left *frontal eminence* at 5 o'clock in the afternoon, returning several times at *short intervals*, and alternating with the sensation as if a *convex button* were pressed upon the part near the vertex. This same sensation, which ceased immediately upon the parts being touched, and returned again as soon as the contact ceased, was experienced several times in the right *mastoid process*, in the left *parietal bone*, and *under the right clavicle*. In the evening he perceived a painful *little tubercle* in the middle of the left *eyebrow*, and, after he had gone to bed, a digging-tearing pain was experienced in the *muscles of the right side* of the *nape of the neck*, extending momentarily as far as the right scapula, and being relieved by contact, accompanied by roaring in the left *ear* and *creaking when swallowing saliva.* On the following morning, after waking, *pressure* and *tension* in the left and afterwards also in the right *orbit.*

21st. Took fifteen drops. In the afternoon, the well-known *pressure* as with a *convex button* in a region of the left *parietal bone.* At 7 o'clock in the evening, H. suddenly experienced a momentary pressure as of *a nail which had been driven in*, in the left *frontal eminence* (while walking in the street), and after returning home and entering the room, a *luminous disk* of the size of a pea *hovered before his eyes;* it shone like a fire-fly (lampyris noctiluca).

22d. No medicine was taken. In the evening he experienced a transitory pain in the left *frontal eminence as of a nail which had been driven in.*

23d. H. concluded his provings with seventeen drops of the 60th dilution. At 10 o'clock in the forenoon, *drawing-sticking* pain in the left *temporal muscle, increased by mastication* and *diminished by contact.* This pain continued for two hours, and in the open air as well as in the room. At the same time H. experienced a beating tearing with sensation of heat in the right frontal eminence, and a pinching pressure in the dorsum of the left foot, occurring frequently during the day.

24th. On waking, *drawing pain* in the left *frontal eminence* (this pain had made its appearance already in the evening after lying down), and *profuse sweat about the genital organs.* In the forenoon, while walking in the open air, headache in the forehead over the left eyebrow, extending as far as the right side of the forehead. In the evening, a continuous *drawing* and *tension* below the *mastoid process* of the right side, accompanied with occasional *drawing* in the left *frontal eminence* towards the temple, and with roaring in the left ear.

25th and 26th. No symptoms observed; but on the 27th, a few moments after waking, H. had a complete *hemicrania* in the left side of the forehead.* It was a violent, drawing pain, commencing directly over the left upper eyelid, extending perpendicularly upward through the middle of the left eyebrow, and dividing in the left frontal eminence into a number of threads and rays which penetrated deep into the brain. This symptom lasted a few minutes, and disappeared as rapidly as it came.

Feb. 13th. On this date, clear Thuja symptoms having been constantly present in the intermediate period, H. discovered a painless *nodule* near the borders of the hairs on the left side of the nape of the neck, disappearing again on the following day, except a small rough place.

16th. A tubercle was observed on the inner side of the right thigh

* H. had never had any hemicrania before.—*Mayrhofer.*

an inch and a half from the perinæum, which *felt like a wart* and looked dark-red, of the size of a hemp seed, the tip having a *dingy white appearance*, and the base being surrounded with a *bright-red areola* of some three or four lines wide; it was somewhat painful when touching or moving it, and was filled with pus on the day following. A few days afterwards it changed to a brown scab, which came off spontaneously.

The most remarkable thing in the provings of Huber, is the length of time during which he observed the effects. Even as late as the 10th of March, forty-six days after he had taken any of the drug, he distinctly, although feebly, felt several of the effects of Thuja. The symptoms of the head lasted longest and were most frequent, especially the sensation as if *a nail had been driven in* in the angles of the parietal bones; as this sensation ceased, an *itching gnawing* was experienced in the same region, which induced him to scratch. The sensation as of something alive in the abdomen, and the *seeing of a luminous disk* shining like a fire-fly, lasted as long. This was sometimes perceived in the daytime, but most frequently at twilight in the room. Afterwards this luminous circle, which followed the movement of the eyeball, and was hovering at various distances now before one, now before both eyes, assumed a more elliptic form, and had a dark violet or blackish nucleus in the centre. Sometimes the disk was of the size of a millet or hemp seed only, but always luminous on the edge.*

D.

W. Huber, brother of the former prover, surgeon at Kleinzell, proved the Thuja on six persons; on himself, on two females, one of whom was his own wife, and on three of his children.

W. HUBER'S PROVINGS OF THUJA ON HIMSELF.

W. H. instituted three provings on his own person.

(25.) *First proving, with dilutions.*

1845, April 19th. W. H. commenced with the 30th dilution, taking every morning before breakfast 100 drops, and descending in the scale of the dilutions, until he had reached the first on the 18th of May, when the first proving was concluded. After taking the 21st dilution, he for the first time experienced a slight pressive headache over the right *superciliary eminence;* after the 20th dilution, violent pressive

* We may be permitted to remark, that in our opinion the 60th potency would not have excited so many symptoms, if the provings with the massive doses had not gone before. If the organism has been once thoroughly impregnated with large doses, the least quantity of the drug excites a new reaction as long as the first disturbance is not entirely counterbalanced.—*Mayrhofer.*

headache commencing in the region of the posterior and inferior angle of the left *parietal bone* and extending as far as the right *frontal eminence.* The pain only lasted while the prover remained in a state of rest: every movement diminished it and it returned immediately after the movement ceased. This pain became especially violent after the 19th dilution. It commenced half an hour after taking the medicine, and lasted all day. Even on the day following he was awakened by it at 5 o'clock in the morning and was compelled to rise, after which it ceased; the head, however, remained stupid and full. This was accompanied on the same day by frequent attacks of a boring pain in the *region of the bladder*, with painful *drawing up of the testes.*

From the 1st until the 12th of May, W. H. took from the 18th to the 7th dilution. The headache continued with more or less violence; on the last day it was accompanied with roughness of voice and a scraping sensation in the throat, which, however, continued only a few hours.

From the 13th to the 18th of May he took from the 6th to the 1st dilution. The headache gradually disappeared. In the place of this, H. had almost daily attacks, and sometimes several attacks a day of the boring pain in the region of the bladder, with painful *drawing up of the testes*, which was accompanied with occasional urging to stool. All these phenomena were but slightly marked during the last period of the proving, and disappeared in a few days after the medicine was discontinued.

(26.) *Second proving, with small doses of the tincture.*

June 18th. W. H. took 10 drops of the tincture before breakfast, increasing the dose every day by 10 drops.

During the first days the above described headache again made its appearance, but it was less violent and ceased entirely after the fourth day. On the 5th day, an hour after taking the drug, he experienced a sensation in the right side of the throat as though it were about to inflame; during the whole of that day he experienced stinging pains when swallowing, which disappeared again entirely in the subsequent night. No symptoms made their appearance from the sixth to the tenth day, except nausea on taking the drug; this nausea was excited even by the mere sight of the medicine.

(27.) *Third proving, with large doses of the tincture.*

July 7th. W. H. took 200 drops of the tincture, and repeated that dose on the 7th, 9th and 12th of the same month.

Every time he took the dose, he felt nauseated and disposed to vomit. The above described headache appeared again immediately after taking the first dose, but it never reached the violence which it had while proving the attenuations, although it continued until the

15th of July. The giddiness and the obtuseness of the head, on the contrary, were more violent. These symptoms were accompanied with *want of disposition to do anything*, *ill humor* and *inclination to anger*, pain in the throat during deglutition, and sour-smelling sweat almost every night. These phenomena continued in greater or less intensity during the proving, and even a few days beyond.

H. thinks that the scarcity of his symptoms is owing to the constant exercise which he was obliged to take during the period of the proving.

W. HUBER'S PROVING OF THUJA ON HIS WIFE.

H.'s wife made two experiments with Thuja.

(28.) *First proving, with dilutions.*

From the 19th of April to the 18th of May, Mrs. H. swallowed 100 drops of the various dilutions, from the 30th to the 1st, at the same time and in the same order as her husband, without experiencing any other symptoms, except slight vertigo and some headache in the forehead.

(29.) *Second proving, with the tincture.*

The second experiment was likewise instituted simultaneously with that of her husband, from the 18th to the 28th of June, with this difference, that, whereas he took progressively increasing doses, she took 10 drops a day for ten days in succession.

The prover was but little affected by those doses. On the fifth day after commencing the proving, several *wart-shaped excrescences*, of the size of a poppy-seed, made their appearance on both hands, gradually increasing during the proving, and amounting in number to sixteen. At the conclusion of the proving they varied in size according to the different periods when they had made their appearance. Their shape was that of a truncated cone; their surface was smooth, and they appeared to be seated in the epidermis.*

A fortnight after concluding the proving of Thuja, the warts ceased to grow. The largest warts were of the size of a small pea, and their formerly smooth surface had become rough and split. The remainder were smooth and of various sizes, according to their respective ages. They remained in that condition until about the middle of August, when the larger ones became depressed in the centre, and resembled a little pit surrounded by an elevated ridge. This ridge disappeared gradually, together with the wart. The smaller warts disappeared without going through this process.

* Huber's wife had formerly been troubled with warts, and, when she commenced the proving, she had one on the dorsum of the left hand, which had been in existence for several years.—*Mayrhofer.*

On the 10th of September eight warts still remained, and on the 11th of December (more than five months after the proving had been concluded,) all the warts had disappeared except a small one on the third joint of the left little finger.

(30.) HUBER'S PROVING OF THUJA ON THREE OF HIS CHILDREN.

Three of the children of Dr. H. likewise proved the dilutions of Thuja, from the 30th down to the 1st; two boys, of five and ten years, and a girl of seven. No symptoms were discovered in any of the children, except warts of the above described shape on the hands, of which the elder boy had six, the younger five, and the girl three.

On the 14th of September, after the results of the proving had been sent in, new warts continued making their appearance in the elder boy, and on the 11th of December he still had twenty-two warts of different sizes; while on that day the warts of the younger boy had all disappeared but one. No further information has been received in relation to the three warts of the girl.

(31.) HUBER'S PROVING OF THUJA ON A FEMALE AFFECTED WITH WARTS.

The prover is 40 years old, of a stout-make, middle-size, and sanguine temperament. Her menses appeared early, she married at the age of 20, and has five healthy children. Except during the periods of pregnancy and lactation, her menses were very profuse for three or four days; her health was constantly good. Three years ago she was attacked with horny warts, one on the tip of the left ring-finger, two in the palm of the left hand, and one in the palm of the right hand; they troubled her a good deal in her domestic affairs; while washing, either in cold or warm water, they became cracked and exhibited deep painful rhagades on the surface.

Being informed that she might possibly get rid of her warts by proving the Thuja, she consented to undertake it. From the 3d of May until the 30th of June, she took six drops of the mother-tincture every day, and from the 1st to the 26th of July, ten drops a day.

The prover living at a distance, H. could only see her occasionally, and he recorded the following observations at those intervals.

May 11th. The prover complained of frequent attacks of vertigo and diminished sleep. Her mood was *anxious*, and the menses, which appeared on the 6th, were inconsiderable and lasted only one day.

19th. Her complaints were the same. The vertigo frequently made its appearance when sitting or lying down; during the day she frequently experienced a transitory tremulousness over the whole body.

26th. The above-mentioned phenomena continued, especially the *anxiety*. The woman thought she could not continue the drug, because she had almost entirely lost her appetite, and suffered constantly from a sweetish taste; even streaks of blood were occasionally seen in the saliva, and the warts became still more painful. She consented, however, to continue the drug.

June 3d. The former symptoms continue. Moreover, *wart-shaped excrescences* of the size of a poppy-seed were discovered on the dorsum of either hand, six on the left, four on the right. In the daytime she is frequently attacked with *chilliness*, feels very weak, and has a slight *leucorrhœal discharge*, which she never had before. The old, horny warts are very painful when touched, or while she is at work, but the new ones are painless.

10th. The *chilliness* has been almost constant since the 3d, the prover has no appetite, is quite unwell, faint, debilitated as by fatigue, without being able to state what ails her. The warts looked as if split up, and exhibit deep, painful rhagades, especially while washing. To her great dismay, *the new, painless warts*, became larger every day. The leucorrhœa lasted until the 8th, when the menses made their appearance, which, however, lasted only a *single day*, and consisted in the discharge of a small clot of black blood of the size of a hazelnut. On the 9th, the *leucorrhœa* re-appeared. It is but scanty, but obliges her to wash herself frequently in the daytime. It is mild, yellow-green, and leaves spots of a similar appearance on her linen.

16th. The *leucorrhœa* increases. Every day she feels *a pain as if bruised*, at times in the *shoulders*, at times in the *thighs*. When stepping she feels an ulcerative pain in the soles of the feet, and they sweat constantly. The horny warts become more painful every day, and the skin around them becomes slightly *reddish*. The new warts are painless, almost as large as the old warts, of the shape of truncated cones, have a smooth surface, and appear to be seated in the epidermis only. Besides these warts, traces of new warts are perceived on the dorsa of the hands and on the fingers.

26th. The pain in the shoulders and thighs ceased six days ago, the ulcerative pain in the soles of the feet continues, the leucorrhœa and the chilliness continue likewise. The painful old warts are still surrounded with a red areola, and the rudimentary traces above mentioned have been developed into ten new warts of the size of poppy-seeds.

30th. The ulcerative pains in the soles of the feet have ceased. The other symptoms continue.

July 8th. Having taken ten drops of the tincture every day, she has felt worse, ever since the first dose. She complained of being *faint*, *chilly*, *anxious*, and that she had lost her appetite. This condition continued until the 7th, when the menses appeared, after which the pains diminished. The menses lasted only *one day*, and consisted in the discharge of three clots of black blood, of the size of a hazelnut. *The leucorrhœa continued after the menses.*

18th. The last 10 drops had affected the prover very much. The frequent chilliness with debility were now accompanied with *difficult breathing*, short and hacking cough, and momentary *palpitation of the heart*. These symptoms were especially troublesome in the daytime:

the nights were quiet: the old warts presented the same appearance as before: the new ones (the first crop) assume an irregular shape, and exhibit a *rough surface.* The most recent warts (the second crop) had become somewhat larger, and traces are even perceived of a third crop. The leucorrhœa continues, and the prover thinks she has become thinner during the period of proving.

26th. All the symptoms continue in an increased degree. The difficulty of breathing and the feeling of anxiety attending it are especially troublesome. The appetite is almost entirely wanting; every meal causes pressure at the stomach. The debility is worse. The prover looks pale and sickly. Her dresses have become loose. There are four sets of warts: the oldest are still surrounded with red areolæ; the next have a rough surface and an irregular shape; the smaller warts of the second crop have smooth surfaces, and the shape of truncated cones, and lastly the warts of the third crop, which are very small, from the size of a poppy-seed to that of a millet-seed.

As she not unreasonably feared that continuing the experiment would produce further trouble, and increase the number of her warts, she put an end to the proving on the 26th of July.

All the symptoms continued with diminished violence until the 3d of August. The warts remained unchanged, except that the last crop seemed to have ceased to grow.

On the 7th of August, the menses made their appearance; they were somewhat greater than the last time, and lasted a day and night. On their appearance, all the other symptoms diminished, even the old warts became less painful, and the red areolæ paler. All the recent excrescences remained unchanged.

18th. Most of the symptoms had disappeared; she had a good appetite, her breathing had again become easy and the leucorrhœa had ceased. The old warts had become smaller and less painful, and they ceased to crack during washing. The three subsequent crops continued unchanged. By the 30th of August the health and good looks of the prover had entirely returned. The old warts had ceased to be painful, had much diminished in size, were even scarcely raised above the skin; several of the new warts had disappeared without leaving a trace, and the remaining ones were much diminished.

Sept. 8th. The old warts had almost entirely disappeared, and the recent warts likewise.

The menses, which appeared on the 5th of Sept., lasted three days, and flowed as before the proving.

Dec. 11th. One hundred and thirty-eight days after the conclusion of the provings, the old horny warts had disappeared without leaving the least trace in the epidermis. Of the recent warts nothing was left at that time except a very small trace of one only.

E.

F. LACKNER'S PROVING WITH THE TINCTURE (32.)

Frederick Lackner, student of medicine, twenty-two years old, of a melancholy choleric temperament and a robust constitution, had dysentery when a boy, also scarlet-fever and measles, was frequently affected with worms and toothache, and had a violent ophthalmia when he was sixteen years old, which left a great disposition to congestion to the head and eyes, continuing to the present time. For the last four years L. has enjoyed excellent health.

1844, Oct. 10th. He commenced the proving of Thuja with 6 drops of the tincture, which he took in the morning. They caused eructations, colic towards noon, and diarrhœa.

11th. 8 drops had the same effect. 12th. 10 drops, after which the colic became exceedingly painful; it diminished gradually after a copious evacuation. In the hypogastrium the prover experienced a sensation as of *pressure*, especially directly above the *symphysis pubis*.

13th and 14th. L. took 12 and 14 drops, and no medicine on the 15th. On all those days the colic was less, but the *sensation of pressure in the hypogastrium* from within outwards remained the same.

16th and 17th. 16 and 18 drops, the colic and diarrhœa increased.

18th. 20 drops; had slight colic and felt drowsy the whole day.

19th. 25 drops, after which he experienced a constant gurgling in the bowels.

20th, 21st and 22d. 30, 35 and 38 drops, which increased the colic and diarrhœa.

23d. 40 drops. After the lapse of two hours the colic became so violent, that he was scarcely able to stand straight, and had to sit with his trunk bent forward. These pains lasted upwards of an hour, and diminished after a copious evacuation accompanied with emission of a quantity of flatulence. In the evening the pains became again more severe, without, however, reaching the former degree of violence. His sleep was restless and full of dreams.

24th. No medicine was taken, and the colic abated and the sleep became more quiet.

25th and 26th. 45 and 50 drops, which again brought on slight colic, which was considerably increased on the 27th, after taking 55 drops.

L. now discontinued the proving for three days. On the 28th the colic kept increasing and disturbed even his sleep; it was accompanied with distention of the abdomen and constipation. On the 29th in the morning he had eructations; towards 10 o'clock great nausea with accelerated pulse, debility of the limbs as from weariness, and cold sweat over the whole body. This condition improved during a walk, by the raising of a quantity of wind. The colic, on the contrary, increased until noon, but abated towards evening. In the morning and after dinner he had a copious fluid evacuation. The appetite was less, the sleep restless and disturbed with dreams. On the 30th, in the morning, he had a scanty liquid evacuation; the colic was very slight and the appetite diminished.

On the 31st of Oct. and on the 1st of Nov. he took 60 and 65 drops, which did not produce any new symptoms, but on the 2d of Nov., after taking 70 drops, he had again colic and diarrhœa, which became so violent on the following day, after another dose of 75 drops, that he was scarcely able to stand straight at noon. While driving home, the colic, which was now accompanied with headache and chilliness, became almost intolerable. After it had lasted almost an hour, it abated somewhat after a very copious liquid evacuation, which was accompanied with copious emission of flatulence: but again increased towards evening.

Nov. 8th. L. continued taking the Thuja, and, nevertheless, increased the doses by five drops every day, so that at this date he took 100 drops.

The most constant symptom was the colic, which increased from morning until noon, intermitted after dinner, but re-appeared in the evening and continued until midnight; this was accompanied with the *sensation of pressure in the hypogastric region.*

9th. 110 drops. During the day he had colic; in the evening *burning* in the *eyelids* and *the sight was less distinct;* in the night pain in the head and eyes, pressure in the pit of the stomach, and hurried breathing. He did not sleep till towards morning, after which the symptoms disappeared.

10th and 11th. 120 and 130 drops, after which he experienced a *burning* in *the eyelids* with *obscuration of sight;* the sleep was interrupted and restless. The same symptoms appeared on the 12th, after taking 140 drops. In the evening the pupils were dilated. On the 13th no medicine was taken; 150 drops, which were taken on the 14th, were not followed by any new symptoms.

15th. 160 drops. After dinner he suddenly felt a *shrill ringing* in the right ear, which, after a few hours, as suddenly changed to a dull *buzzing* and *groaning*, the latter sensations gradually changing to a *noise as of a bubbling liquid*, which continued all night. In the evening and night he emitted a large quantity of *flatulence* and *yellowish wine-colored urine;* his sleep was disturbed by *voluptuous dreams;* in the morning he felt excessively drowsy, and was loth to leave the bed. No alvine evacuation.

16th. 170 drops. The whole day he emitted a quantity of flatulence without any motion of the bowels; his mood was especially cheerful; he slept quietly at night.

17th. 180 drops. These caused the *emission of an excessive quantity of flatulence* day and night. In the morning he had a scanty evacuation with some colic.

18th. 190 drops, after which he had a scanty papescent stool (after dinner) and then *a violent burning at the anus.* In the evening he had colic and emitted a quantity of flatulence.*

* The colic which is occasioned by Thuja seems to originate primarily from the distention of the bowels produced by flatulence.—*Mayrhofer.*

19th and 20th. 200 and 210 drops, which occasioned nothing but colic and a liquid evacuation.

21st. 220 drops. These occasioned a papescent stool in the forenoon. In the evening, moderate colic, and, during the night, *constant desire to urinate* and emission of a *large quantity of light-yellow urine.* Every urination was followed by a violent *burning pain* in the *urethra*, and in the *fundus of the bladder.* In the morning he had a hard stool and soon after violent colic.

22d. 230 drops, after which the colic lasted all day, the desire to urinate likewise; the pain after urinating was, however, less.

23d. 240 drops, after which he discontinued the drug until the 30th. During this period of time he observed the following symptoms: every day, after dinner, he had a papescent stool with emission of a quantity of flatulence, hoarseness and secretion of mucus in the fauces obliging him to spit; *obscuration of sight with dilatation of the pupils and burning of the eyelids.*

30th. 150 drops, after which, he discontinued the drug until the 7th of Dec. The same symptoms appeared as on the previous days, but in a less degree, and they disappeared, finally, altogether.

Dec. 8th, 9th, 10th and 11th. 260, 270, 280 and 290 drops of the tincture; the only symptom occasioned by these doses, was a slight colic.

12th. 300 drops. At noon he felt a slight colic; in the evening he suddenly felt a violent pain in the whole abdomen, as if all the bowels were pulled towards a point behind the umbilicus. This was accompanied with distention of the abdomen, headache and accelerated pulse. This colic lasted six hours, and abated gradually after a liquid evacuation accompanied by an emission of a large amount of flatulence.

13th. 310 drops. The colic continued until evening; on the 14th, after taking 320 drops, he experienced all day occasional shooting stitches in the abdomen. Took no medicine on the 15th and 16th, and had no symptoms.

From the 17th to tho 24th of Dec. inclusive, L. took a dose daily, increasing every dose by 10 drops, so that on the last day he took 400 drops.

The symptoms elicited by this prover were meagre and one-sided. He was attacked with colic every day, noon and evening, which increased from day to day, and became extremely violent on the 23d of Dec. and on the 3d of November. The colic abated considerably on the emission, during a walk, of a considerable quantity of flatulence upwards and downwards, and after a copious liquid evacuation at noon. In the afternoon and evening he occasionally suffered from sticking, gurgling, rumbling and shifting of flatulence in the abdomen, and he had a sleepless, restless night.

24th. These symptoms abated; on the two subsequent days when L. took no medicine, he complained of nothing but debility.

27th and 28th. 410 and 420 drops did not occasion any new symptoms; on the following days, 430, 440 and 450 drops occasioned no other symptoms than the constant rumbling and shifting of flatulence in the abdomen, accompanied with shooting stitches in all the parts of the body.

Persuaded that the Thuja had been prevented from manifesting its proper effects upon the organism by the rapid succession of large doses, L. discontinued the proving for a few days, and even during the first days of January, 1845, perceived traces of the last named symptoms.*

January 8th and 9th. No symptoms being any longer observed, L. took 460 and 470 drops, without any results.

10th. 480 drops; two hours after taking the drug, he had eructations, desire to vomit, and a peculiar feeling of qualmishness in the pit of the stomach; these symptoms continued until midnight, and were accompanied with constipation, restless sleep, and vivid dreams.

11th and 12th. 490 and 500 drops, which occasioned the following symptoms: drawing and tearing in the pericranium, at times in the region of the vertex, at times in that of the occiput; one scanty stool every day; confused dreams about the most absurd things. On the evening of the last day, *burning* and *stinging* in both eyes and eyelids, with injection of the cornea; these symptoms continued on the 13th after taking 510 drops.

14th and 15th no medicine was taken. On waking on the 14th, he was for a long time unable to open his eyelids. They were painful and closed again involuntarily. After rising he felt debilitated all over, especially in the upper arms and thighs; *clouds* and *streaks* (*muscæ volitantes*) were hovering before his eyes the whole day, accompanied with *indistinctness of sight*, which continued the next day.

16th and 17th. 520 and 530 drops occasioned a warm feeling in the region of the stomach; 540 drops, which he took on the 18th, occasioned a feeling of qualmishness, eructations, and the emission of a quantity of flatulence.

No medicine was taken from the 19th until the 6th of Feb. inclusive. On the first day the region of the stomach was very sensitive even to the least pressure, especially in the evening; there was a frequent and continuous rising of wind from the stomach, and continual emissions of copious flatulence from the rectum. These symptoms gradually abated on the following days, and finally ceased entirely.

Feb. 7th and 8th. 550 and 560 drops; the only result obtained was eructations tasting of resin, accompanied with aversion to the drug, which became so invincible that he had to conclude his provings after having taking 15,920 drops of the undiluted tincture in the space of 122 days.

* The development of the effects of a drug is most certainly prevented when the doses taken are relatively so large as to excite vomiting, diarrhœa, profuse sweat or enuresis; by means of these processes the drug is carried out of the body, and is thus prevented from penetrating the organism and manifesting its physiological action upon those parts of the organism to which it stands in physiological relation. —*Mayrhofer.*

This indefatigable prover deserved a better result: the drug in him principally affected the primæ viæ, producing violent flatulent colic, diarrhœa, and enuresis, by which revulsions the development of the specific effects of Thuja was prevented.

F.

Jacob Landesmann, chief physician to the battalion of Grenadiers, under Major Blankardt, made two experiments upon himself with Thuja.

(33.) *First proving with dilutions.*

The unquestionable effects which L. had experienced from a few drops of the first dilution of Bryonia, induced him to commence the proving of Thuja with the smallest doses of the higher dilutions, and to descend by gentle degrees to the lower.

After he had discontinued taking Bryonia for three weeks, and had felt free from any drug-symptoms for two, he took, from the 4th to the 20th of Sept., 1844, regularly every morning, one hour before a milk breakfast, three globules moistened with the 27th dilution of Thuja, (1 : 100 prepared by himself five years before).

Sept. 4th and 5th. L. remarked no change in his sensations.

6th. In the forenoon, *drawing tearing* in the right arm, lasting several hours.

7th. The same sensation.

8th. Drawing, sticking pains in the right index and middle fingers.

9th. A renewal of the drawing tearing in the right arm, in the morning; later, at about half-past ten, debility and lameness in the right forearm, and violent trembling of the right hand, in which the veins swelled without any apparent cause. This appearance lasted half an hour, and disappeared while writing.

10th. *Violent itching on different parts of the skin*, particularly on the breast, with a sensation as if the skin at those spots was pierced *with many very fine needles*, which irresistibly obliged him to scratch. On the evening of the same day, there came on, without cause, a heavy cold preceded by dulness of the head and frequent sneezing.

11th. At 10 in the morning, a sticking pain in the ring-finger of the left hand; towards noon, *stinging itching* on the breast again, and on both sides of the neck, and at 9 in the evening, drawing pains in the left shin-bone.

12th. A slight pain was observed in the right side of the pharynx, extending to the ear, somewhat aggravated by swallowing.

13th. The morning pain in the neck had entirely disappeared, but returned in the afternoon, with feeling of dryness and increased thirst, and wholly vanished again in the evening.

The remaining days presented no new symptoms. It is particularly to be remarked, however, that the *catarrh* was troublesome through the whole of this proving, and had *this peculiarity*, that it often completely disappeared for hours together, and then suddenly returned without cause, with renewed severity, and with much sneezing.

From the 20th to the 28th, L. took every morning six globules moistened with the sixth dilution, which had no other effect than that they seemed to sustain the still continuing catarrh.

From the 29th Sept. to the 3d Oct., L. took again the 27th dilution, and five drops besides every morning, but without effect.

Oct. 4th, 5th, and 6th. He took every morning five, and from the 7th to the 17th, ten drops of the sixth dilution. Whereupon, besides the still continuing catarrh, the following symptoms appeared:

5th. In the afternoon, *cutting pains* in the *vesica* for some minutes.

6th. In the morning, sticking, cutting pains in the left side of the neck, as far as the left ear, which soon disappeared again.

7th. In the afternoon, drawing pain in the left middle finger.

8th. Repeated drawings in the left great toe, and at night *lascivious dreams with a pollution.*

From the 9th to the 12th, except the constant catarrh, no symptoms.

13th. Dryness in the throat; soreness of the breast, with aggravated catarrh, and in the night *confused lascivious dreams.*

14th. In the morning and at noon, a feeling of stoppage in the left ear, with diminished power of hearing, each time lasting several minutes.

15th. In the morning, distinct, violent stitches from the anus into the region of the left iliac bone.

16th. At various times, drawings in the left little finger.

From the 18th to the 22d Oct., L. took, every morning, fifteen, and from the 22d to the 29th, thirty drops of the first dilution.

18th. The catarrh, which had remitted, became worse with frequent sneezing. Afterward on the same day in the afternoon, a *sharp lancinating* pain in the left frontal eminence, and soon after, sharp tearings in the inside of the right ankle.

19th. Were perceived at several times, tearings in the little finger of the right hand, and in the evening dulness of the head in the forehead.

20th. Frequent *quiverings* of the *lower lid of the left eye.*

21st. Again, frequent quiverings of the same *eyelid;* further, *drawing* in the little finger in the right hand, and restless sleep with *lascivious dreams.*

The following days passed without symptoms. But on the 26th, frequent quiverings came on in the afternoon and evening, *pulse-like jerks in the muscles* of the right arm, especially in the deltoid. L. was, also, the whole day, causelessly excited and inclined to be angry, contrary to all his previous habits.

28th. At about half past ten in the forenoon, while walking, he was attacked with such deadly hunger, that he came near fainting, and was obliged, at a very unwonted time, to eat something in a neighboring tavern. This symptom made the more impression on him, as it was repeated in the evening of the same and of the following day. He had likewise, in the right nostril, a feeling of soreness or ulceration, which was aggravated by pressure upon the ala, but disappeared on the following day.

29th. L. took forty drops of the first dilution, but was prevented by circumstances from pursuing the experiment from that day. No further symptoms developed themselves which could be attributed to the drug. The catarrh lasted until the middle of December, and the prover has much less hesitation in ascribing it to the power of the drug, because a catarrh had never lasted him so long before.

(34.) *Second proving, with the tincture.*

Feb. 1st. L. began a new experiment with the tincture of Thuja, of which he took on the first day ten drops and increased the dose daily by five drops, so that on the 15th of the month he had reached eighty, and had taken in the whole 675 drops.

Not the slightest change in his feelings followed any dose of the tincture.* From this circumstance, the prover concluded that his susceptibility to the remedy was by this time exhausted, and in the conviction that continuing to take it in increasing doses would produce conditional symptoms, depending more upon the quantity than the quality of the drug, he discontinued the proving in order that he might no longer defer the more grateful result of an experiment with a remedy more accordant with his constitution.

(35.) G.

Dr. and Prof. Liedbeck, from Upsala, aged 42, of a sanguineo-bilious temperament and narrow build, often suffering from catarrhs and hemorrhoids, made an experiment with Thuja during his residence in Vienna.

1844, Sept. 14th. He took, at about five o'clock in the afternoon, a teaspoonful of the undiluted tincture. Thereafter, eructations with the taste of the remedy and, an hour later, transient pain in the forehead and in the left side of the face, a sort of twitching.

15th. After having taken sixty drops in the morning; eructations tasting of the drug, then a repeated transitory *stitch* in the left frontal eminence, and a sensation of dryness in the mouth—after another sixty drops taken the same afternoon, *a gloomy, melancholy state of mind* came on, which was still apparent on waking next morning.

16th. Seventy drops; followed by eructations, strong aversion to meat, which had already been perceived on the preceding day, difficult swallowing, without any apparent cause, in the throat, stitches in both

* We can render no satisfactory account whatever, why it is, nor under what conditions it happens, that in certain cases attenuations produce more powerful effects upon the organism than the concentrated drug, and in certain other cases, precisely the reverse occurs; and so long as this veil is not lifted, so long will the contest about the superiority of the high and low potencies remain undecided.—*Mayrhofer.*

sides of the thorax under the mammæ, both during respiration and when not respiring. The melancholy frame of mind continued. These symptoms disappeared in the course of the following day, excepting the stitches in the thorax, which often returned and did not seem to be connected with the respiration.

25th. L. took 140 drops of the tincture of Thuja. Eructations followed, and a feeling as though perspiration was about to break out.

26th. The same symptoms followed a like dose. It is to be observed, that the prover thinks that he passed ***more urine*** during the experiment than at other times.

The departure of our northern brother in the faith unfortunately prevented the further prosecution of the experiment.

H.

Dr. Maschauer instituted two experiments upon himself with the Thuja.

(36.) *First proving, with the tincture.*

1844, Sept. 21st. M. began the proving with ten drops of the tincture taken early, fasting. He perceived no effects but an unpleasant taste.

22d and 23d. Each day ten drops; followed in the afternoon of the first day by rumbling in the abdomen with emission of flatulence, ***copious limpid urine*** and constipation; on the second day, scraping in the throat and inclination to cough. In the afternoon, the uvula seemed to be lengthened, and the tonsils were vividly reddened, but the swallowing was not worse.

24th and 25th. Thirty drops; on the first day dryness of the palate with inclination to cough, sidelong stitch in the lower half of the left breast; in the evening aching in the forehead with failure of the sight —at night ***frequent urination.*** On the following day, continued scraping in the throat with frequent cough, the headache and increased urination also persisted, and were accompanied by a ***stitch*** in the left ***testicle.***

26th. Forty drops. The scraping in the throat much less; at noon, a double stitch in the breast; want of appetite with great thirst and dryness of the mouth; at night ***copious urine, with itchings in the urethra.***

27th. When nothing had been taken, restless sleep, interrupted by straining cough; the urine continued increased.

28th. M. took fifty drops, and discontinued the dose for two days. Effects, nauseous taste; eructations with smell of Thuja; frequent hawking with the sensation as if the throat were sore, continuing the whole three days. In the evening, headache in the vertex, remaining until midnight; ***itchings in the urethra when urinating;*** restless nights.

Oct. 2d and 3d. M. took on each day 60 drops on an empty stomach. On the first day frequent hawking with cough; in the afternoon stitches in the lower part of the left breast, and debility, with feeling as if beaten in the limbs. On the second day, soon after taking the dose: dryness of the tongue; throughout the day much thirst and *itching in the anus;* in the evening considerable headache which lasted until midnight; constipation. On the third day, *itching in the anus* passing into a severe *burning* after a hard evacuation; *scraping in the throat* compelling him to cough, accompanied by *itching in the urethra.* During the whole three days frequent and copious urine, especially at night.

4th and 5th, M. rested. The itching in the anus appeared at times in both days, and the evacuations ceased.

6th. 70 drops. The itching in the anus and the hawking and cough again became worse; the latter with oppression of the chest, which seemed somewhat to embarrass the breathing; also, copious urine, hard stool, and restless sleep.

7th and 8th. 80 drops each day. On the evening of the first day, a repeated, violent stitch in the left side of the chest; on both days, frequent raising of mucus with cough and reddened tonsils without pain; disagreeable *itchings in the urethra and anus.*

9th. After taking 100 drops, lasting pressing headache in the forehead with *burning in the eyes,* which were pained by the light. Continuance of the *itching in the anus and the redness of the tonsils: copious urine,* failure of an evacuation, (M. was accustomed to have a regular passage every day in the morning,) and a restless night. On the three following days, he took no medicine, and the above symptoms, except *accasionally the itching in the anus,* disappeared.

13th. M. took again 100 drops. In the afternoon, *itching through the whole urethra during urination,* and headache on awaking after a restless night.

14th. 120 drops. The headache continued all day. In the afternoon, a violent stitch in the left side of the chest, increased by inspiration. Afterward, a hard evacuation with subsequent *burning in the anus;* the *urine* was copious, rest good.

15th. 140 drops. Two hours after, a violent evacuation with bellyache and *burning in the anus;* in the evening, headache in the forehead; at night, another evacuation and rumbling in the abdomen; also, general debility and *copious urine, with itchings in the urethra.*

16th. 140 drops. Shifting of flatulence with constipation; scrapings in the throat with cough; in the evening, headache followed by a restless night. During the three following days, no medicine being taken, the evacuations became again regular, but the *urine* remained *increased,* and the sleep was restless.

20th. After taking 160 drops, no evacuation, but a strong urging towards it, with *itching in the anus* and *into the urethra; the urine still copious:* in the evening, headache, which lasted until about midnight; after that, quiet sleep.

21st. Another 160 drops, (taken fasting and diluted with water, as was always done); swelling in the region of the stomach, diminished by emissions of flatulence; in the afternoon, a hard stool and *itching during urination;* in the evening, a return of the headache. On the two following days, no dose was taken and no symptoms were perceived.

24th. 180 drops were followed by these symptoms: uneasiness in the region of the stomach with eructations of the drug; scrapings in the throat with frequent cough; in the afternoon, headache with ***burning in the right eye***, which disappeared on repeatedly washing it with cold water; ***copious urine***, especially at night.

25th. M. closed his proving of the tincture, with 200 drops. After two hours, a sudden debility, with painful lassitude, with pain in the calves of the legs; then, an internal chill in the whole body, with dry and hot skin, which compelled him to lie down. He could not, however, keep warm in bed, and the debility increased to such a degree that he could with difficulty move his limbs. At about ten o'clock in the evening this chill first began to disappear, merging in a dry and burning heat, and towards morning, *a sweat broke out over the whole body.* He had no appetite, much thirst, passed no urine during the whole day, and had during the access of heat a full, quick pulse and intolerable headache. On the morning of the following day, he passed a small quantity of dark-red urine; the sweat continued until noon, and the prover could not leave his bed on account of his extreme weakness. A chill came on again in the evening, followed by a sleepless night.

27th. The debility continued; he had no appetite, his tongue was furred, and he urinated copiously.

28th. For the first time, M. felt better, but could not bring himself to continue taking the tincture of Thuja; for the simple smell of the drug disgusted and horrified him.

29th and 30th. ***The itching in the anus*** was again perceived and the *copious urine* persisted.

Nov. 8th. The prover first considered the action of the Thuja to be exhausted, as all the vital functions were then favorably re-instated.

(37.) *Second proving with the first three dilutions* (10 : 90).

Forty days after the last dose of 200 drops, M. began his second proving.

Dec. 5th. He took ten drops of the 3d dilution, and increased the dose daily by ten drops until the 15th of the month, without noting the least variation in his ordinary sensations.

From the 16th to the 23d, M. tried daily ten drops, morning and evening, of the second dilution—with a similar want of result. From the 24th to the 27th, he took twice a day ten drops of the first dilution. After doing this three days in succession, the well known *itching in the **anus*** developed itself and was especially troublesome in the forenoon.

28th. After twice taking fifteen drops of the same dilution, a slight *stitch in the urethra, increased urinating* at night, and dampness at *the anus.*

30th. M. took in the morning 30, and in the evening 15 drops of Thuja of the first dilution; afterwards uneasiness in the stomach, eructations of wind, bitter taste; in the evening, violent headache, lasting until ten o'clock; *copious, limpid urine, itching and sweat on the anus.*

1845, Jan. 2d. He observed, after 30 drops, from time to time, *stitches in the urethra, with urgent desire to urinate,* loss of appetite, vertigo, and headache in the forehead in the evening.

From the 3d to the 10th, M. took daily 30 drops of the first dilution in the morning, and 20 in the evening. The constant symptoms were; *urgency to urinate,* with stitches in the *urethra* and *itchings in the anus.*

This very promising experiment was unfortunately broken off in consequence of the death of a person nearly connected with the zealous prover.

I.

I (Dr. Mayrhofer) proved the *arbor vitæ* upon myself and on my wife.

On myself I instituted four experiments.

(38.) *First proving, with the first two dilutions.*

I began the proving of Thuja with the second dilution, making no change in my manner of life.

1844, Sept. 8th. At 3 o'clock in the afternoon, I took 50 drops without experiencing the slightest change in my sensations; 100 drops taken early, fasting, on the 9th, produced no further effect, nor did 150 more taken in the evening of the same day, nor 200 drops taken on the 10th.

I tried then, on the 11th, at 6 o'clock in the morning, 100, and in the evening 200 drops of the first dilution, without observing any morbid phenomena.

Second proving, with the tincture in increasing doses.

1844, Sept. 12th. The want of susceptibility of my tough system to the power of the dilutions determined me to try the undiluted tincture, of which, on this day, I took 50 drops morning and evening each, but waited yet in vain for any signs of life in Thuja.

13th. After 100 drops taken early and fasting, I first perceived, during the day: *swelling of the hemorrhoidal veins, with tenesmus, itching and burning in the anus.* In the evening, on repeating the

100 drops, I had two slight passages, ending with discharge of mucus, itching, and burning.

14th. In the morning 100, and in the evening 200 drops. The *itching and burning in the anus* increased, and were especially troublesome in the evening after a stool.—During the night, *more frequent and copious urine* than formerly, and, immediately after urinating, I felt a renewed inclination, whereby a few drops were discharged without pain.

15th. 200 drops, taken both morning and evening, produced no new symptoms.

16th. At 6 in the morning, 300 drops. Immediately afterwards, nauseous taste and confluence of much saliva in the mouth. After a quarter of an hour, dull headache over the whole frontal region (lasting an hour). At six in the evening, a stool, with subsequent *burning in the anus*, and shortly after a reiterated discharge of mucus, attended with *very violent stitches in the rectum* in the direction of a line from the anus to the sacrum. As the stitches ceased, the itching and burning returned, and lasted until ten o'clock.

17th. 300 drops. *Itching and burning in the anus* remained the prominent symptom, lasting till midnight and preventing sleep. Three stools followed, ending always with discharge of mucus; the *urine* was plainly *increased*, and after urination the *inclination returned, attended with the voiding of a few drops more.*

18th. At about six in the morning, 600 drops were taken in a glass of water, with the following result: Eructations of the drug for some hours, confluence of saliva in the mouth, headache in the frontal region, and in the evening three stools, with subsequent *itching and burning in the anus* and *irritating stitches up the rectum.* On the following day, on which I took no dose, I frequently felt flying stitches under the right shoulder-blade, and in the evening had three stools with the accustomed accompaniments.

As in the course of the 20th, the following day, I perceived no drug-affections, I took 400 drops at about nine in the evening. Before midnight sleep was destroyed by the emission of much flatulence, by *itching and burning in the anus, accompanied by flying stitches in the rectum and by repeated urination;* sleep, however, came on after midnight, and on awaking I found myself better than I could have expected after a bad night. I took no medicine on the next three days; regularly every evening *the itching and burning in the anus* set in; every day also I had two stools ending with a discharge of mucus.

23d. In the evening, 500 drops. Increased warmth in the face with dull confusion in the head (effect of the alcohol); unrefreshing sleep, interrupted by terrible dreams (of the dead) and by *frequent urination.* On the following morning dull confusion in the head with general debility. Through the day *flying drawing pains* in various parts, especially in the hands, and in the evening a return of the *itching and burning in the anus.*

From the 25th to the end of the month I ceased to take the drug, and made the following observations: On the evening of the 26th, three round red spots of the size of a lentil, which itched and obliged me to scratch, appeared on the inner surface of the right forearm near the wrist. The itching became *burning* when they were scratched. On the following morning they had disappeared without leaving a trace; on the 28th, I remarked a painful *tubercle* of about the same size in the neighborhood of the anus, on the raphé of the perinæum, which likewise disappeared in a couple of days. *Flying drawing*, now here, now there, and troublesome *itching in the anus*, especially in the evening, developed themselves every day, gradually however, wearing off.

Oct. 1st. At five in the afternoon, 500 drops; followed by nausea eructations of the remedy and (after half an hour) *itching and burning in the anus.* During the night, *discharge of much flatulence* *copious urine;* at six in the morning of the following day an evacuation with burning in the anus; through the day felt well.

2d. On taking 500 drops, the constant *burning and itching in the anus* reappeared, and the night's rest was as usual disturbed by *frequent urination* and restless dreams. On the following day, no other symptoms were perceived except debility and occasional flying *stitches in the rectum.*

4th. I took, at about three in the afternoon, another 500 drops. In the evening dull confusion of the head and *burning in the anus;* on the following night *abundant urine, much flatulence*, and dreams. On the following day I felt pretty well again; while urinating, however, I made the unpleasant discovery that the glans penis was entirely covered with a *greenish-yellow, ill-smelling secretion,* and after I had cleansed it, I observed on the dorsum of the glans, near the hinder border, four *tubercles* about the size of a flaxseed, with a *vesicle* on the summit, and in the sulcus, near the attachment of the foreskin, was a small eroded spot, surrounded by a red circle, about the size of a lentil.

6th. Nevertheless, I again took 500 drops of the tincture; upon which the symptoms already described again appeared, and the *tubercles* on the glans had increased by two. The *urine*, since the large doses of Thuja, had become turbid, and, in cooling, deposited a flocky, mucous cloud. Urination was performed without pain, but a sensation was often experienced, while seated, as if the *glans had been bruised.*

7th. No new symptoms were developed by a fresh dose of 500 drops, except that the *vesicles* of the elevations before described were broken, and left behind little painless *erosions*, surrounded by a red margin, and yielding the secretion alluded to.

During the three following days no medicine was taken, and the *protuberances became flatter, the circle paler*, and at last the *sore spots* disappeared also. Pains, at one time *drawing*, at another *tearing*, were repeatedly felt, especially in the extremities, for the most part while at rest, but in the right tibia also while walking, so as to make me limp.

11th. At three in the afternoon, 600 drops. Besides the usual phenomena, I noticed on the following day, *granular, elevated red spots on the glans penis, which was uncommonly sensitive*, and on the 13th the *sebaceous glands of the prepuce appeared swollen and inflamed;* but, on the 14th, the inflamed spots were paler again, the clustered, prominent *tubercles* flatter; and on the 15th the appearance of the prepuce and glans was again natural.

16th. At three in the afternoon I drank 1000 drops in a pint of water. Immediately afterwards, nausea with vomiturition and confluence of saliva in the mouth. After an hour, headache in the frontal region with heat in the cheeks; and half an hour later, general feeling as if beaten, with a chill over the whole body in so remarkable a degree, that I was obliged to go to bed, although it was only six o'clock in the evening. The night was disturbed by many dreams and frequent urination. On the three following days, no medicine being taken, I felt uncommonly debilitated. I was especially annoyed by the *itching and burning in the anus*, attended by several violent *stitches in the rectum* (particularly in the evening). I also had, at times, *drawing pains in the hands and feet*, which still continued even after eight days, growing, however, weaker and weaker. No change was perceptible in the glans penis, but I felt a burning pain in the perinæum, the *raphé* of which *was more prominent* than usual, and one inch from the anus *a tubercle of the size of a pea* appeared, which increased for three days, became moist, smarted in walking, and then day by day became smaller and disappeared in about ten days.

(40.) *Third proving, likewise with the tincture.*

Nov. 8th. After I had desisted for three weeks, and felt myself pretty free from the effects of the drug, I began a new proving, by taking 300 drops of the tincture at four o'clock in the afternoon; whereupon the well-known Thuja symptoms made their appearance, as *transitory drawing*, perceptible now here, now there, *itching and burning in the anus, copious urine, sensitiveness of the glans*, &c., &c.

9th. 300 drops in the evening. In the night, increased sexual desire, which, during the whole course of the preceding proving, had been rather diminished than exalted.

10th. On the following day, soon after waking, I was annoyed by an *itching, burning pain in the hollow below the os coccygis*, lasting all day. The same phenomena recurred on taking 300 drops in the evening. Three days subsequently the *glans became sensitive*, and the sebaceous glands of the prepuce *swollen* as before on the 12th of October. On the fourth day I remarked *a red tubercle* between the scrotum and the right thigh; violent *itching in the hollow* below the os coccygis was again very troublesome, and the *anus became as sensitive*, after a slimy discharge, as though *the skin were cracked and chapped there.*

19th. When most of the Thuja symptoms had ceased, I took at about three o'clock in the afternoon 1200 drops of the tincture (in weight one ounce and two scruples) in a pint of water. The effect of this draught was at first the drunkenness induced by alcohol; heat in the head and face, uncertain gait, reeling of surrounding objects, &c. In the evening, a general feeling as if beaten, which drove me to bed at eight o'clock. Sleep was interrupted, as before, by dreams and *frequent occasion to urinate.* On the following days, besides the occasional drawing in the limbs, I was annoyed by most constant Thuja symptoms, *itching and burning in the anus with tenesmus*, especially in the evening.

23d. *Deep-red spots* showed themselves on the glans, and *the inner surface of the foreskin was inflamed and swollen.*

24th. The fifth day after the large dose of Thuja, a *slight burning pain* was perceived in the glans, which, on examining in the furrow behind the corona, was entirely covered with a *thin, yellowish, ill-smelling secretion*, on the removal of which *two deep-red spots* were discovered which appeared to be eroded, and from which the fluid alluded to transuded.

25th. The two spots had increased in size, run together, and were covered with *granular elevations*; the *glans was rendered uncomfortable*, but urination was performed without pain.

26th. The whole *furrow* as far as the frænulum *was sore* and covered with *papillæ of the size of a poppyseed.* The secretion from the glans was very copious.

27th and 28th of the month, the secretion was diminished in quantity, but some twelve or fifteen *reddish excrescences* arose on the hinder border of the glans, the largest of which was about the size of a flaxseed, and the inner surface of the prepuce was full of *granular tubercles.* On the next day, the elevations on the glans disappeared, as well as the sore spots in the furrow, with a steady diminution of the purulent discharge; the sebaceous glands of the prepuce remained, nevertheless, for some time swollen and prominent.

(41.) *Fourth proving with the oil of Thuja.*

Dec. 1st. At about three in the afternoon, I took three drops of the oil of Thuja on a lump of sugar; the oil had been obtained (one drachm from four pounds of leaves) by the distillation of the tender twigs of the tree; it tasted exceedingly sharp and caused eructations for several hours. In the night *frequent urination*, with very *hasty, incessant urgency*, and on the following day redness of the *glans at the aperture of the urethra.* After taking ten drops of the oil in the evening, the eructations continued into the night.

3d and 4th. A dull pain developed itself in the *left testicle* as though it had been *bruised*, and was perceptible both when seated and when walking. On the 6th an *eroded spot* appeared again in the middle of the *furrow of the glans*, which discharged *a pus-like fluid.*

7th and 8th. The *discharge from the glans* had attained its former height. The whole furrow was covered over with pus, so that it was necessary to cleanse it often.

9th. After moderate use of wine, the condition was still worse. *The inner surface of the prepuce* was *sore* in spots, *highly inflamed* at the frænulum, the *glans* was sensitive and painful when walking.

I was now content with this painful present, and closed my proving of Thuja. The *discharge from the glans* was first entirely cured, after several alternations of better and worse, at the end of four weeks. *Itching and burning in the anus* lasted the longest, and was still felt at times after the lapse of months.

I must here repeat the observation, that during the whole duration of the experiments with Thuja (unica nocte exempta) the sexual impulse was diminished even to indifference. According to the results above detailed, the chief operation of Thuja is upon the genital and urinary systems. It was especially in the parts under the influence of the *plexus pudendo-hæmorrhoidalis* that its effects fastened themselves, and were produced in objective phenomena. Its influence on the muscles was of very short duration in my case, and it left the respiratory and digestive organs entirely undisturbed.

(42.) *Proving of Thuja on my wife.*

1845, June 17th. Maria Anna M., 35 years old, sanguineo-melancholic temperament, tall and slender form, mother of six healthy children, began the proving of Thuja, four months after the birth of her last child, by taking 200 drops of the second dilution. This was at about three o'clock in the afternoon. She experienced no effect from the dose, nor from another of 200 drops of the first dilution.

19th. In the afternoon, she took 30 drops of the tincture, and on awaking next morning, complained of *painful tension in the left side of the neck*, darting upwards to the occiput and downwards to the scapula, and preventing her from turning her head.

20th. On which day she took nothing, the tension seemed somewhat to remit, but returned in greater severity on the 21st, after taking 40 drops of the tincture. In the evening also there came on a *crushing pain* in the inner side of the left wrist, in the head of the radius, which last was plainly swollen and painful to the touch.

22d. In the afternoon, she took 50 drops. In the evening she felt *tension in both knees and heels*, especially when rising after being long seated. The *stiffness of the nape* of the neck continued.

23d. The same symptoms continued on taking 60 drops. She compared the *tension in the knees and heels* to a feeling as if the feet had been rendered stiff by over exertion in walking. She took nothing on the last days of June, and the *tension in the nape of the neck* and in the *knees and heels* diminished, but did not altogether cease.

July 1st. After a pause of eight days, she continued the proving, by taking 70 drops of the tincture. The tension over the patellæ and in the heels (at the point of attachment of the tendo Achillis,) immediately increased. The rest at night was good, and no change was perceived in the urine or stools.

3d. 80 drops were taken in the afternoon as usual, upon which a dull, stunning headache, in the frontal region and vertex, came on, which, however, did not last long.

5th and 8th. Nothing new was produced by 90 and 100 drops. The *tension in the knees and heels* continued, but was only troublesome while walking, not while sitting; *the tension in the nape* was still occasionally sensible, especially in the morning.

9th and 10th. 120 and 140 drops of the tincture having been taken, no new developments took place, and the prover, stiffened in *neck and feet,* concluded her experiment.

12th. The menses appeared at their regular period, but were weaker than ordinary.

The poverty of symptoms in this proving is worthy of remark in connection with the uncommon duration of the phenomena which did appear. The stiffness of the left side of the neck, and the tension over the knees and in the heels, diminished only very slowly, often disappeared, and then suddenly set in again, and first completely vanished at the expiration of three months.

K.

Dr. Reisinger instituted on himself three experiments with Thuja.

(43.) *First proving with increasing doses of the tincture.*

1844, Nov. 5th. Dr. R. took in the morning 10 drops of the tincture, and increased the dose daily until he arrived at 100 drops, which he then repeated every other day, until the 10th December, without experiencing the slightest influence. Various hindrances prevented the prosecution of this experiment.

(44.) *Second proving with the tincture, in massive doses.*

1845, March 1st. R. recommenced the proving of Thuja with 100 drops of the tincture, and added 100 drops every other day, so that on the 15th the dose was 800 drops. The sole symptom which he ascribed to the drug, was a tolerably strong, jumping, sticking pain in a hollow tooth of the left under jaw, which had never ached before. This pain appeared only upon the day of taking the drug, and about three to four hours after its administration. But this very probable symptom of Thuja disappeared again under the subsequent remarkably large doses.

15th. After taking 800 drops, R. perceived in the evening a slight oppression of the chest, with inclination to cough.

17th, 19th, and 21st. 1000, 1200 and 1500 drops produced no effect whatever.

R. now discontinued the doses for eight days, and waited, but in vain, for the after effect of the remedy.

29th, 30th, and 31st. He took, each day, 1500 drops of the tincture, and remarked afterwards, slight vertigo (effect of the alcohol), perpetual eructations, dryness of the pharynx, frequent hawking up of mucus, and *pressing, tensive feeling in the lungs*, that became more perceptible and sticking on taking a deep inspiration. The other functions remained normal.

April 1st. Encouraged by this impunity, R. took from the 1st to the 5th of April, in daily increasing doses, 1600 to 2000 drops of the tincture, without perceiving the slightest change in his sensations, except a feeling of dulness and confusion in the head.

9th. R. drank at one draught *two ounces of the tincture.* Of the subsequent symptoms, the increased warmth in the stomach and whole frame, the vertigo, the headache in the whole frontal region, and the violent thirst, are rather to be set to the account of the alcohol; Thuja will have the credit of the following; swelling of the veins, especially of the arm; eructations of wind, smelling of the drug; oppression of the chest with some pain on inspiring; frequent hawking up of a tough mucus; restless sleep with confused dreams, and excited sexual impulse.

(45.) *Third proving with dilutions.*

As was to have been expected, no results followed an experiment instituted by R. with the first twelve dilutions (1 : 99). He began with 100 drops of the first dilution, and took daily the same quantity of the succeeding dilutions in regular order, closing his resultless experiment with 100 drops of the twelfth. He had now taken some 25,000 drops of the Thuja tincture, and was well weary of it, but not sick.

Dr. Reisinger's proving of Thuja confirms the opinion, that for the production of a drug disease as well as for the origin of a natural sickness, two conditions are necessary, a noxious influence, and a natural susceptibility. Where the proper soil, the sensitiveness of the organism to the special influence of the drug, is wanting, there no symptoms of disease will spring up, even under the exhibition of full doses of the remedy, and the scattered seed, instead of ripening into full sheaves, will barely bud, or at most give but a very sparing harvest.

L.

Dr. Sterz made two short experiments with Thuja.

(46.) *First proving with the tincture.*

1844, Oct. 13th. He took the tincture every forenoon between ten and eleven o'clock, upon a lump of sugar. He began on the 13th Oct., 1844, with 5 drops, took 10 on the 14th, and increased the dose each day by ten drops, until, on the 19th, he took 60 drops, but perceived not the slightest effects.

20th. An hour after taking 80 drops, a sensation of roughness in the throat came on and lasted until midnight.

21st. 100 drops. Immediately after the dose, feeling of roughness on the tongue, the hard palate, and in the throat; at noon sensitiveness of the gums of the molares; at seven in the evening, colic-like pain in the hypogastrium and movings in the bowels as if preceding a diarrhœa, which, indeed, came on very violently at half-past eight with severe bellyache: the pains then remitted, but the hypogastrium remained tender for several hours. His sleep was quiet after midnight, and towards morning *much flatulence* was discharged, the *throat* was still rough and the *fauces dry*. He was frequently obliged to hawk, and throw off white, tough mucus. After ten o'clock in the forenoon he took a fresh 100 drops, upon which, frequent eructations with nausea; at noon, dull confusion in the forehead, which disappeared at midnight; in the evening a copious evacuation, with discharge of much flatulence. All the morbid sensations had vanished on the next day after a quiet night's sleep.

(47.) *Second proving with dilutions* (10: 90).

Dec. 7th, 8th, 9th, and 10th. No effects were perceived from 200 drops of the 15th dilution, (the dilutions were prepared with one part of alcohol and four of distilled water,) taken daily, nor from the same quantity of the 12th dilution taken on the 11th.

12th. S. took morning and evening 200 drops of the 12th. At noon *feeling of dryness on the palate*, and the next day *drawing* in both thumbs on awaking.

13th. 400 drops of the 12th. Thereupon roughness of the palate and drawing in the right thumb, which last continued all day.

14th. Nothing new was developed by 400 drops of the 8th dilution. The drawing in the right thumb extended into the wrist-joint. On the 15th no dose was taken, and except dryness of the throat no symptoms appeared.

16th. 400 drops of the 6th dilution, which were repeated three days after, on the 19th; after which, scraping and roughness in the throat, and drawing in the right knee.

After a pause of twenty-eight days, S. also experimented with the 4th and 2d dilutions.

1845, Jan. 16th, 18th, 19th, and 21st. He took 400 drops each day of the 4th; and on the 5th, 6th, 7th and 8th of February 200 drops of the 2d. The following weak symptoms appeared: feeling of dryness in the throat, with frequent hawking and spitting of a tough white mucus and confluence of much saliva into the mouth; the taste was injured by it, and the food tasted as if it had not salt enough.

M.

Dr. Wachtel proved Thuja only in the dilutions.

(48.) *First proving with the 3d dilution* (10 : 90).

1844, Dec. 10th. Our associate, so remarkably sensitive to the effects of Thuja, began his proving by taking 30 drops of the 3d dilution about an hour after breakfast. He observed, in the forenoon, a sudden thrust from before backwards in the right half of the chest; at noon, complete loss of appetite; in the afternoon, *itching and biting in the prepuce;* afterwards, tearing pressing in the upper part of the right thigh and left arm, which greatly resembled the effects of Bryonia, with this difference, that the pain produced by Thuja seized the middle of the affected member, was confined to a small spot, and was mostly in the muscles; while that produced by Bryonia seemed to prefer the joints and tendons. In the evening, he perceived maddening (! Ed.) twitching in the right frontal eminence. An hour later, this pain attacked the right eyeball much more violently, but shortly disappeared, leaving behind a sensibility of the eye to touch of the hand, which remained a long while. The sleep of the following night was good; but immediately on waking, the same pain reestablished itself in the right eye.

11th. 10 drops of the same dilution, producing a return of the chest pain of the day before, but this time in the left half. Afterwards, an unsatisfactory, hard stool, wlth subsequent *itching and biting in the anus.* In the afternoon, *drawing* through the whole length of the outer surface of the thigh (of which side? M.); in the evening, pressing pain in the frontal and occipital regions; *itching* in the corona of the glans when walking (for half an hour). His sleep was good and comfortable, with lively and pleasant dreams. Feeling of health on awaking, except weariness and lameness in the feet. On the 12th, no striking symptoms followed a repetition of a similar dose; W. only remarked in the middle of the left parietal bone a *spot* of the size of a dime, *sensitive* to the touch, and a *drawing* from the crest of the right *iliac bone to the upper part of the thigh.*

13th. *Pressing in the occiput* was the only symptom after taking 10 drops of the 3d dilution. On the 14th, after a similar dose, *pressing in the forehead*, lasting all day.

W. now discontinued the Thuja from the 15th December, 1844, until the 7th January, 1845, inclusive, in order to see how long the effects of the drug would continue; and acknowledges his astonishment at the duration of its action. During this time, he observed the following symptoms:

16th. Violent *drawing and pressing in the sacral region* for two hours in the forenoon. On the 16th, while writing, *drawing pressing* in the right thumb (for five or six minutes); then in the index, later in the middle, and finally in the little finger. In the afternoon, the same sort of pain appeared in the left arm, shifted then to the upper part of the thigh of the same side, soon after appeared in both the mastoid processes of the temporal bones, then in the frontal eminences, where the pain took more of a digging-twitching character, and finally reappeared in the extremities. This wandering about of the pains continued through the following day. On the 18th, for several hours in the forenoon, the pain remained in the neighborhood of the left wrist; and during the whole afternoon, in the upper part of the left thigh.

19th. While lying down, the *pressing in the sacrum* was fixed in the same spot for a whole hour. It was diminished and disappeared on motion; but afterwards appeared while lying in bed, in *the lower part of the left thigh*, in the same spot where it had already appeared once before. The prover remarked this day, on the edge of the upper lip, two small, dark-red, burning spots, of the size of a lentil; on which, during the three following days, little elevations were developed, which dried up and fell off. Later, two new spots appeared, which ran the same course. He observed, in addition, feeling of stiffness on the left side of the nape of the neck, which had been already perceived during the first days of the experiment, but had been attributed from the beginning, by the prover, to an uncomfortable position in bed.

24th and 25th. W. was often tormented by a very painful tearing *drawing* in the left side of the chest, in the neighborhood of the fifth and sixth ribs. This pain appeared when standing and sitting, disappeared when moving, and was rather diminished than increased by a deep inspiration.

26th. *Crawling drawing in the left zygoma*, which left behind for a long time a feeling of dulness. This symptom appeared again on the 27th, on the same, and afterwards on the right side. In the evening, *drawing tearing in the* mastoid process of the left temporal bone, and then in both *eyeballs*, where the pain ceased.

28th. The prover was annoyed through the whole day with a *crawling, pressive pain* in the left side of the sternum, which was *confined to a spot* about the size of a dollar, remained the same in rest or motion, and finally left the feeling as though the *spot was sore*.

After three weeks, isolated symptoms were still perceived. The pains were, for the most part, *drawing, tearing or crawling*, seldom pressing, and least of all, sticking. They were mostly *confined to a small spot, seldom continued long, frequently changed their location*, and came on *distinctly when at rest* as well as during motion.

(49.) *Second proving with the* 12*th dilution.*

1845, Jan. 8th. After W. had almost ceased to perceive the symptoms produced by the proving of the 3d dilution, he took, at seven o'clock in the morning of this day, three ounces of the 12th dilution. An hour and a half afterwards appeared (weakly marked) the characteristic *tearing drawing* pains, sometimes in the *frontal eminences* and in the *occipital protuberances*, sometimes in the middle of the left arm and thigh (only when at rest). The *crawling and drawing* in both zygomata, and in the left upper maxillary bone, came on instantaneously, and disappeared again as rapidly as it had appeared.

9th. Rather violent drawing in the right shoulder, and later, without the slightest cause, cutting and griping in the left side of the abdomen.

10th. No abnormal sensation was perceived; but on the 11th, extraordinarily violent *tearing* in the left *concha*, and soon after in the left *eye*, which ended with a *darting stitch* through the middle of *the eyeball. Copious urine* also came on.

12th. The prover remarked in the region of the heart a *small spot*, sensitive to the touch, *with pain, as if it were sore*, and on the following day a similar spot immediately upon the vertex, upon which the skin was somewhat reddened. At ten o'clock he went to bed in good health, but after half an hour was suddenly seized with *anxiety*—after which a slight perspiration broke out; whereupon he fell asleep, but continually started up again. Finally, *drawing pains* in the arms and feet, and especially in the *small of the back*, came on. These having ceased, he had quiet sleep till morning.

14th. W. found himself tolerably well; only general weakness and frequent accesses of drawing pains in different parts of the body annoyed him. In the evening, the general debility increased, and he was obliged to go to bed at seven o'clock. After some minutes *his feet became as cold as ice*—he became again *anxious*. It was a very striking symptom that in no position of the body, whether sitting or lying, could he feel the pulsation of his heart. *Slight shiverings*, which spread themselves by little and little over the whole body, came on. At last, after a quarter of an hour, he experienced a *trembling of the heart*—after which *a general sweat* broke out, so that in the course of a minute the whole body was wet. This was followed by dozing for an hour, unrefreshing, and disturbed by frequent starting and horrible images. When he awoke from this, he was tormented with *drawing and tearing pains* in the hands and feet, and when these last suddenly disappeared, the *anxiety* and *heart trembling* returned. It was only at the expiration of a quarter of an hour that his heart again beat regularly; but then *drawing tearing pains* in the epigastrium, in the hypochondria, on the chest, but worst in the small of the back, came on, ending in a slight perspiration, and finally in sleep.

On awaking, W. was very weak, and every part of his body felt as though it had been bruised; the head, however, was free from pain; the weariness, too, nearly disappeared in the course of the day.

15th. The prover went to bed later than usual. After he had lain quietly for a quarter of an hour *his feet began again to become cold, anxiety* again came on, and in an instant, in place of the regular beat, he felt a *trembling of the heart.* The sweat that then broke out was interrupted by the prover's being called to a patient: on his return, at the expiration of an hour, he slept tolerably well until morning.

16th. During the day *drawing pains, now here, now there;* weariness, with apparent loss of sensation in the limbs; in the evening, after lying down, *cold feet again,* with *anxiety and palpitation,* but less in amount and of shorter duration.

Isolated symptoms were still remarked by the observant prover, six weeks after the three ounces of the 12th dilution had been taken. The following were daily visitors: *the drawing pains* in the hands and feet, in the sacral region, and between the shoulders. The *crawling drawing in the zygomata, and the tearing in the occipital protuberances and in the petrous portion of the temporal bone* were oftenest perceived. No chest or abdominal symptoms appeared. But *wartlike excrescences* frequently appeared on the back of the right hand,* on the *chin and other places.* A *furunculus,* behind the right ear especially, continued a long while, and formed a scab, from which exuded a glutinous moisture. This soon dried and fell off, when another formed; it was sensitive to the touch, and lasted four whole weeks.

Finally, W. repeats the observation, that the symptoms of Thuja came on almost exclusively during rest, remained but a little while, and were either rendered worse or caused to break out afresh, by the use of spirituous liquors, except the customary beer.

This interesting result authorizes the conclusion, that individual susceptibility for a particular remedy plays a very important part in the proving of drugs. While *Reisinger's* constitution, unsusceptible to the influences of Thuja, remained almost unmoved by massive doses, that of *Wachter,* especially subject to Thuja, produced with the smallest doses the most abundant harvest of symptoms.

N.

Dr. Watzke instituted four experiments with Thuja, and of all the drugs which he has assisted in proving, Thuja seems to have found the least sensibility to its specific effects in him. He experienced no regular drug sickness, although isolated Thuja symptoms were clearly developed.

* These *excrescences* deserved a fuller description.—*Ed. Aust. Journal.*

(50.) *First proving with dilutions gradually descending.*

1844, Nov. 26th and 27th. "I took," says W., "on these days, twice in the forenoon, six drops of the 12th dilution, and during the two following days the same dose in like manner of the 9th, and observed a strict diet. Whether the symptoms which then appeared were certainly produced by the Thuja or not, I do not know; but of this I am confident, that they were such as I had never before experienced, and such as almost constantly returned when I subsequently experimented with larger doses of the drug.

"There appeared, especially during the time of proving, repeated, *short, dry cough*, without throat symptoms or pain in the chest. The *hypogastrium* appeared the whole time somewhat *inflated* and sensitive to pressure, and even to *the jar of the foot on the ground.* It seemed to me as if I perceived the *vesica to be larger*, and I was obliged to urinate oftener than usual; but I had neither pains in the urethra, nor was the urine at all changed.

"From the 2d to the 14th December, I took nearly every day a dose of Thuja; until the 6th, six drops of the 9th; until the 10th, six drops of the 6th; and on the 13th and 14th, six drops of the third dilution.

"Although during this time I did not altogether observe a strict diet, still some certain symptoms of Thuja manifested the working of the drug; *certain*, because they were renewed with renewed intensity under the larger doses.

"These symptoms were, *dry cough, pain in the patellæ, frequently returning* whether sitting or walking; *a twitching as if a tendon were slowly drawn out and then suffered to return;* a similar pain while sleeping; the outer malleolus of the right foot was painful while walking, as if after a false step; circumscribed pain in the inner side of the thigh, as if after a long walk; *swelling in the region of the hypogastrium with frequent urgency to urinate.*

(51.) *Second proving with small increasing doses of the tincture.*

"From the 19th December, 1844, to the 2d January, 1845, without changing my ordinary mode of life, which was not confined to a very severe diet, I took, at about noon of every other day, a dose of the tincture of Thuja, beginning with 10 drops, and increasing it each time by 10, until, on the last named day, I arrived at 80 drops.

"The abnormal sensations which I experienced during the duration of this experiment, were the following: contractive pain in the right temple, pretty severe, often returning and always lasting several seconds; pressure in the right eyeball; biting in the corner of the right eye, once at about five o'clock in the evening (without any cause affecting the eyes), the surrounding objects, which I wished to regard, suddenly swam before my eyes; I could not see clearly, much less read. This lasted nearly a quarter of an hour. Sensitiveness of isolated spots on the thorax; feeling of weight, and frequent cramp-like constriction in the chest; dry cough, increasing in a direct ratio with the duration of the experiment, becoming constantly more troublesome, and finally obliging me to lay aside the proving for a while; *sensitiveness and feeling of inflation in the region of the vesica with frequent urgency to urinate;* violent itching in distinct points on the inner side of the thigh *and on the parts of the genitals covered with hair; sensibility of the glans* and darting stitches through it; remarkable *indifference to the opposite sex;* several times, on awaking, drawing pain in the great toe: a feeling in the little toe as if the skin were lacerated in spots; weariness of the lower limbs; especially remarked in the lower part of the thigh."

(52.) *Third proving with steady doses of the tincture.*

"From the 16th to and including the 20th January, I took daily 100 drops of the tincture without noticing any new symptoms; those developed under the previous proving again appeared with less violence, except the dry, frequently returning cough, which rendered me so anxious about my health that I was induced to discontinue the experiment."

(53.) *Fourth proving with large increasing doses of the tincture.*

Feb. 5th. I took 150 drops of the tincture; on the 6th, 300; on the 7th, 450; on the 8th, 600; on the 9th, 700; on the 10th, 900: each time between ten and eleven o'clock in the forenoon.

"These doses produced nothing new; they simply caused the most of the symptoms developed by the second experiment to return, more markedly, and with greater force. The last dose of 900 drops was followed, during the whole afternoon, by frequent eructations of food with the taste of the drug, and several times by violent, nearly watery, but painless diarrhœa.

"Were these last two symptoms the result of accident? or was the organism so loaded with matter incapable of being assimilated by means of the previous large doses, that it was obliged to get rid of it by the shortest route? and had it already by that means lost the capability of further developing in itself the characteristic symptoms of Thuja?"

(54.) *Let the last proving reply to these queries!*

Feb. 25th. I took in the forenoon *two*, and on the 27th *three tablespoons* (about 1350 drops) *of the tincture*, at the same time observing a strict diet.

"If these enormous doses gave me no drug disease regularly classified in any nosographic system, they at least produced in me the firm conviction, that I could be very regularly and earnestly sick on taking the medicament in that quantity. The goal, which I had proposed to myself in this experiment, lay now at last in view! Why did I not, then, attain it? I confess, I had not the courage for it. The energetic attack which the drug had already made upon my thoracic organs, frightened me back. Already had my first experiment with the dilutions pointed out to me this unpleasant tendency of Thuja, although but slightly, and I found it advisable to break off the second and third provings almost from the beginning.

"The somewhat numerous symptoms that constitute my last proving began to appear for the most part some hours after the dose, and confined themselves principally to the first twenty-four or forty-eight hours; but nevertheless, they did not run an acute course, nor vanish, like meteors, after a single appearance, but returned separately during the period of from 8 to 14 days. They seemed to have a chronic character, and a marked, though irregular periodicity.

"*It was more especially upon the thoracic organs*, as in the former provings, on the *muscles, the head, especially the occiput*, and *upon the organs of generation*, that the Thuja exerted its influence. The peculiarity of the muscular pains was, that they generally affected the *middle* instead of the tendinous portions of the muscle. Most of the symptoms came on *during rest*, many of them *on waking* in the morning.

"To prevent a tedious and unnecessary repetition, I confine myself to a description of one day, the 27th of February, which was one of the richest in symptoms. At 11 o'clock in the forenoon, I had taken three tablespoonfuls of the tincture.

"Immediately after the exhibition of the dose, the head felt cloudy; I felt my spirits excited and became lively and loquacious (effect of the alcohol?). Soon I perceived a slow-drawing, sometimes darting pain in the right half of the face, from the temple to the teeth; then the whole became sensitive, and increased in sensitiveness with the subsequent symptoms, in the course of the afternoon. The occiput was externally warmer to the touch in a particular spot, corresponding with which I felt heat and pressure in the brain. At times dull stitches ran through the brain, generally in the direction of the eyebrows, and from the eyeball to the occiput.

"*The chest smarted internally, as if sore, especially during the dry cough which appeared from time to time. In some spots I had the feeling, as if the thorax from without, and the corresponding portions of the lungs from within, were strongly and durably constricted;* a feeling which returned frequently and strongly on the following days, especially during rest, induced frequent deep sighing, and annoyed me not a little.

"There were spots here and there on the thorax and extremities, painful *as if from a thrust* and especially during movement. In the other spots I perceived a stitch, leaving behind an itching, as if they had been bitten by fleas or ants; in the forearm several times a coursing and gurgling, as of single drops of blood rolling one after another. I had frequently, for a minute at a time, a pain which in the axilla, in the dorsum of the foot, and on various points of the external chest, was pinching and pressing; in the patellæ and heels was stinging, and in the external ear compressing.

"Violent twitching came on in isolated muscular parts, which was strongest in the middle of the upper part of the right thigh and of the left arm. In the ends of the fingers and toes, the twitching was finer and more transient. This muscular twitching was frequently repeated on the following days in different parts, and was one of the most troublesome symptoms; for example, it still came on on the 13th of March, and lasted for almost ten minutes in the chin.

"*The stinging pain in the heel* often returned, and was especially troublesome in walking, (for a quarter of an hour.) *The inner side of the upper thigh and the parts of the genital organs covered with hair*, were very unpleasantly affected with *itching and scraping*, frequently lasting from 5 to 10 minutes. *Frequent stitches darted through the glans*, and *the whole member, especially the glans*, was constantly sensitive. An uncomfortable sensation of fulness in the region of the bladder forced me to frequent urination; the quantity of urine did not seem increased, and its quality was perfectly normal. My digestion and evacuation seem to have been left nearly or quite undisturbed. The symptoms of the fourth proving, (eructations of food and diarrhœa,) must be considered as the result of accident.*

"The most lasting and most troublesome symptoms in my case, as may be gathered from the foregoing account, were those which affected the muscles and the chest. *The dry cough, the constriction in spots on the thorax* and in the corresponding parts of the lungs, (frequently returning, very irritating and annoying, compelling frequent deep inspirations and ameliorated by wine and beer,) first entirely disappeared in the course of about eight weeks. The striking *indifference to sexual intercourse*, by no means customary to me, continued during the whole experiment, and, in fact, still longer."

O

Dr. Wurmb instituted five experiments with Thuja; four with the tincture, and one with dilutions.

* Although Thuja has produced gastric symptoms in various provers after the exhibition of large doses, yet, it must be considered as established as the general result of all the experiments, that gastric affections are the effects not of the quality but of the quantity of the drug; effects, which may result from the administration of any of the remedies in enormous doses.—*Mayrhofer.*

(55.) *First proving with small doses of the tincture.*

1844, Sept. W. took, from the 17th, until and including the 21st, at about 5 o'clock in the evening of each day, a coffee spoonful of the tincture of Thuja; omitted it on the 22d; took the same dose at the same hour on the two following days; omitted it on the 25th; and from the 26th to, and including the 30th, again repeated it. The following were the results.

18th. In the morning after urinating, *burning in the urethra; very painful stitches from the urethra to the anus; pressing in the region of the neck of the bladder, with urgency to urinate.* These feelings, which the prover thought similar to those usually perceived at the beginning of a clap, or after drinking new beer, lasted about twenty minutes.

19th. Soon after the dose: *tearing* in the outside of the right ankle; then in the left elbow; then *drawing* in the inner side of the upper thigh, and finally *tearing* in the second joint of the right thumb. On the 20th, soon after dinner, violent *pressing* in the left *temple*, which continued all the evening, but in a less degree. During the proving, the stools were softened, more copious, and took place from two to three times a day.

(56.) *Second proving with larger doses of the tincture.*

Oct. After a cessation of eight days W. took from the 8th to and including the 14th, at five o'clock in the evening of each day, two coffee spoonfuls of the tincture; with the following result:

11th. Soon after the dose, *feeling of roughness in the throat*, lasting some hours; pressing in the right *side of the chest*, particularly noticeable when breathing deeply, and when bending the body: at seven in the evening, drawing in the first joint of the right thumb, especially during rest, instantly disappearing on moving the finger, and returning as quickly on the cessation of the motion. This symptom continued nearly an hour; several times *drawing* in the third joint of the right ring finger, and *pressing* to the left under the short ribs.

12th. The *pressing pain* appeared at the lower extremity of the right *side of the chest*, after getting up; it was somewhat violent at first, but decreased very much during the day, without, however, entirely disappearing. In the morning a very copious soft stool. In the evening, on going out, after taking the drug, vertigo, *drawing* in the inner surface of the right thigh, in the right knee, in the right calf, in the bend of the elbow, *in both popliteal spaces*, especially the left. The feeling of roughness in the throat was less than the day before.

13th and 14th. The sexual impulse was exceedingly importunate (without any known cause). He thinks he passed more urine than usual.

15th. *Frequent*, and on every occasion *copious urination.*

16th. The *prominences* of the right *elbow* were painful, as if after a *severe knock*, and this feeling did not entirely disappear until the 18th.

(57.) *Third proving with large doses.*

Oct. From the 20th to the 30th, W. took daily at nine in the morning, and five in the evening, two coffee spoonfuls of the tincture, and observed as follows: On the 22d, in the morning, after getting up, painful *drawing* in the second joint of the left thumb, (only during rest) for about two hours. The same feeling, but not lasting, and much weaker, appeared in the course of the forenoon, in almost all the finger joints (but only during rest). For an instant, this drawing appeared in the inner side of the left foot, as far as the sole. In the morning he had the usual, and at eleven o'clock a papescent, stool. At six in the evening, sudden drawing on the inner side of the left foot in the metatarsus.

23d. No evacuation. In the evening, before going to sleep, *drawing* in the left side of the neck. Restless night. He awoke at two o'clock, and for an hour could not go to sleep; then fell into a sleep which was interrupted by frequent waking. He had besides a feeling of stoppage in the right nostril, with frequent sneezing and *chilly feeling* in the feet, which were externally warm to the touch.

24th. Immediately after getting up, a very troublesome *drawing* in the *left side of the neck* and in the left shoulder, which only disappeared in the afternoon.

At ten o'clock in the forenoon, *drawing* in the right heel, and half an hour later, in the right index finger (disappearing instantly on movement). The symptoms of the nose continued, with dull confusion in the head. As W., according to his own observations, is but little sensible to changes of temperature, and can trace no cause for this cold, he thinks that these symptoms must be ascribed to Thuja.*

25th. The cold, with its accompaniments, sneezing, dull confusion in the head, &c., continued. At about eleven in the day, transient drawing in the index finger. Two hours subsequently, a similar drawing in the left superior maxillary bone. At eight in the evening, troublesome drawing in the left side of the hypogastrium (for a couple of minutes), which spot was also painful to the touch.

26th. The catarrh is still present, only somewhat diminished in degree. In the forenoon, sudden drawing in the left thumb and right little finger (immediately disappearing on movement and as quickly returning in rest). At about ten in the forenoon, drawing in the hypogastrium on the left side, and tenderness on pressure. At about two in the afternoon, troublesome clawing in the sternum, *frequent short dry cough, and increased discharge of urine.* Frequent waking at night; towards morning, a pollution.

27th. On rising, drawing in the right thumb; at ten in the forenoon, drawing and pressing in the hypogastrium, on the left side, particularly when touching it; during the day, drawing, now here, now there, and

*It is certainly a property of Thuja, for the catarrh came on in the same way with several of the provers.—*Mayrhofer.*

frequent hacking cough; in the afternoon, drawing in the right arm and forearm; towards evening, painful drawing in the right great toe; at six in the evening, pressing in the middle of the sternum.

28th. Perfect health.

29th. Immediately after the dose, drawing in the lower incisors; about eleven, drawing in the right thumb; at five in the afternoon, drawing in the left superior maxillary bone; in the evening, feeling of roughness in the throat and frequent short, dry cough.

30th. In the forenoon, drawing in the right superior maxillary bone, in the inner side of the left forearm, and in the fingers of the right hand; feeling of roughness in the throat, and frequent dry, hacking cough. The catarrh, which had vanished, showed itself anew by an increased secretion of mucus from the nose. Copious urine.

31st. Increased urination: the catarrh worse.

Nov. 1st. In the morning, a loose stool, and after it a troublesome pressing in the anus, which remained the whole day. The catarrh became very severe, and one or the other nostril was almost constantly obstructed. At three in the afternoon, sneezing, succeeded by very violent sticking in the lower part of the right lung, which lasted until eleven in the evening, when, although very severe before, it disappeared at once. This sticking was greatly aggravated by sneezing, deep breathing, and coughing (but not by movement). Pain, as if the parts were sore, in the region of the ribs on touching them. At four in the afternoon, drawing in the fingers of the right hand, and afterwards in the right elbow.

2d. Drawing in the right calf the whole day. The catarrh reduced to a minimum. At four in the afternoon a hard, scanty stool, and *pressing and itching in the anus* for almost the whole evening.

3d. The running from the nose is again pretty copious; frequent sneezing; at about four in the afternoon, sneezing, and then some painful stitches in the side of the chest, within.

4th. At six in the morning, very severe stitches in the lower part of the right side of the chest; about five in the afternoon, drawing tearing in the right knee.

(58.) *Fourth proving with large doses.*

Dec. From the 7th to the 14th, W. took every day at about 9 in the morning, a tablespoonful of the tincture.—Effects:

7th. A pollution in the night, and after, a troublesome burning in the urethra.

9th. Want of appetite, especially in the evening. On the 10th, a pollution in the night.

11th. Feeling of roughness in the throat, which soon went off; then for an hour, a feeling in the throat as if there were a painless tumor there. At four in the afternoon, a papescent stool, and transient drawings often flitted about, now here, now there, especially in the upper part of the thigh. Urine increased.

12th. Pressing in the left breast, after the sensation in the lower lobes of the lung, especially when breathing deeply—frequent urination; no evacuation.

13th. *Chills*, even in the warm room; in the evening, well; no evacuation.

14th. On waking in the morning, *drawing in the left side of the neck;* then drawing in the upper part of the left thigh (lasting two minutes and rendering walking painful.) Two stools followed, one hard and unsatisfactory, afterwards another papescent, and which left behind a long continuing burning in the anus.

15th. In the forenoon, three papescent stools (at six, nine, and eleven o'clock.) Dinner nauseated him. *Chills* even in the warm room, and apprehension of becoming sick. At six in the evening these symptoms vanished, and the feeling of health was restored.

16th. Sudden drawing here and there, especially in the fingers of the right hand; no evacuation; at four o'clock in the night a pollution.

17th. Sudden drawing in the limbs.

18th. In the morning, a hard, unsatisfactory evacuation; drawing in the limbs—at one o'clock, feeling of dryness and sense of constriction in the throat. It was the same sensation that is perceived when one is for a long time exposed to the heat of the sun without drinking. In the night a pollution.

19th. After rising, *burning in the external canthi and in the urethra:* drawing pain in the inner side of the left fore-arm, during the whole forenoon, particularly when the arm was at rest. The feeling of dryness and constriction in the throat appeared again in a slight degree. Drawing in the inner side of the left upper thigh, in the right knee and in the right hip. At six in the evening, a very unsatisfactory stool after much straining.

20th. Feeling as if the *eyelids were swollen* and a foreign body were in the eye; drawing now here, now there, in the extremities; in the evening, pressing towards the back in the chest, with oppressed breathing; no stool.

21st. In the forenoon, an unsatisfactory stool; drawing in the extremities, especially on the inner surface of the upper part of the left thigh and forearm (only while at rest.)

22d. In the afternoon, another unsatisfactory stool, drawing in different parts of the extremities, not lasting long, but frequently quite troublesome.

(59.) *Fifth proving with dilution.*

1845, January. After a pause of five weeks, W. on the 27th, 29th and 30th, took each day, about six in the evening, two tablespoonfuls of the 12th dilution of Thuja, and on the 10th of February, at about five in the evening, he took three ounces of the same dilution. The dilutions were prepared with distilled water.

30th. He first perceived, soon after taking the drug, feeling of dryness in the throat, lasting two hours; in the evening, drawing in the right thumb and forearm; then in the left thumb and in the teeth of the right superior maxillary bone. The increased secretion of mucus obliged him frequently to blow his nose.

31st. In the morning, frequent sneezing, stoppage of the right nostril, alternating with running. This catarrh lasted a couple of hours, then suddenly vanished; it appeared again for a little while in the evening, and ceased suddenly as if cut off.

Feb. 1st. The same symptoms.

10th. Immediately after the dose, feeling of dryness in the throat, which lasted all day.

11th. Feeling of dryness in the throat the whole evening; pressing in the left side of the chest, particularly troublesome in the region of the ribs; several times, drawing in the lower incisors, and in the first joint of the right index finger; violent *itching* in the lower part of the sacral region; at night, sticking from the right velum palati into the internal ear; the secretion from the Schneiderian membrane increased.

27th. As a closing experiment, W. drank three ounces of the 30th dilution (prepared with distilled water) at one draught. This was at about five in the afternoon; he perceived no result whatever.

This persevering and energetic experiment is not so rich in results as the quantity of the remedy swallowed would have led us to expect. Whether a want of susceptibility to the action of drug must bear the blame, whether this might have been overcome by still more massive doses, or whether dilutions taken for a greater length of time would have given a better result, cannot be determined. We may be permitted to remark, however, that the proving of drugs is no such light matter as it might appear to be. Both the idiosyncrasy of the prover and of the drug play so important a part, that a successful proving is often an entirely accidental windfall for the susceptible prover, while the boldest experimenter, with the very best will and the greatest devotion, if unsusceptible, can only obtain a scanty and one-sided result.*

P.

Dr. Ferdinand Zeiner, forty-two years old, of a delicate constitution and phlegmatico-sanguineous temperament, healthy from childhood (except the usual diseases of that period), for the last two years frequently troubled with hæmorrhoidal affections, instituted four experiments upon himself with Thuja. (It was his first essay with drugs.)

* The opponents of Homœopathy have made use of this diversity of result as an argument against the system. They forget, however, in so doing, that the susceptibility for drugs (drug-diseases) runs parallel with the susceptibility for natural diseases; and that, if there be constitutions which a particular disease, for example, variola or syphilis cannot infect, there must also be constitutions which cannot be rendered sick by a particular drug. It is only after repeated trials on individuals of the most diverse constitutions, and under the most varied influences and conditions, that we can obtain a true notion of the character of a remedy, resting on sure and broad foundations.—*Mayrhofer*.

(60) *First proving with the tincture in small doses.*

1844, Nov. 7.—Without making any alteration in his ordinary mode of life, Z. took, in the forenoon, at about nine o'clock (two hours after breakfast, *café au lait*), one drop of the tincture in water.

Immediately after the dose he experienced vertigo, soon disappearing, *scraping in the throat*, slight griping above the navel, sticking in the right temple, numbness of his left foot, and feeling of weakness in it in walking up and down the room; *feeling of coldness* over the whole body. One hour after, the griping drew from the umbilical region towards the right groin, and occasioned there flying, often-returning pressing. The vertigo, scraping in the throat, and lame feeling in the left foot still continued.

Two hours after having taken the dose, the vertigo and griping in the abdomen disappeared in the open air, but single stitches were repeatedly felt in the right groin and between the sacrum and anus. Frequent urination in the course of the day.

At six in the evening, inflation of the abdomen for an hour, which disappeared by eructations. An hour afterwards (ten hours after taking the drug) *single stitches* were perceived *in the anus*, alternating with burning in the prepuce.

At about nine in the evening, the prover's smell* was exceedingly, almost intolerably, increased, so as to become perceptible to those about him. The night's rest was good; but soon after walking, *the stitches in the anus* came on, and the *biting in the prepuce* also was troublesome for an hour.

8th. At nine in the forenoon, Z. took another drop in water; some minutes after, griping above the navel, and during the first hour; *single stitches* in the right *frontal eminence*, scraping in the chest, forcing him to cough, and *quivering* in the upper *eyelid*, *pressing* in the right *side of the forehead*, *biting* on the upper surface of the *glans* and in the prepuce, feeling of weariness in the sole of the left foot when seated.

At ten in the forenoon, another drop. Soon after, he felt *shivering in the back*; the *feeling of weariness* in the left foot, the *sticking* in the *right side of the forehead* and the griping in the abdomen continued. Towards eleven, *drawing in the left testicle* and frequent eructations of wind. At two in the afternoon (four hours after the dose) *the itching on the prepuce* became almost intolerable. Z. also observed during the day *frequent urgency to urinate*, with passage of a copious urine. Stools regular on both days.

9th. At nine in the forenoon, Z. took four drops on sugar; soon after, slight vertigo, griping about the navel, *itchings on the prepuce*, scraping in the trachea, obliging him to cough; with *quivering* of the right upper *eyelid*, *burning* in the *left eye* near the internal canthus, compelling him to rub it, *weakness of the eyes*, *single fine stitches in the*

* Olfactus an transpiratio?—M.

temples, feeling of weakness in the left *foot* when seated, pressing in the small of the back. At two in the afternoon, increased secretion of sweet saliva (lasting five hours), *drawing in the left testicle, urgency to urinate, with copious urine, swelling of the cervical glands,* pains in the small of the back. On the following day, on which nothing was taken, he felt in the forenoon, the pains in the small of the back, *quivering in the right eyelid* and *feeling of weakness in the left foot;* in the evening, *burning in the orifice of the urethra* and *frequent stitches in the anus.*

11th. Eight drops of the tincture. Soon after taking the dose, quivering again in the right upper eyelid, *feeling of coldness with numbness of the left foot, solitary stitches* in the shoulders, and *frequent chills over the whole body.* At three in the afternoon, a *general chill; drawing in the left testicle,* in the left thumb, *in the occiput; sticking in the temples,* in the right *side of the forehead* and in the *left knee;* pressing in the sacral region.

12th. Z. took nothing. In the evening, sticking now in the left knee, now in the head, and now in the elbow and finger joints; then, *general debility,* with such *weakness in the feet* that he thought he should fall. On the following day, he observed a *red spot* on the inner *surface of the prepuce* which itched violently and disappeared after twenty-four hours.

(61) *Second proving with the third dilution.* (5 : 95).

Nov. 25. After omitting the drug for fourteen days, Z. commenced again at nine in the forenoon, by taking four drops of the third dilution on sugar. Soon after, he perceived griping about the navel, *itchings* on the right *knee,* on the left shoulder, on the *scrotum,* and divers other places, and *burning on the inner surface of the prepuce.* After an hour: violent *drawing in the testicles;* vertigo; *greatly increased secretion of saliva* (of a metallic taste) lasting two hours, with *swelling of the salivary glands.* In the afternoon from four to five o'clock, *sticking pains in the glands of the groin.* During the whole day, *slight chills* in a warm room; *increased urgency to urinate.*

27th. At nine, A. M., eight drops of the third. After a quarter of an hour, *itchings on the prepuce,* griping about the navel, *sticking in the left side of the forehead,* pressings on the right shoulder; *weakness of the eyes,* particularly observable when writing. After an hour and a half, renewed *increase of saliva* (of an acid taste) during two hours; *sticking* in the *anus* and violent stitches in the left side of the chest, which frequently returned throughout the day; continual slight *chills and increased secretion of urine.*

28th. The symptoms of the preceding day were repeated after taking twelve drops of the same dilution.

(62.) *Third proving with the tincture in strong doses.*

Dec. 17. Z. ceased taking the drug for eighteen days, and commenced again by taking fifteen drops of the undiluted tincture, whereupon, in the course of the day, he observed the following symptoms: *pressing in the forehead, frequent stitches in the frontal eminences, sticking, at one time* in the right, at another in the left side of *the chest,* griping about the navel; *scraping in the throat, intolerable biting in the anus, drawing in the left testicle, obscuration of the eyes* while writing.

18th. Twenty drops of the tincture. Soon after the exhibition of the dose: staggering while walking in the air; *pressing in the middle of the forehead, sticking in both frontal eminences* (lasting the whole day, and continually increasing); *general debility and weakness in the feet:* sticking in the shoulders and in the right knee; *stitches in the region of the groins,* often repeated during the day, with the feeling *as if the inguinal glands were swollen; intolerable itching in the anus,* lasting almost the entire day; *hasty urgency to urinate, with copious urine.*

19th. No medicine. On awaking, *sticking pain in the left frontal eminence,* as well as violent *pressing between the shoulders,* which feeling had entirely disappeared eight days before; frequent twitching in the middle finger of the right hand. The *itching in the anus* appeared but seldom.

20th. After twenty-five drops; dull confusion in the head, weakness in the feet when walking; stitching in the forehead and in different parts of the body, especially in the shoulders, arms, and legs; in the evening, *spitting of much saliva.* The *itching in the anus* is almost gone; the *tongue and palate* are very sore.

On the following three days, no dose.

21st. On awaking, sticking in the left shoulder, and in the course of the day *flying stitches in the glans;* there was also *an increased secretion of saliva.*

22d and 23d. The whole of the symptoms gradually disappeared, and the prover no longer perceived the troublesome *itching in the anus* which had so much annoyed him during the whole continuance of the experiment.*

24th. Z. took thirty drops. During the first two succeeding hours: *burning and itching in the anus,* griping about the navel, painful constriction in the hypogastrium, weakness in the feet, cracking in the knee-joints, *drawing* in the *right groin* and *pressing in the renal region.* At six in the evening: *pressing in the forehead, sticking in the left frontal eminence,* acid taste with *increased secretion of saliva,* swelling of one (which ?—M.) of the cervical glands (tonsils ?—M.)

(63.) *Fourth proving with the 12th dilution.* (10 : 90)

1844, January 4th. After having rested ten days, Z. took ten drops

* In my case this itching in the anus was the most durable symptom, and disappeared after the lapse of several weeks.—*Mayrhofer.*

of the 12th dilution. During the first two hours, he observed during rest: transient griping about the navel, *repeated stitches about the anus*, which continued to increase in violence during the day, eructations of wind, sticking in the left side of the chest, on the left scapula and right temple, *failure of the eyes* when reading, transitory *chill* over the whole body with cold hands in a heated room, pressing, at one time in the right, at another in the left arm, drawing in the fingers, pain (of what sort ?—M.) in the nape of the neck, stitches in the left side of the forehead, *numbness of the sole of the left foot* while sitting, *crawling in the toes*, extraordinary weakness in the left foot when going out, slight reeling, pains in the small of the back, and *increased secretion of saliva.*

At four in the afternoon, *drawing in the left testicle* with feeling of weight in it, *urgency to urinate with copious passing of water.*

During the three following days, no medicine being taken, frequent pressing in the forehead, sticking pains in the frontal eminences and temples, pressing between the shoulders.

8th. Fifteen drops of the 12th. During the first two hours: *pressing and sticking in the forehead, sticking in the shoulders, stitches in the anus, numbness of the left foot, drawing in the left testicle, feeling in the testicles as if they moved*, drawing in the fingers and pressing in the left upper arm.

All these symptoms disappeared while walking in the open air.

9th. No dose. *Frequent itching on the glans and prepuce*, alternating with *stitches in the anus*, and *the urgency to urinate was frequent and hasty.*

12th. The proving was concluded by taking twenty-five drops of the 12th dilution. Thereupon he observed: *pressing* in the middle of *the forehead*, sticking pain in the right axilla, *increased salivary secretion*, which lasted all day, *stitches in the inguinal glands, itching in the anus, flying stitches in the glans, weakness of the eyes* when reading, pressing between the shoulders and *crawling* in the toes of the left foot, which were painful in treading. In the afternoon, while seated, feeling of lameness in the left foot. At seven in the evening, when walking, uncommonly violent stitch between the *coccyx and the anus.*

13th. After waking, sticking in the left side of the chest, lasting all day.

On discontinuing the drug, all the abnormal manifestations disappeared.

Dr. Zeiner accompanies his beautiful and instructive proving with the remark, that during its whole period, the sexual desire was completely asleep; and he further made the observation, in accordance with the experience of other provers, that the greater part of the drug-symptoms were most clearly developed during rest.

Q.

The boldest and most indefatigable prover of Thuja was Prof. von Zlatarovich, who took in 155 days, 42,260 drops of the tincture in large doses. He proved it not only on himself, but also upon a female.

1.

Zlatarovich's proving upon himself.

(64.) *First proving with increasing doses of the tincture.*

1844, Sept. 6th. Z. began his proving with six drops of the tincture, which, as also the succeeding doses, he took in the morning, fasting. On the three following days, he took eight, ten and twelve drops, and experienced no effect. On the 10th, after taking fourteen drops, he first perceived, in the evening, a transient *pain in the vertex, as though the bone were repeatedly pierced with a needle near the sagittal suture.*

11th. No effect after sixteen drops.

12th. After eighteen drops, in the evening, *pressing and burning in the hemorrhoidal vessels* (? Ed.) and frequent violent sneezing, which returned on the morning of the 13th, after twenty drops.

From the 14th Sept. to the 5th of October inclusive, Z. increased the dose daily by two drops, and observed the following results:

Sept. 14th. After dinner, frequent violent sneezing without catarrh, (a thing very unusual with him).

15th. In the morning, several times, *short, dry, barking cough.*

16th. In the afternoon and evening, *pressing* in a small spot *under the sternum,* which gradually extended to the scrobiculus.

17th. At night, and on waking, several times, *short, interrupted, convulsive cough,* which is excited by an inclination in the larynx, and leaves an unpleasant dryness in it. At noon, moderate appetite, head somewhat confused, especially in the forehead, *the throat dry and rough,* and some difficulty in swallowing. In the evening he felt very weak and unwell, with heaviness and tension in the feet, so that walking was painful; the head ached in that part of the anterior half which was covered with hair, as though compressed: nevertheless, a very good night succeeded.

18th. Of the catarrhal symptoms, nothing is left except a little roughness in the throat. This also disappeared by noon, and he felt well again. Until this point in the experiment, the sexual impulse had been much exalted.

19th. A good night's rest was followed by a day destitute of symptoms.

20th. On rising, inconsiderable cough and roughness in the throat, disappearing by noon. In its place appeared troublesome *dryness and sensitiveness of the nose,* as at the commencement of a catarrh. This sensation extended by degrees into the frontal sinuses, and the *eyes* also became sensitive. These catarrhal symptoms disappeared again during the afternoon. At the commencement of dinner, a *jerking constrictive pain* was felt in the hairy portion of the head, and in the afternoon painful *tension* in the right *popliteal space.*

21st. In the forenoon, dull confusion of the head; slight *burning* in the stomach, and in the left external canthus. At two o'clock, violent *burning in the eyes and eyelids;* frequent sneezing. The roots of the hair of the left eyebrow are sensitive when passing the hand over them. At dinner, burning tearing in the whole left side of the face, apparently in the periosteum. After dinner, general uneasiness for a couple of hours. In the evening *burning pressing pains in the left eye*, on the whole upper surface of the globe, aggravated by the touch; sensitiveness of the left temple; slight *drawing in the nape*, and repeated sticking from the nape to the right ear and axilla. After supper, dull confusion in the head for an hour. On lying down, the right leg was so painful, that he was obliged to place himself on his left side, contrary to his usual habit, and so to lie during the whole night.

For several days the skin on the vertex has been sensitive to the touch, and shines so clearly through the hair, that the prover was afraid he was becoming bald.

22d. On awaking, some headache in the forehead; after rising, the same feeling in the left nostril and right frontal sinus came on that had been experienced two days before; but now the right nostril was entirely free from it. At noon, frequent blowing of thick mucus from the nose. The whole right leg was painful. *Repeated urgency to urinate,* even when there was but little water in the bladder. In the evening, all the morbid symptoms had vanished, except that a little spot upon the vertex still remained sensitive to the touch.

23d. No symptoms; two liquid stools which were evacuated soon after taking the dose, seem to have prevented their appearance.

24th. He had no other symptoms to-day, than a slight *burning in the hæmorrhoidal* vessels, and copious secretion of mucus from the nose.

25th. In the morning, dull confusion in the head, especially in the region of the forehead and temples, which an hour after began to increase and extended over the vertex, but subsequently entirely disappeared; *slight burning in the canthi.* After dinner, *general weariness* with slight headache in the forehead. In the evening, *tension in the extensor muscles* of the extremities and trunk, now here, now there; subsequently heat.

26th. Normal feelings during the day. In the evening, *drawing* and *sensation of weariness, with apparent dullness of feeling* in the limbs, especially in the upper and in the forearm near the wrist; *dull confusion in the head*, especially in *the forehead.* Intellectual exertion soon fatigues; tobacco smoke is not as agreeable as at other times; frequent yawning.

27th. In the afternoon, slight dulness in the head; no other symptom.

28th. In the night, frequent cough with raising of thick mucus. After dinner, general uneasiness, restlessness, swelling of the abdomen, feeling as if beaten in the upper arms. In the evening, good health. The cough ceased in the day.

29th. On awaking, *the glans is very sensitive;* drawing back the prepuce causes pain; frequent *dry hacking cough.* Soon after the dose, general uneasiness and stretching of the limbs. In the evening, frequent violent sneezing and tickling in the nose.

30th. In the morning frequent sneezing again, with increased secretion of mucus accompanied with *frequent dry hacking cough.*

Oct. 1st. During the day, frequent *dry hacking cough:* in the forenoon, when walking, some *itching in the hæmorrhoidal vessels:* after dinner, strong inflation of the abdomen.

2d. In the forenoon, violent *itching and pressing in the hæmorrhoidal vein.*

3d. In the forenoon, *on the upper lip, an elevated, red, violently itching spot,* which compelled him to scratch, but was gone without a trace at the expiration of an hour.

4th. In the morning, frequent violent sneezing, in a short time ends with dulness of the head: after dinner, extraordinary distention of the abdomen, which seriously embarrassed the respiration.

5th. No symptoms after taking sixty-four drops.

6th. Seventy drops. At night, *much flatulence* was discharged. In the morning sneezing; burning in the skin of the right lower leg. After breakfast, frequent eructations with the taste of Thuja; *frequent short, dry, interrupted cough; slight chill.* In the evening, sudden, cramp-like *twitching of the under lip,* and here and there *in circumscribed spots on the skin.*

From the 7th to the last of October, he increased the dose daily by five drops, so that on the first day he took 75, and on the last 195 drops. The following were the results:

7th. No symptoms.

8th. An hour after the dose, *squeezing in the hæmorrhoids.*

9th. No symptoms.

10th. *Discharge of bloody slime from the anus,* as well by day as at night; frequent discharges of *flatulence,* which were always accompanied by some moisture. Towards evening, uncommonly strong appetite, which must be appeased; subsequently, *pressing in the hæmorrhoidal vein* when seated.

11th. No symptom worthy of mention appeared during the whole day, but in the evening, after much conversation in company, a pressing headache began in the forehead, extended gradually towards the vertex, and slowly disappeared.

12th. One hundred drops. Slight drawing behind the right ear, and some constriction in the ear; ache in the forehead, which, after an hour, merged in the sensation as if a wedge were driven into the temple. Sneezing did not aggravate the headache, but motion of the head and swallowing had that effect. At the same time, cheerful disposition and inclination to intellectual exertion. In the night very good sleep.

13th. Uncommonly comfortable and easy.

14th. In the morning, transitory *burning in the anus.* At noon, tension in the whole right leg, while walking. After dinner, slight sensitiveness in the skin under the hair on the forehead, where the cool air at the open window was exclusively felt.

15th. At noon, frequent violent sneezing.

16th and 17th. No symptoms.

18th. In the afternoon, burning and pressing in the stomach, lasting several hours.

19th. Several small, painless *tubercles* appeared *upon the head.* The hair comes off on the vertex.

20th. In the morning, raising of tough mucus; in the forenoon, *itching in the perinæum* when seated; slight drawing over the left eyebrow.

21st. At noon, great dulness of the head; drawing in both thighs. In the evening, pressing in the forehead and in the right temple.

22d. On waking, ache in the forehead, which disappeared again after half an hour. After a normal evacuation, *burning and drawing in of the anus.* At noon, drawing in the lumbar muscles, while walking.

23d. At noon, drawing again in the loins. The lumbar vertebræ are somewhat painful when leaning forward in sitting; *feeling of soreness in the perinæum.*

24th. No symptom during the whole day.

25th. In the morning, on rising, drawing from the loins towards the nates. After dinner, very violent *itching in the anus.*

26th. At night, increased secretion of mucus in the larynx and trachea.

27th. Slight pressure in the hæmorrhoidal vein; in the evening, slight drawing in the left upper arm.

28th. *Drawing, now here, now there:* but worse on the *left side of the body: burning* in the external *canthi.*

29th. In the morning, slight heat and redness, with burning on the upper lip; drawing in the left arm.

30th. On awaking, frequent violent sneezing with tickling in the nose, and *burning in the eyes,* as though a catarrh were coming on; drawing in the right forearm.

31st. In the forenoon, *itching and burning in the hæmorrhoidal vessels,* when walking; *internal shuddering and feeling of cold* the whole afternoon, with dull confusion in the head. *In the sulcus inter nates, a clammy moisture is secreted.*

Nov. 1st. The dose was omitted; *drawing* in the limbs, particularly in the right forearm, aggravated by movement of the limb; *coldness* in the hands and feet; drawing in the whole right leg; pressing in the left side of the chest.

2d. Two hundred drops. In the morning, *roughness in the throat* with continual inclination to hawk, and with a deeper tone of the voice, which disappeared again after breakfast. At noon, *burning and feeling of soreness in the anus.*

3d. Two hundred and five drops. In the forenoon, drawing in the right elbow joint, and *squeezing in the hæmorrhoidal vessels.*

4th. No dose. At noon, violent *itching and squeezing in the hæmorrhoids : tension in the extensors* of the right arm, when writing. In the afternoon, normal state. In the evening, a renewal of the violent squeezing and pressing in the anus: *very earnest frame of mind*, in spite of the cheerfulness of those around him; a small *suppurating boil* on the back.

5th. Two hundred and ten drops. At noon, *drawing* in the right lower leg, especially on the outside towards the ankle, and in the right hand, particularly in the thumb. In the afternoon, from four to six o'clock, severe burning and pressing in the stomach.

6th. Two hundred and twenty drops. In the forenoon, burning in the stomach for an hour. At noon, flying stitches on the right side near the sternum for a quarter of an hour.

These stitches had this peculiarity, that instead of being aggravated, they disappeared on taking a deep inspiration, and returned again only on the succeeding expiration. In addition, slight tension in the extensors of the right hand, and drawing in the dorsum of the right ring finger.

7th. Two hundred and twenty-five drops; and he daily increased the dose by five drops until—and including the 16th of November, when he took two hundred and seventy drops—in the morning, *discharge of copious, inodorous flatulence*, and a hard unsatisfactory stool; tension in the bend of the right elbow, when writing.

8th. In the forenoon, pressing and burning in the stomach for an hour. At noon, he perceived a sensation as if the lower part of the thorax were surrounded with a bandage, which sensation disappeared in the afternoon. In the evening, a very disagreeable pressing in the region of the heart, confined to a small spot.

9th. Immediately after the dose, rolling and rumbling in the intestines; afterwards, frequent *dry hacking cough ; tension* in the right hand, especially in the thumb; the same in the outside of the right thigh, extending into the knee, particularly when walking and bending. In the forenoon, the right knee-joint was painful when seated, but the pain soon disappeared, and was succeeded by a feeling of cold in the knee. A transitory pressing and tension in the heart then came on, and on its ceasing, the coldness in the knee was again perceived, but in a less degree. All these symptoms were gone at noon. At half-past one, on closing the eyes, a feeling of vertigo, (an obscure designation! M.) The power of thought was increased, but rather for analytical than synthetical reasoning.

10th. Half an hour after the dose, rumbling in the intestines, with slight griping; frequent coughing up of mucus.

11th. In the morning, *roughness in the throat*, and frequent *hacking cough.* The *upper lip* somewhat swollen, and *burns.* After a loose stool, *burning in the anus.* After dinner, dull confusion of the head; afterwards, *heart-burn.* These symptoms disappeared in the open air. In the evening, slight *burning in the eyes.*

12th. In the morning he felt well. At noon, dull confusion of the head; *burning and dryness* in the right *nostril*, up as high as the frontal sinuses; *slight burning in the right eye;* oppression in the lower part of the thorax; frequent short, *dry hacking cough.* He feels much better in the open air than in the room; the indefinite feeling of uneasiness, however, cannot be exactly described. In the evening, the knees were painful while walking, as though bruised; the weight of the body seems to him to be too great for the legs.

13th. *At night he urinated more than usual.* In the morning, after rising, frequent raising of mucus, leaving behind a feeling of sensitiveness in the larynx: *discharge of copious inodorous flatulence.* After dinner, drawing behind the right ear, with single *stitches in the mastoid process of the temporal bone.* When this symptom had disappeared, as it soon did, short accesses of *crawling and running* on the left side *of the occipital bone* came on; also, *burning and pressing in both eyes.*

14th. On waking, aching in the forehead, which disappeared by degrees after rising, but returned at about half-past nine, became heavy and pressing, and only vanished after four hours; after which, pressure on the vertex, as if a weight lay there. To these were added, weariness and uneasiness in the whole body, *coolness and flying shudderings over the back.* At noon, his food had a disagreeable bitter-sharp aftertaste, which was recognised, especially at the root of the tongue and in the fauces. The uneasiness became less after dinner, but even black coffee left behind an unpleasant after-taste.

15th. Soon after the dose, constriction about the navel and slight pressing in the lower border of the right orbit, soon going off; but the orbital edge remained sensitive to the touch, and to the closing of the eye for a quarter of an hour. Afterwards, tension in the right ankle while walking. The respiration is not altogether free; the thorax is raised during inspiration, with somewhat more difficulty than usual, and a short, *dry hacking cough* frequently comes on: a *violently itching tubercle* makes its appearance *upon the upper lip*, near the right corner of the mouth.

16th. An hour after the dose, oppression of the chest; troublesome breathing, drawing between the shoulders, burning and pressing in the stomach, increased by movement and by speaking. Constriction of the anus after two papescent stools. Also, heaviness and lameness in the right arm, and slight *drawing* in the right *masseter*, with *confluence of saliva into the mouth.*

From the 17th to, and including the 29th, he ceased to take the Thuja, and observed the following symptoms:

17th. In the night, *drawing* in the right *upper arm, axilla, and shoulder*, preventing his lying on that side. In the morning, these pains became intolerable, but by warmly wrapping up the painful parts, they gradually diminished, and finally entirely disappeared, leaving behind a feeling of lameness in the arm. At about half-past nine, the tearing in the shoulders and upper arm returned in *frequent short attacks.* After dinner, general weariness and universal feeling of discomfort. In the evening he feels generally better, but the pain in the shoulder is again very violent, and in the right arm; especially in the forearm there is a condition bordering upon *paralysis, with feeling of coldness.* Before going to sleep, *very gloomy frame of mind.*

18th. At ten in the forenoon the pain in the arm came on in short accesses, was sensible until noon, but was milder than the day before, and ceased entirely in the afternoon. The mind became more cheerful again.

19th. The pain in the arm is entirely gone, and Z. feels well the whole day.

20th. At noon, slight drawing in the small of the back, *drawing* in the left *groin* and frequently *a dry hacking cough.* No trace of the pain in the arm.

21st. Burning in the whole nose, which seems to feel as if swollen, with increased sensitiveness on the septum, on which several *vesicles* are to be seen. The *upper lip* is likewise sensitive. In the afternoon these symptoms have disappeared again, and the vesicles on the nose are dried up. On the two following days no drug symptoms were observed.

24th. In the evening of the 24th and the whole forenoon of the 25th an exceedingly troublesome headache came on, which was seated in the upper surface of the vertex, was heavy and pressing, and from time to time in single stitches and thrusts. The brain was apparently unaffected, but the *head* externally was somewhat *sensitive* to the touch, as were also the eyes. Cool air diminished the pain; when it was at the worst, he supported his face in the concavity of his hand, and for some time rubbed his forehead, eyes and face, whereupon the pain entirely disappeared, and in the evening his head was wholly free, except a slight crawling and running on the places before indicated. On the four following days, no symptoms.

(65.) *Second proving with massive doses of the tincture.*

Nov. 30th. 300 drops of the tincture. Two hours after, slight *tearing in the nape*, and distension of the abdomen by flatulence.

Dec. 1st. No medicine was taken. In the morning he remarked upon the forehead over the root of the nose, a *red streak*, which did not itch nor present any appearance of roughness, and was visible until noon. He had a feeling over the crest of the right ilium, on touching it, as if it had been bruised. At noon, a transient drawing came on in the first joint of the right thumb which was, in consequence, somewhat less easily moved.

2d. 300 drops. In the forenoon, the *red streak* was again visible upon the forehead, but no other especial symptom manifested itself the whole day.

3d and 4th. 300 and 310 drops produced no effect.

5th. 320 drops. There appeared *in the sulcus between the nates,* not far from the *anus, a painful spot,* which felt sore for an hour.

6th. No drug and no symptoms.

7th. 330 drops. Immediately after the dose, flying stitches in different parts of the body; frequent *dry hacking cough;* afterwards, raising of mucus; in the afternoon, pressing and burning in the stomach for an hour; then, transient feeling of pressure in the heart and single stitches in the lower half of the right side of the chest. Not the slightest trace is perceptible of the hæmorrhoidal congestion, which was usual during the earlier days of the experiment, and this the prover considers as a curative effect of the drug.

8th. No dose and no symptoms.

9th. 340 drops. In the afternoon, slight burning and pressing in the stomach during an hour. In the evening *general weariness* and uneasiness, with dull confusion of the head; drawing in the joints of the hands and feet. The abdomen was incommoded by a supper which was eaten with hearty appetite.

10th and 11th. 350 and 370 drops produced no symptoms.

12th. 380 drops. In the morning, a small, painless, non-itching *tubercle near the raphé of the perinæum;* the eyes on waking were glued with mucus. In the afternoon, relaxation and sleepiness. In the evening, inclination for exertion; frequent slight *drawing from the mastoid process* of the right temporal bone downwards. Afterwards single, flying, very painful *stitches from the depth of the right ear* through *the external ear.* An hour after, when the ear-ache had disappeared, a violent stitch drove suddenly through the left temple as if an awl had been forcibly thrust into the brain. The pain lasted but a few seconds, but the spot remained for some time sensitive.

13th. 400 drops. In the morning, feeling of fulness with stoppage in the right ear and frequent sneezing, which returned in the evening, soon after which pretty violent *itching in both nostrils* towards the point of the nose, after a short continuance of which, *a secretion of a thin mucus* followed. Also, sticking drawing on the inner surface of the left forearm towards the wrist, nausea mounting from the abdomen, with slight inclination to vomit.

Z. made the observation that the morbid feelings produced by Thuja are aggravated during rest; and by remaining quiet, symptoms are developed which disappear on motion in the open air.

14th. No dose and no further symptoms except tension in the flexor surface of the right leg and inflation of the abdomen.

15th. 410 drops. In the afternoon a couple of transient tearings in the tendinous expansion on the right side of the neck.

16th. 420 drops. During the whole forenoon a very unpleasant sensation of cold, the external temperature being + 1 R. (34° F.). The *hands and feet are icy cold* and the skin of the hands is purple. At noon, before dinner, for a little while *oppression of the chest with difficult respiration* and slight pain in the anterior surface of the stomach on taking a deep inspiration, as though from external pressure. In the afternoon and evening, these symptoms were gone.

17th. No drug and no symptoms.

18th. 430 drops. Soon after the dose, tenesmus and a hard, very unsatisfactory stool; also, transitory pressure on the chest; *burning in the urethra* towards the bulbus for several minutes; in the evening, something of a headache; at night, quiet sleep.

19th. No dose. On awaking, violent pressing headache in the vertex, which went off by degrees while he was still in bed, and disappeared entirely after he had arisen. Breakfast did not relish; and while at table, slight vomiturition; to which were added general weariness and faintness, with pressure and sensitiveness in the eyes.

20th. 450 drops. Not a trace of a symptom appeared in the forenoon; even the eructations with the taste of Thuja, which formerly were sure to come soon after taking the drug, did not once manifest themselves. In the afternoon, general malaise, with a sensation as if a chill were about to come on. Dull confusion of the head for half an hour.

21st. No dose. In the morning, *burning in the skin of the right lower leg;* slight sensitiveness in the vertex and right eye; *feeling of soreness at the anus.* Towards noon, throbbings in the right temple, when rising from a seat. Dinner was devoured with a veritable canine appetite. Two hours afterwards, general malaise, frequent *dry hacking cough*, and slight dulness of the head. In the evening, *pressure* in the hæmorrhoidal vessels when sitting. A painful inflamed tubercle makes its appearance on the right side of the forehead, and the neck appears as if swelled, so that the loose neckcloth is troublesome. Serenity of mind.

22d. No dose and no symptoms.

23d. 500 drops. In the morning, before the dose, short, *dry, troublesome cough*, without the former catarrhal symptoms. After it had gradually become quieted, by taking sugar moistened with water, violent burning in the stomach came on, which lasted until he got up. In the forenoon, uneasiness and sensitiveness to the cold air; at noon, troublesome drawing in the right radius, along the forearm as well as in the hand, into the little finger. In the afternoon, *heart-burn.*

24th. In the afternoon, when passing his water, slight *burning in the urethra.*

25th. In the morning, on walking, he had a violent erection, with strong desire for coition; but notwithstanding the existing voluptuous feeling, there was no emission, which is not usually the case with him.

He felt besides, weight and tension in the right leg, and in the evening, *burning in the eyes*, especially in the internal canthi.

26th. He felt perfectly well, and so on the 27th he again took five hundred drops. On awaking (before the dose), the sexual impulse was again active, and on this occasion, with normal results. After the dose, in the forenoon, violent *tension in the right lower leg*, on which the skin was painful as though *sore* and *ulcerated*, which sensation was lessened after dinner. In the afternoon again, a very violent erection. Afterwards, a delightful feeling of corporeal well-being and inclination to intellectual labor. In the evening, his foot was entirely without pain, and a *short, dry, interrupted cough* was excited by tobacco smoke.

28th. 500 drops again. In the forenoon, when walking in the open air, slight transient colic. As he came in at night from the cold air into a room, he felt a very violent stitch in the right ear, from the external part inwards to the internal, which compelled him to hold his breath, and left the ear sensitive for a while.

29th. No dose. In the morning another but less severe attack of the pain in the ear came on. He had a sensation in the ear, as if the free access of the air were prevented, but without the slightest diminution of the hearing. In the forenoon, the ear was well again; but after dinner he had the feeling in it as if the external organ were filled with water, similar to the sensation felt when one dips his head under the surface. *Drawing and tension in the occiput.* The right lower leg was twice painful during the day.

30th. 500 drops. Immediately after rising, the pain in the right lower leg again established itself. A spot next to the tibia, near a varicose dilatation, smarted as though it was *sore*, was very *sensitive* to the touch, and the *skin over it* was slightly *reddened.* In the forenoon, burning and pressing in the stomach. At noon, but little appetite. In the afternoon, strong inflation of the abdomen; burning in the stomach; *dry, short, hacking cough*, and *peevish humor.* In the evening, the right lower leg was again painful upon its upper surface, as if sore.

31st. No dose. On rising, after a very good night's rest, the pain in the leg again made its appearance. The spot which we noticed yesterday is still sensitive, but no more reddened. The ear, which for some days has not felt altogether right, is now entirely recovered. In the afternoon, *heart-burn.* In the evening he felt well.

1845, Jan. 1st. After a good night's sleep, he awoke with a very severe pressing headache, which, at the commencement, was confined to the vertex: after a while extended to the frontal eminences and eyes, and again returned to the vertex and disappeared. In the morning, he hawked up a thick tenacious mucus from the larynx. Although no Thuja had been taken, still the burning in the right lower leg developed itself in the forenoon, as did also, for a little while, a reminiscence of the earache of the 29th December. In the afternoon, severe burning on the inner side of the right lower leg was again troublesome. In the evening, the head and ear were entirely relieved. But when he especially directs his attention that way, the head and earache threaten to come on again, which is not the case when he intentionally fixes his mind upon the other suffering parts.

2d. 500 drops. In the forenoon, frequent eructations of wind preceded each time by painful constriction of the stomach. Instead of the right, the left ear has, to-day, a touch of the sticking pain. The right lower leg is still sensitive in the spot upon the tibia, heretofore indicated.

3d. 500 drops. Heaviness of the right leg, with *burning* on the whole inner surface of the lower leg. At two, in the afternoon, slight searching and griping about the navel. In the evening, great drowsiness.

4th. No dose. In the morning, after much straining, a very hard evacuation, followed by *pain in the anus.* At the same time, borborygmus, and three hours after, a couple of liquid stools, with subsequent *burning in the anus* (over an hour). Pressing and burning in the stomach, two hours after dinner. The right foot is less painful than yesterday. Several *inflamed tubercles* are visible on the face.

5th. 500 drops. In the morning, frequent hawking up of thick mucus. The burning in the right lower leg is drawing nearer to the ankle. After breakfast, a very unpleasant sweetish salt taste, especially in the back part of the mouth and on the root of the tongue. At ten, in the forenoon, pressing and burning in the stomach for a quarter of an hour; afterwards repeated coughing up of mucus. In the evening, heaviness and burning again in the right lower leg. The hinges of the under jaw crack when he yawns; a wholly unusual occurrence.* In the night, the whole right leg up to the hip-joint was painful, heavy, and less movable. The pain was drawing and tensive.

6th. 500 drops, after which the dose was omitted for six days. The following were the results: Soon after the drops, *burning in the throat*, obliging him to hawk; then slight raising of thick mucus; *frequent sneezing*, with obstructed nose and *roughness in the throat.* These catarrhal symptoms became more severe in the evening, and were accompanied by aching in the forehead, with weight and pressure in the eyes, and were followed by a very restless night.

7th. According to the report of his wife, he has slept very uneasily, has constantly rolled about in bed and moaned. On waking, his throat is entirely coated with phlegm, and after hawking, the larynx and trachea are painful. Then, general malaise both of body and mind; his head aches in the forehead, *his eyes burn, his nose is obstructed, and his voice is hoarse.* At noon, he felt better when walking in the open air, but when at rest the aggravation again returned. There was much *flowing from the nose, his feet were cold*, and the general feeling of illness sent him to bed early in the evening. It was, however, a long time before he could get warm, and dulness of the head, frequent

* Compare Dr. Huber's proving.

cough, stoppage of the nose, and, in short, all the symptoms of a slight catarrhal fever set in.

8th. This morning he felt very uneasy, and very weak, and lay in bed until ten o'clock. Afterwards he felt better. At noon, buzzing in the head, which feels dull, frequent *dry cough*, *pressure in the hæmorrhoidal vessels;* for the rest, good appetite. After dinner, burning in the stomach lasting until evening, when a short, jerking, dry cough took its place. Nevertheless he was incomparably better in the evening than on the previous day. The febrile symptoms came on again at night, but ceased after midnight, whereupon quiet sleep succeeded, and towards morning perspiration broke out.

9th. During the night burning in the stomach. On awaking, frequent *dry hacking cough*, and somewhat deeper and hoarser voice. At noon, buzzing and roaring in the head, and feeling in the extremities as though they had been bruised. In the evening, troublesome *dryness in the nose* up into the frontal sinuses.

10th. In the night, grumbling and rumbling in the intestines. In the morning, frequent *coughing up of thick mucus.* On rising, *burning in the eyes.* At noon, a great improvement over the preceding day; in the afternoon, at one o'clock, while sitting, *single flying, very painful stitches in the anus*, as if from a fine needle. These stitches returned from time to time, but not in so frequent a succession as at the beginning. Troublesome *dryness in the nose.* After dinner, great inflation of the abdomen, to which was added roaring in the head. On movement in the open air, these symptoms disappeared.

11th. On awaking, frequent *coughing up and blowing from the nose of thick mucus;* subsequently, a return of the troublesome *dryness of the nose with sensitiveness of the eyes.* At eleven in the forenoon, violent *pressure in the hæmorrhoidal vessels.* In the evening, the earlier catarrhal symptoms returned, accompanied by *sensitiveness of the eyes and frequent dry cough.*

12th. No symptoms to-day, except a frequent dry cough.

13th. 500 drops. In the forenoon, *squeezing* and *pressing* at the anus; in the afternoon, he felt well. No cough came on, notwithstanding he smoked and spoke much. After supper, *flying tearing in separate jerks* from the angle of the under jaw to the os hyoides pretty deep in the integuments.

14th. 500 drops. Again troublesome *dryness in the nose* with tickling; then griping in the intestines, burning in the right lower leg, and after a very well relished breakfast, a bitter sharp-salt taste in the mouth, particularly about the root of the tongue. In the forenoon, the dryness and pressure in the nose and frontal sinuses so increased, that he was very much incommoded by it in his lecture. At noon, *a catarrhal flowing came on, and disappeared again entirely in an hour after.* Soon after the pressure on the root of the nose, and copious secretion of mucus returned. The pressure on the root of the nose afterwards drew off towards the ears, where it produced tension in the auditory passages and stoppages of the ears. This symptom vanished again, after some time, and in place of it transitory *pressure in the hæmorrhoidal vessels* was perceived. After supper, pressing and burning with occasional painful constriction of the stomach.

15th. 500 drops. Immediately after the dose, *dryness and tension in the nose*, with the feeling as if the *whole mucous membrane were swollen;* the taste in the mouth alluded to yesterday also appeared. These symptoms disappeared after an hour. At two in the afternoon, emission of sparing and exceedingly dark colored urine, causing *burning in the urethra.*

16th. A mucous cough set in in the morning; no dose was taken, and with this exception no symptoms were perceived.

17th. 500 drops. In the morning, frequent *coughing up of thick mucus.* At noon, while sitting quietly in the room, the familiar troublesome, *dry feeling in the nose* appeared, which was much ameliorated in the open air, but returned, though less violently, on coming into the house again. The nose first became moist after he had smoked a cigar. He noticed, in addition, two painless *tubercles* about the size of a hempseed in the *sulcus between the nates* not far from the anus. In the evening he perceived *some painful spots on the head*, at most the size of a penny. The pain seemed to be seated in the bone itself.

18th. 550 drops. On awaking, he felt his head all over, but could not detect yesterday's sensitive spots: the tubercles near the anus were also missing. In the forenoon, frequent *cough*, with *raising of thick mucus;* in the afternoon and evening, short *dry cough.*

19th. 575 drops. Discharge of much loud *inodorous flatulence*, and frequent raising of *thick mucus with slight cough.*

20th. 600 drops. In the morning, frequent violent *sneezing, with cough and raising of mucus*, and slight *burning of the eyes.* He remarked, on accidentally touching *the raphé of the perinæum, that on the right side it was sharply prominent, and felt thickened as if the skin were indurated*, without being in the least painful. *Violent heartburn* an hour after dinner, lasting a couple of minutes, then lulling for several minutes, then returning, and so coming on in *frequent accesses.* Through the whole day, the *nasal secretion was tolerably copious*, and *thick mucus* was thrown off by *frequent coughing.* Pressure in the stomach was occasioned by roast meat eaten in the evening. He also perceived, here and there, a slight drawing under the skin in the tendinous expansions, and on making certain movements with his head a *creaking* in the *cervical vertebræ.* This symptom had already been frequently observed by the prover without any particular attention being paid to it, but to-day it was troublesome in a much greater degree.

21st. No dose. He slept remarkably well during the night. In the morning he coughed up mucus once or twice. Towards noon, a very unpleasant, pressing headache came on in the vertex, which diminished in the afternoon, and disappeared in the evening. At six in the evening, slight burning in the stomach and frequent coughing up of mucus.

22d. 600 drops. Thereafter, frequent slight *coughing up of mucus.*

At noon, burning in the lower border of the right nostril, which was sensitive to the touch (for half an hour).

23rd. 620 drops. During the whole forenoon he could not get warm, and twice, while walking, spat blood, the origin of which he supposed to be in the cavity of the mouth, but could not trace it with certainty. In the afternoon, burning and pressing in the stomach (for an hour); in the air, *tearfulness of the eyes.*

24th. 650 drops. In the morning slight *coughing up of mucus;* otherwise, he felt well all the forenoon. Afterwards, in the room, a watery, *catarrhal flow* came on, and after dinner, frequent, *short dry cough.* For a long time, the urine, on emptying the chamber, has been found thick and turbid, with a sediment at the bottom of the vessel.

25th. No dose. In the forenoon, an especial feeling of malaise with general discomfort. He frequently coughed up thick mucus, and had pain in his stomach and heaviness in the right foot.

26th. 700 drops. During the night, excellent sleep. In the morning, immediately after the dose, emission of flatulence both upward and downward. He subsequently observed slight burning on the inner side of the right lower leg. After breakfast, weakness in the stomach with confluence of saliva into the mouth. While seated at his writing-table he felt the influence of the drug spreading through his system, and he had no doubt that if he remained quiet, manifold symptoms would soon make their appearance, but he was obliged to go out, and the development of the effects of Thuja was always hindered by bodily movement. At ten in the forenoon, slight burning in the stomach and in the eyes, slight squeezing about the anus, and short accesses of drawing in the right arm and leg. In the open air he felt well. After eating ices, scraping sensation in the throat, unpleasant taste in the mouth, and constriction in the region of the os hyoides. In the evening, tobacco-smoke, reading and writing by candlelight produced either burning in the eyes or cough, an intimation that the catarrhal symptoms were the effect of the operation of the drug.

27th. On waking, the eyelids were slightly agglutinated. Some thick mucus was thrown off by slight coughing, and after a papescent stool, slight burning in the anus was manifested.

The dose of 725 drops produced, after breakfast, an unpleasant, resinous, constrictive taste in the mouth. As he was much in the open air no other symptom was developed except frequent sneezing.

28th. In the morning, *coughing up of thick mucus* again. Immediately after taking 750 drops, tearing in the tendinous aponeurosis on the skull (for some minutes); in the forenoon, frequent light *cough with raising of thick mucus;* at noon, great excitement in the genital organs, especially *tickling in the prepuce and glands.*

Z. remarks: "In my case, Thuja operated in a striking manner upon the hæmorrhoidal vessels; for I felt in them, at times, congestion, and then again, such a slimness, I might say emptiness, that it attracted my observation even when I was not paying attention to that quarter; and this alternation of sensations frequently took place twice or three times a day."

29th. 775 drops. No symptoms the whole forenoon. After dinner, sleepiness, *feeling of coldness*, especially *in the feet;* a boring stitch on the right side of the under-jaw; a couple of erections, and on the emission of some very dark colored urine, *burning in the urethra;* late in the evening, when visiting the privy, two flying, very painful stitches low down in the left side of the chest.

30th. In the morning, he several times coughed up thick mucus. After taking 800 drops, *burning in isolated spots* under the skin, particularly on the right side of the chest. Towards noon, while walking in the open air, *a sudden, flying stitch darted through the urethra*, came out from the bulbus, pressed almost to the middle of the urethra, and was so violent that he was unconsciously obliged to bend over. At five in the evening, a laming drawing of short duration in the right shoulder and in the thumb of the right hand; soon after, tearing in the palm of the hand near the wrist (for half an hour). At half past eight, he was seized in the street with general malaise and such universal debility, with weakness in the stomach, that he took a small glass of cordial at a coffee-house. After a while he felt better again, but about 10 o'clock he felt an indisposition by no means easy to describe in words; his mind was at the same time wholly undisturbed. It was a long time before he could go to sleep, and he awoke in the morning earlier than usual.

On the 31st and the two following days he took no medicine.

31st. In the forenoon, *burning in the anus; at 7 in the evening, violent heartburn.* Notwithstanding the shortness of the preceding night's rest, he felt, all day, no tendency to somnolency. The urine was voided very seldom. On the following night, a good sleep.

February 1st. In the morning, frequent *hawking up of mucus, sneezing, slight agglutination of the eyes*, and burning in the *right lower leg.*

2d. After rising, *drawing tearing* in the right arm, especially along the course of the ulnar nerve, in the right thigh, in the right zygoma, and in the right side of the chest. After a little while, these symptoms passed off and appeared, but weaker, in the left side of the body.

3d. In the morning, coughing up of mucus and a single sneeze. An hour after 850 drops, *dulness in the head*, on the *right side of the forehead*, continuing an hour, and *dryness of the nose.* After dinner, slight bnrning in the stomach, heaviness and weariness of the legs with dulness of the head, and indisposition to any kind of intellectual labor. *The eyes secrete much gum;* the face is wan and the appearance bad all day.

4th. No dose. In the morning, slight dulness of the head; *short drawing tearing, now here, now there, but always on the left side of the body.* In the evening, *burning of the eyes* as if the room were smoky (for an hour). Subsequently, debility of the legs, and on writing, a return of the burning of the eyes. The secretion of urine is very sparing; and the urine itself soon becomes thick and turbid by standing, and deposits a copious, clayey sediment.

5th. 875 drops. Thereupon, *emission of much flatulence;* slight pressing on the inner side of the right knee; transient drawing in the left ancle, afterwards in the right thumb, and finally on the radial side of the right upper arm, where the pain disappeared after half an hour; slight griping in the intestines, with the feeling as though they were pinched with the fingers in a circumscribed spot, now here, now there: on smoking a cigar, the dryness of the nose, which had been already often remarked, came on, and the mucus hawked up had an unpleasant, sharp, resinous taste. These symptoms vanished in the open air; but in walking against the wind, *his eyes continually watered*, which had already been frequently remarked to be the case, but had not been specially attended to by the prover. After dinner, great inflation of the abdomen (for an hour) and a couple of gripes in the intestines. In the evening, slight *itching and pressing in the anus.*

6th. 900 drops of the tincture. Immediately after the dose, two sneezings, which seemed to be excited by a vapor rising from the stomach into the nose; then a couple of *short, dry coughs*, and slight burning on the dorsum of the right foot. The eyes were somewhat agglutinated and watery in the open air. During the lecture, his voice was hoarse with frequent inclination to hawk. On coming into the room from the open air in the afternoon, he had, for some time, painful thumping and roaring in both ears. An evacuation, followed by violent pressing, was unsatisfactory.

7th. 925 drops. Immediately afterwards, discharge of flatulence upward and downward, burning externally over the lower ribs of the right side; then, burning in the stomach, with eructations with the taste of Thuja during the whole forenoon. Burning in the stomach again at dinner, which was eaten with appetite (for an hour). For several days past he has noticed that while he is smoking a cigar, seated at the writing table, he is obliged to cough, dry and interrupted, which was not usually the case. In the evening, on eating fish, pressing and burning in the stomach.

8th. 950 drops. Soon after, inclination to cough, and burning in the throat on the left side near the larynx, which afterwards extended towards the left ear, with more of a feeling of soreness, and soon after disappeared. Slight constriction and compression of the lower half of the chest, and transient stitchy pains on both sides of the thorax extending to the armpits. Towards noon, *burning at the anus*, and in the right leg. He felt well in the air. After dinner, slight *burning in the urethra when urinating.* In the evening, *burning and stinging in the edges of the eyelids* (even the smoke of tobacco burns in the nose), *with sticking in the nape over the joint of the atlas* (for half an hour). The following night, he slept well, and *sweat*, on awaking, *so strongly on the inner side of the thighs and legs*, that the skin was completely wet, while the rest of the body was dry. (Compare Dr. Huber's proving.)

9th. Z. concluded his second experiment by taking 1000 drops of the tincture. After the dose, burning in the stomach (for half an hour); then, *feeling of coldness* over the whole body, in a warm room, especially in the hands; rumbling and slight griping in the intestines; somewhat later, *creeping shudderings*, particularly in the *back*, with hot face; heaviness of the eyelids, with slight *burning of the eyes* and heat in the right ear. The breathing at the same time was easy, and the passage of the air through the nose free. The temperature of the open air 3° R. (39° F.) affected him so unpleasantly that he trembled from head to foot with cold. After dinner, transient pressing headache in the vertex; *laming drawing* in the right *armpit*, *coming on by fits;* occasional drawing in the right thumb.

10th. His voice was hoarse during his lecture, and his throat so choked with mucus that he was frequently obliged to hawk. After dinner, *burning of the eyes* again, and somnolency also; slight compression and crawling externally on the occiput. After a short and very refreshing nap, burning in the stomach, eructations of wind, discharge of flatulence, frequent *dry cough.*

11th. In the morning, after a hard scanty stool, *pressing and burning at the anus;* also, soreness in the bend of the right arm when extending it (the whole forenoon); pressing headache on the vertex and in the temples (the whole evening); *feeling of coldness*, especially in the hands and feet, and on the anterior surface of the thigh down to the knee, when seated in the warm room.

12th. In the morning, coughing, with raising of mucus. In the forenoon, there was a return of the soreness in the bend of the arm, but in a less degree than yesterday.

(66.) *Third proving with the 10th dilution.*

Z. now instituted an experiment with the diluted Thuja.

On the 12th of February he tasted the 10th dilution, which had been provided for the proving, in order to ascertain if he could discover the taste of Thuja in it, which was not the case. Thereafter, in the course of scarce a couple of minutes, the same troublesome *dryness in the nose* came on which had been perceived on the third of the month, and remained for half an hour. In the afternoon, he perceived burning and pressing in the stomach (for an hour).

13th. 10 drops of the 10th dilution, which had been previously shaken for five minutes with two ounces of distilled water. In the afternoon, *burning in the stomach* (for an hour), and in the evening, *pressing in the hæmorrhoidal vessels.*

14th. The same dose. After dinner, sleepiness, and on lying down on the couch, instead of the expected slumber, painful, *cold running* from the *nape*, over the *back*, down to the sacral region, which were increased by every movement of the body, and soon disappeared after rising.

15th. For the last time, Z. took 10 drops of the 10th dilution immediately before breakfast (café au lait). Shortly after he perceived a sharp taste in the mouth, and had eructations with the taste of Thuja.

He remarks at this point: "I must confess that I am not in a situation to account for this symptom. How should it be possible for ten drops of the 10th dilution of Thuja, drunk in two ounces of water, followed by a breakfast of bread and coffee and the smoking of cigars, to affect the gustatory nerves?" *

The drawing in the right shoulder also came on for a little while. After dinner, he was again annoyed by the dryness in the nose, already often described, and burning on the tongue; in the evening, burning in the stomach.

16th. An entirely new symptom made its appearance. As he was going to dinner, there *was a sudden sparkling before his eyes*, and a multitude of *black shining points swam before them*, so that he could not clearly make out surrounding objects. After a while this symptom disappeared; first from the right eye.†

26th. Eleven days after the closing of the proving. In the evening, *tearing and laming drawing in the left axilla*, which on the following day extended to the right shoulder, where it remained an hour. On the same day he perceived, for a short time, a constrictive feeling in the back between the scapulæ, which somewhat hindered respiration, and also motion of the arms. Afterwards he had a *feeling* in the internal *canthus of the right eye, as if a grain of sand* had fallen into the eye; this continued until bed-time, and rendered the movement of the eyelids somewhat painful, though no objective alteration in the appearance of the organ could be detected.

28th. The eye was entirely restored; but in the morning, a pressing headache in the region of the vertex came on for a short time, and returned in the evening, accompanied by burning in the stomach. No other effects of the Thuja were remarked by Professor Von Zlatarovich. ‡

Q.

(67.) *Zlatarovich's proving of the tincture of Thuja on a young woman.*

Catharina Ratmayer, 23 years old, unmarried, thin, of a nervous excitable constitution, suffered when a child from scaldhead, and from worms. She was chlorotic from her twelfth to her nineteenth year. The catamenia first appeared in her fifteenth year; but during the first year, they appeared very irregularly, and even at the present time, are

* In our opinion, this taste of Thuja is to be attributed, not to the ten drops of the 10th dilution, but to the 40,000 drops of the mother tincture which had been previously taken, which had penetrated, and, so to speak *thujacised* the whole body. A new reaction followed the new and almost immaterial dose, and that might disengage a perceptible portion of the previously taken mass.—*Mayrhofer.*

† Compare Dr. Huber's proving.

‡ We must give this bold and persevering experiment the highest tribute of our acknowledgment and admiration.—*Mayrhofer.*

sometimes absent for two or three months, especially on any violent mental excitement. They appeared last on the 23d of September, and continued for six days, which has been their usual duration for some time past. She has suffered for a year with accompanying cramps in the abdomen. She has had for some years a flat, dry tetter on the chin and lips.

1844, Oct. 17th. She began the proving of Thuja with ten drops of the tincture, taken fasting in water, in the morning. Two hours after she perceived heat and vertigo (for half an hour).

18th. 15 drops. In the forenoon, pressing in the stomach.

19th. 20 drops. After dinner, transitory *coldness over the whole body.*

20th. 30 drops. She felt well during the day. In the evening, *chilliness for several hours*, passing into heat on lying down.

21st. 35 drops. No symptoms.

22d. 40 drops. In the following night, pain in the stomach, with nausea and vomiturition (for an hour).

23d. 45 drops. Pressing headache through the day, beginning on the right side, afterwards extending over the whole head.

24th. 50 drops. In the forenoon, eructations with the taste of the drug and slight headache for a couple of hours.

25th, 26th, and 27th. 55, 60, and 65 drops. No symptoms.

28th. 70 drops. *Coldness all day;* cutting above the navel, extending into the sacral region; before bed-time, difficult respiration with pressure on the chest, by reason of which she could not get to sleep for a long while.

29th. 80 drops. In the morning, on waking, very violent pressing aching in the forehead, lasting all day. The menses, which should have appeared on the 25th, came on, for the first time, to-day, but unattended with colic.

The following six days passed without taking any of the drug. During the first two, she had continual headache, copious eructations of wind, and wandering, drawing pains in the hollow teeth. On the 1st of November she was well. On the 2d she had, in the morning, a three hours' headache, at one time in the right, at another in the left temple, and again in the vertex. On the 3d, the catamenial flow ceased; it had been less than usual.

4th. 85 drops. After breakfast, exceedingly violent colic, and transient cutting and rumbling in the intestines.

5th. 90 drops. A return of yesterday's colic, but less violent; accompanied by *weariness and general weakness*, with heaviness in the feet and general feeling of discomfort. She felt as if she were threatened with a severe attack of illness.

6th. She awoke with a very violent headache, and took 95 drops. During dinner, very severe, but very transitory colicky pains came on suddenly, and also frequent *creeping coldness*, as during a fever.

On the following two days, 100 and 105 drops produced no symptoms.

9th. 110 drops. In the forenoon, *feeling of coldness;* in the afternoon, *frequent feverish alternations of cold and heat.*

10th. 115 drops. Slight headache all day.

On the next two days, 120 and 125 drops produced no symptoms.

13th. 130 drops. She felt all day weak and debilitated.

14th. 135 drops. Violent tearing on the left side of the head, and in the teeth of that side.

15th. 140 drops. For four hours after the dose, she was as if stupefied, sleepy and weak; the rest of the day well.

16th. 145 drops. She then ceased taking the remedy for sixteen days. During this time the results were as follows:

On the day of the dose, stupefaction again and sleepiness, which did not last so long, however, as on the previous day. In the afternoon, frequent eructations of wind, and pressing in the stomach, which extended through the throat into the fauces. Late in the evening, on going to bed, tearing on the right side of the head, and itching over the whole skin, especially on the abdomen, as if she were covered with an eruption. Painful *inflamed tubercles* appeared on various spots on the body.

17th. In the forenoon stomach-ache and melancholy state of mind; in the afternoon, more cheerful humor. This alternation of humors has already manifested itself for some days past.

18th. In the forenoon, pains in the stomach; *hawking up of mucus; stoppage of the nose,* with nasal sound of the voice, *biting on the whole body;* in the evening, sticking in the head, and transient tearing in the left hand.

19th. In the afternoon, tearing in the teeth of the left side, and afterwards a very restless night.

20th. Very severe catarrh with increased secretion in the air passages, painful swallowing, and sticking in the head.

These symptoms disappeared by degrees on the following days, and she continued the proving on the 2d of December, by taking 150 drops. Soon after the dose, stupefaction (effect of the alcohol? M.) and extreme drowsiness during the whole day.

Dec. 3d. 155 drops. Stupefaction, sleepiness and frequent eructations of wind.

4th. 160 drops. After dinner she was very thirsty, and so inflated that she could not bear the pressure of the strings about her body.

5th. 165 drops. The same symptoms.

6th. No dose. Extreme melancholy.

7th. 165 drops. After awaking, very violent headache, lasting all day and disappearing on the next day on which the dose was omitted.

On the next three days, 170, 175, and 180 drops produced no symptoms.

12th. 185 drops. After dinner, extreme thirst; in the evening, colic.

13th. 190 drops. Colic with two fluid evacuations, great thirst and *cold over the whole body,* with drowsiness.

14th. No dose. She awoke with sticking in the left side of the head, which soon went off; but the head was dull all day. She had also *drawing from the head over the nape and the back to the sacral region*, and complained of *general weakness with heaviness and coldness of the feet*, and in the evening, of general burning heat, whereupon restless sleep followed.

15th. She awoke with headache, and took 195 drops. In the evening, *coldness in the back with alternations of heat.* She has made the observation for several days past, that on bowing, she has sticking in the left side of the head, even if she were not just then suffering from headache.

16th. She closed the proving with 200 drops. The headache with which she awoke lasted three hours, and after it had ceased, sticking pain came on when bowing, but on the right side of the head. After dinner, pressing in the right side of the chest, during the whole afternoon, accompanied in the evening by sticking, which extended into the sacral region. During the whole day, *coldness*, especially in the *back*, with general weakness and sensation of weariness. In the evening, manifest fever symptoms developed themselves, as: headache, heat of the skin, full, accelerated pulse, besides sticking in the right hypocondrium (especially during respiration), which extended into the sacral region. She went to bed on this account, and general heat came on, succeeded by quiet sleep.

17th. There was no fever, but she felt weak. She has had no evacuation for two days past, and no appetite; a bitter mucous taste in the mouth. The pains in the chest are completely gone; borborygmus is frequent in the intestines; in the evening, sticking in the head, and pressing in the left side of the chest. These symptoms are diminished by an evacuation. The sleep was disturbed during the night by heavy, harassing dreams.

18th. In the morning, headache and *cough, with copious excretion of mucus; catarrh* and bitter taste the whole day, *thirst with alternations of heat and cold*, the latter *especially in the dorsal and sacral region*, with hot head and face. On going to bed, *pressing on the chest, with difficult breathing* and sticking in the side. Before midnight, *coldness;* towards morning, *warmth;* finally *perspiration.*

19th. On rising, violent sticking in the head, especially on moving; great accumulation of mucus. In the forenoon, *alternations of heat and cold.* Towards noon, the headache became very severe, and remained so for half an hour; there came on then, *drawing in the small of the back* (aggravated while seated), *stoppage of the nose, burning of the eyes*, frequent eructations of wind, *difficult*, almost panting *respiration*, violent *cough*, with *raising of mucus.* In the afternoon, slight colic, with borborygmus and inflation of the abdomen. In the evening, *general chilliness* without thirst. The pulse beat at the rate of 100 in a minute, was full and hard. Several *inflamed tubercles* appeared in the face. Her food tasted insipid.

20th. During the night, in which she continually suffered from *se-*

vere coldness, the catamenia appeared, ten days earlier than usual. In the morning, she felt very ill; her head was dizzy as if stupefied, her mouth tasted very bitter; all her teeth seemed to be loose; she frequently coughed up mucus as thick as lard. In the forenoon, she felt pretty well. Towards noon, *alternations of heat and cold* came on, with *weakness* to the extent of falling. In the afternoon, she felt well again except a slight headache. Catamenia very scanty. She observed for several days past, that she becomes hot at dinner, and her body is covered with perspiration.

21st. During the night, she slept extremely restless. So bitter was the taste in her mouth that she was obliged to get up in the night and rinse out her mouth with water. She awoke at about three in the morning, and could sleep no more on account of heat. Afterwards, a chill came on, and in the morning a very violent headache, lasting all day. Before dinner, she felt weak and sleepy, and was *cool over the whole body*. She felt better in the evening.

22d. In the morning, headache, but less than yesterday; frequent spitting of saliva and mucus, with hollowness at the stomach and insipid taste. General feeling of discomfort; she looks very ill, is weak, *depressed* in body and *mind*, and is somewhat bloated in the face. Towards noon, an attack of coughing, with raising of tenacious mucus, vomiturition and strangling; after this she felt ill and weak for half an hour, and had a return of more violent headache. At noon every thing tasted insipid. In the afternoon, when walking, great heat, weight upon the chest, breathlessness and occasional dry cough, with sticking in the head. In the evening, *coldness in the back*, with accompanying heat in the head, with great drowsiness and thirst; at night quiet sleep.

23d. In the morning, bad taste in the mouth; less sticking in the head than yesterday; she feels very hot and weak, and is frequently obliged to sit down to rest, although she insists upon it that she is better to-day than for some days past. She coughs very little, and has shorter breath than usual, with weight on the chest; her urine is copious, she has had no evacuation for two days. In the evening, chill again followed by heat, thirst and sleepiness. Pulse 120, full and hard; she is very low spirited.

24th. The same symptoms appeared, accompanied by *tearing in the hands;* in the evening, feverish pulse with headache; a good night's rest.

25th. In the morning, headache; also violent *tearing in the nape*, which extended into the axilla (which? M.) and there remained during the whole day. *The upper arms are painful, and so weak* that the patient can, with difficulty, hold them up long enough to arrange her hair; she trembles in hand and foot, looks pale and earthy, is exceedingly out of tune, *sad and disposed to weep;* respiration very short on walking, cough dry, abdomen very much inflated, taste bitter, increased thirst; alternations of heat and cold; pulse not so much accelerated, nor so full as yesterday. A hard evacuation.

26th. The patient feels so weak and powerless that she cannot leave her bed. Her head is very dull; she is as if stupefied and dozes much; her tongue is somewhat furred and half dry; pulse moderately accelerated, full and hard. To these symptoms were added cough and tearing in the left shoulder. This state of things, in connection with a very bad countenance and extreme prostration and depression of spirits, gave Z. reason to apprehend the development of a nervous fever (? M.), and he gave her a drop of *Puls.* 30. She continued the same for the rest of the day; she had occasional naps during the night, but they were disturbed by tearing in the left axilla and slight colic.

27th. In the morning, the same state of things, but in a somewhat diminished degree. Tongue dry at the point. In the afternoon, bitter taste, redness of the face with cool extremities, irritable humor. She had *Cocc.* 30, one drop. In the evening, copious, general perspiration, with diminution of all the morbid symptoms, and tolerably good sleep at night.

28th. In the morning, striking abatement of all the symptoms. The skin is agreeably moist, the pulse less accelerated, the feelings less gloomy; the tongue is still somewhat furred, and the tearing in the left shoulder is still present, but at times, it goes to the right shoulder and nape. She begins to feel a little appetite, and has had two stools; but she still feels very weak, dozes much, and speaks very *slowly and monosyllabically.* She had *Cocc.* 30, one drop in a tumbler of water, with directions to take a tablespoonful every two hours. The improvement continued during the day, and she had a good night.

29th. The pains are considerably diminished; the fever is slight, tongue moist, taste natural, mind cheerful. At night, sleep and copious perspiration. *Cocc.* continued.

30th. In the morning, the patient is exceedingly ill-humored, speaks but little, and keeps her eyes continually closed. For the rest, she complains of no pain, her pulse is but slightly accelerated, and there is nothing further worthy of remark. Z. gave her *Rhus* 24. She sleeps much during the day and has no appetite; the tongue is moist and a little furred; urine copious and yellow. She slept and perspired at night.

31st. With the exception of great weakness and prostration, no morbid symptoms appeared to-day. In the afternoon, the nose bled, after which her head was much relieved.

"It must be observed," remarks Z. in his relation, "that both those about the patient, and she herself had noticed that she was better and worse on alternate days, indications of a tertian type."

"I must confess," pursues he, "that I have no hesitation whatever in considering this whole attack, as it appeared, as caused by the Thuja. Had it been a natural idiopathic affection, there would have been a greater harmony in the symptoms. (? *Ed. Oest. Zeit.*) The febrile symptoms, however, stood in no relation to the extraordinary debility; there were no abdominal pains, no diarrhœa, no delirium, no metorismus, nor any of those symptoms which usually indicate the existence of a typhoid disease." *

1845, Jan. 1st. After a good night's rest, the patient, with the exception of general weakness, which was still present, felt well. Her appetite returned; she was not so depressed in mind as on the preceding days; but her speech is still very slow and drawling. She took *Ignat.* 24. At noon she was for a short time out of bed, and remained well during the afternoon.

2d. The catamenia appeared without any morbid symptoms, but lasted only one day.

15th. For the first time the convalescent went into the open air, which seems, nevertheless, to have been too soon; for on the 16th chills, want of appetite, peevishness, and a small weak pulse again made their appearance. She now took *Nux vom.* (in what dose? M.) An hour after, a shaking chill, lasting half an hour; heat came on over the whole body, preceded by a gradually increasing warmth. She was so weak that she was obliged to remain in bed the whole day. She had a thickly coated tongue, with bitter taste, but little appetite, and for two days past no evacuation. The febrile symptoms were slight. The *Nux* was continued. The next day she was better throughout, tongue cleaner, appetite returned, had a stool, increase of strength. The convalescence now steadily proceeded without any further medication, but it was a full month before she regained her former health.†

R.

(68) *Dr. Zoth's Proving with the Tincture.*

Franz Zoth, medical student, 24 years old, choleric-phlegmatic (? M.) temperament and apoplectic build; at 15 had the typhus; a year ago, was treated for ten days at the medical clinique for an inflammation of the lymphatic glands of the right arm, which had come on in consequence of intoxication with Cyanide of Potassium; in other respects was entirely well.

Zoth's proving produced very few results, notwithstanding he took 5000 drops of the tincture within three months.

1844, Oct. 15th, 16th, 17th and 18th. No effects were perceived from 5, 8, 11, and 14 drops of the tincture.

19th. 17 drops. He perceived single stitches in the right frontal region. On the following two days 20 and 23 drops produced no symptoms.

22d. 26 drops. A cough came on, which he regards as having been possibly caused by an exposure to cold.

* We do not for an instant doubt but that the above described attack was the result of the doses of Thuja; we recognise in the instability of the symptoms, in their evident discordance, and in the irregularity of the course of the disease, the fundamental characteristics of the drug.—*Mayrhofer.*

† What became of the tetter on the chin?—*Mayrhofer.*

The cough continued on the following two days, on which 29 and 32 drops were taken.

25th. 40 drops. To the cough was added swelling of the throat, which continued during the following three days, on which 50, 60 and 65 drops were taken.

From the 29th of October to the 6th of November, Z. increased his dose ten drops each day, so that commencing with 70 drops on the first day, he took 150 on the last.

The prover's diary contains nothing remarkable for these ten days, except that the excretions* were increased in quantity, and were less consistent; which remark will also apply to the previous days.

From the 7th to and including the 22d of November, he continued the Thuja in a similar ascending scale of doses (ten drops a day), and took on the last named day 300 drops of the tincture. (He omitted the dose on the 16th.) The results were as follows:

7th. Painful *throbbing in the base of the glans* (for four minutes); afterwards, pains (of what sort? M.) in the lower half of the spinal column and in the sacrum, continuing and aggravated by bending the body; also in both knees. These pains continued also during the following day, and were attended by great general weariness.

9th. Having taken much exercise this day the pains became less; on the 10th, however, became more violent, decreased by degrees on the following days, and finally ceased on the 16th, on which day he took no dose.

17th. These (undescribed pains! M.) returned again, and were especially violent in both hips, weaker in the sacral region and knees.

18th. They ceased in the sacral region, but continued in the hips and knees.

19th. An eruption upon an inflamed surface appeared on the left side of the chin.†

22d. Violent buzzing in the ears, lasting several hours.

From the 23d of November to the 5th of December, the Thuja was omitted, and all the previously described symptoms vanished.

From the 6th to and including the 20th of December, he again continued the experiment, taking on the first day 310 drops, and daily increasing the dose by five, until he arrived at 380 drops on the last day. He observed no effects.

From the 22d of January to and including the 2d of February, he made a short experiment with dilutions (without saying which! M.) and likewise perceived no alteration in his sensations.

* Urine, fæces, and perspiration?—*Mayrhofer.*

† Its form? It is indispensable, in describing objective symptoms, that their form and duration should be noted with the greatest accuracy.—*Mayrhofer.*

S.

(69) *Dr. Zwérina's Proving with the Tincture.*

Dr. Zwérina, thirty-six years old, perfectly healthy, and of a sanguineo-choleric temperament, proved the Thuja as follows:

1845, January 23d. He began with forty drops of the tincture prepared according to Hahnemann's direction, which he took at nine o'clock in the forenoon, an hour after breakfast, and observed no other result than that during the following night he was obliged, contrary to his usual habit, to rise *three times for the purpose of urinating.* The urine passed was a straw-yellow and amounted to a full measure.

On the following day he took nothing, and observed no symptoms which he could ascribe with confidence to the drug.

25th. Thirty drops, taken early at about nine o'clock. At noon, slight *burning in the urethra,* leaving behind a voluptuous feeling, especially after urinating. The quantity of water passed was again increased during the night; it was clear and straw-yellow. Sensation of great fatigue in the groins. His appetite was small, and his customary morning evacuation did not take place.

26th. To quicken the action of the remedy, the impatient prover took fifty drops morning and evening. Immediately hereafter, *burning in the urethra and copious urine;* the customary daily evacuation absent. *Disquieting dreams, frequent urination,* and four pollutions, disturbed, an unrefreshing night's rest. Sleep came on late, an unusual occurrence with him.

27th. These symptoms did not deter the prover from taking 100 drops this day, fasting. Thereupon he experienced headache in the region of the forehead and eyebrows, such as usually precedes a catarrh; *ill-humor,* lasting all day; want of appetite, with frequent eructations; repeated *shuddering,* beginning at the head; slight *burning in the region of the kidneys,* ceasing after an hour, and followed by still *more copious urine,* accompanied by *burning.* The feeling of fatigue in the region of the groins passed into a *drawing* pain extending into the glans penis, and the *inguinal glands* were perceptibly swollen. A *general feeling of malaise, with internal chills,* came on, and instead of his usual cheerfulness, *peevishness.* For three days he has had no stool.

28th. Notwithstanding this, he again took 100 drops early, fasting, "and now," says he, "for the first time, the drug fairly mastered the health that had so far defied it."

An hour after the dose, the *burning in the renal region* increased, and was accompanied by *drawing along the urethra up to the vesica;* the urine diminished in proportion as the burning in the ureters increased. The glans began *to grow moist* and to secrete *a thin mucus.* In the evening he had a slight chill, attended by *dryness of the throat, with painful deglutition,* vomiturition, and such a feeling of illness, that he was obliged to go to bed before the time. His interrupted sleep was full of *anxious dreams*, and he continued the fourth day costive.

He was now so well satisfied with the pathogenetic effects of Thuja that he dropped the experiment. By degrees his abnormal symptoms disappeared; first the headache, then the dryness of the throat, and lastly the renal affections; on the first of February, after a constipation of eight days, he had a copious, hard evacuation.

According to this proving, Thuja manifested its especial power in the urino-genital system, and it is much to be regretted that so promising an experiment should have been closed after the exhibition of only 360 drops.

T.

The following physiological proving of Thuja, by our associate, Dr. Holleczek, practising physician in Klagenfurt, has only reached us while these sheets are going through the press. It contains, for the most part, only subjective symptoms, and adds scarcely any new lines to the portrait of the Thuja sickness depicted by the experiments already detailed.

Dr. Holleczek has a strong constitution; had an intermittent fever at twelve years old, but was otherwise well until his twenty-second year. He then had a slight attack of pneumonia, and was perfectly restored in a few days by homœopathic treatment. He has had no other sickness. At the time of his first experiment he was twenty-five years old. The symptoms below follow in chronological order.

(70) *First Proving with the Tincture.*

1838, September 2d. He drank at one draught a half ounce of the strong tincture of Thuja prepared according to Hahnemann's directions, having first well mixed it with eight ounces of water.

Violent pressing headache in the region of the vertex; sensation as though something were squeezed out at both ears; heat in the face (immediately); feeling of heat in the whole chest; stitches in the temporal region, in the elbow and heels.

Pressing pain in the occiput; head pains as though the head were stuck through from one temple to the other; slight eructations (all day).

Stitches in the metacarpal bone of the little finger.

Stitches in the scrobiculus cordis; sticking beating in the middle of the right side of the chest; stitches in the cardiac region; pressure under the sternum; sticking in the pit of the throat.

Drowsiness; violent pressing pain in the occiput; feeling, when turning the head one side, as though a piece of lead lay in the brain.

Stitches from the spine through the epigastric region, forward to the pit of the stomach; frequent sticking pains in the right shoulder-joint; repeatedly during the day, a cutting pain, perpendicularly through the middle of the chest from below, upward as far as the pit of the throat;

sticking pains in the forehead; extremely violent sticking pain in the metatarsal bone of the middle toe of both feet; pressure on the right side near the scrobiculus cordis, as if from a foreign body, with frequent stitches, worst in the morning.

Itching on the inner surface of the prepuce; extremely violent pain in the middle toe of the right foot; several stitches in the interior of the right ear; painful, frequently repeated stitches in the right testicle; dreadful tearing pains, which darted like lightning hither and thither through the urethra, with simultaneous violent stitches in the anus (in the afternoon when seated).

Quivering twitching from the ear to the left corner of the mouth, sticking pains in the left shoulder-joint; tearing pains in the metatarsal bones of the right foot; dull sticking pain in the metacarpal bone of the middle finger of the left hand; sticking in the great, fourth, and little toes of the left foot.

Pressure in the larynx; sensation of burning and constriction of the larynx; tearing pains in the under jaw, which began on both sides, in the region of the joint, ran forward together in a line to the chin, united, and instantaneously disappeared.

Painless twitching of the middle finger of the right hand; very painful stitch through the upper part of the left breast from before backwards, which immediately disappeared, and left a feeling of twitching in the spot: tearing pains in the bones of the left fore-arm and wrist, stitches in the point of the third finger of the right hand; sticking in the sole of the right foot, from within outwards; feeling of dislocation in the middle of the spine, increased on the right side by violent bending of the body.

(71) *Second Proving.*

September 4th. The same dose as on the 2d.

Pressing headache on the vertex and occiput, with the sensation as though there were lead in it, aggravated by moving the head and by a false step, with the feeling as though the brain were loosely moving about: when lying on the back, knocking in the chest under the sternum, extending to the sacrum: while lying on the right side, many stitches in the same side of the abdomen, which disappeared on pressure, and returned on walking in the open air; in the evening, when walking in the open air, feeling of fulness and pressure in the occiput; on moving the head sideways, vertigo.

Constant, painful pressures from within toward the nipples; painful pressure in the right abdominal region, which disappeared on making pressure there with the hand, but became sensible again (during the whole day) on taking a deep inspiration, or on forcibly expiring: constant tearing pain in the metatarsal bone of the middle right toe; stitches in both knees when walking.

Cough with the expectoration of mucus when eating; after eating, cough with raising of a tough mucus—sticking headache in the region of the vertex; painful tension in the occiput from one ear to the other.

Little thirst; urine with a penetrating odor.

Stitches in the right wrist joint; boring from without inwards in the region of the right iliac bone; sticking in the middle of the sole of the left foot, from within outwards; a quick drawing, boring pain through the fore-arm and the metacarpal bone of the index finger; painful tension of the hypogastric region with occasional sticking pains, aggravated by deep inspiration (in the forenoon with an empty stomach); painful stitches in the skin of the left elbow.

Pressing in the middle of the chest upwards into the neck, inducing difficult respiration; sticking pains in the region of the heart; constant pressure in the middle of the chest, with sticking pains during the attempt to inspire deeply: frequent creeping chills; pressing pains in the whole upper part of the chest, becoming much more violent by pressure; cutting pain from the spine to the pit of the stomach.

Sensation as though the right side of the scrotum had been bruised; cutting pain deep in the left side of the abdomen; sensation when nodding forwards as if the brain were pressed out at the vertex; sticking in the right thumb, tearing in the right tarsus and great toe; cutting in the left side of the upper lip; dull pain anteriorly in the lower third of the right thigh; sticking in the bones of the lower leg from the tarsus up to the knee; tearing in the scrobiculus; on bending the body to the right side, tearing in the right popliteal space.

Fine sticking in the third joint of the index finger, from within outwards; violent stitches in the anterior extremity of the urethra, without urinating; sticking in the external malleolus, in the hip-joint, in the metacarpal bone of the middle finger, on the inner edge of the foot, in the heel; dull sticking pain in the joint where the thumb and index finger are articulated with the metacarpus; dull sticking in the interior of the right ear.

Twitching of the muscles on the right fore-arm; feeling, when seated, as though the breast were compressed from before backwards, aggravated by stretching the body; painful stitches in the interior of the left chest; dull cutting under the left shoulder-blade; cutting pain on the left side near the scrobiculus.

Stitches in the left testicle (for eight days); when coughing, dull sticking pains in the right inguinal region; violent sticking in the region of the spleen, during a meal; very violent stitches in the toes, noon and evening, on bending the body to the left side (on the seventh day).

Sticking pain in the liver, when walking; sticking pains in the right elbow; sticking in the metacarpal bones of the left hand; oppression of the chest: necessity of frequent deep breathing; dull sticking pain in the left parietal bone; sticking pain in the brain from the neck up to the vertex; stitches through the brain from below upwards, especially when coughing; stitches in the left ala of the nose; vague stitches in the left lung; burning in the forepart of the urethra, without any flowing; drawing sticking pains in the liver; cutting pains in the rectum.

(72) *Third Proving.*

October 31st. *Eight drops of the tincture of Thuja* in a table-spoonful of water.

Sticking in the scrobiculus; sticking beating in the fossa navicularis of the urethra (coming on daily for two weeks, at irregular intervals, and frequently repeated in an hour); sticking in the region of the spleen at indeterminate times, but particularly during dinner and supper (at intervals of four days); an evacuation early every day, with urging, although only a small quantity of thin fæces was quickly passed; afterwards feeling of inactivity in the rectum.

Vertigo, coming on of a sudden after dinner (while looking up); *headache in the occiput;* pressing with *stupefaction* when moving the head to one side.

Corroding aching of the right half of the scrotum.

All the diameters of the chest seem to have become shorter: painful tension in the whole *chest* when inspiring deeply; sensation of want of pliability *of the thorax* and of insufficiency in the inspired air; at night short breath; necessity to assist by breathing deeply.

Violent cutting in the *point of the tongue* and on its under surface; cutting in the upper *eyelid;* quivering of the muscles of *the left thigh* just above the knee; violent pressing pains in the left elbow, as if in the bone.

(73) *Fourth Proving.*

November 15th. *Fifteen drops of the tincture of Thuja* at a dose in a table-spoonful of water.

Sticking in the middle of the *right side of the chest* near the sternum (in a quarter of an hour); stitches like lightning transversely through the chest.

Tearing pain in the *tendo Achillis* on the right side; strong extension *of the right knee* impossible on account of a sensitive, painful obstacle in the popliteal space; the same symptom in the left knee; cutting pains through the chest in different directions; stitches in the right *tendo Achillis.*

Twitching pains under the *heart;* tearing and sticking pain *in all the joints;* stitches through *the whole brain* from below upward.

Burning *when urinating;* burning and sticking in the fore part of the *urethra.*

Cutting in the *right iliac region;* tearing in the *right hip-joint;* tearing in the *left little toe;* violent sticking on the outside of the left knee; violent sticking under the right knee; stitches in the sole and in the palm; itching in the rectum after stool; boring, as of a worm, in the rectum, from within outwards, after an evacuation.

(74) *Fifth Proving.*

1840, January 6th. *Ten drops of the fourth dilution* (5: 95), in an ounce of water.

Vertigo, when seated, returning as though in pushes every minute (after half an hour); sensation as though the brain were raised several times in succession; very painful stitch on the right side near the sternum on the fourth true rib, repeated, in only one spot; dull sticking pain in the left fore-arm, near the elbow; tearing pain in the right shin-bone from the knee down, and from the tarsus up to the knee (subsequently repeated); sticking pain in the right knee, coming from the popliteal space; sticking in the left elbow.

Excessive rumbling in the abdomen; dull sticking from the right ear and under the lobule outward; twitching in the muscles under the left scapula; very painful tearing in the right tibia downwards (the whole day); cutting from below upward on the right side near the sternum.

Frequent eructations; tearing in the left leg downward; pressure on the sternum not affecting the respiration; pressing feeling in the pelvic region on the right side near the linea alba, as if from a foreign body.

7th. Fine superficial sticking in the points of the fourth and little toe; continual, dull sticking pain in the left shoulder-joint; a tearing pain from the ischium through the posterior part of the right thigh, as far as the popliteal space; a cutting through the left half of the under lip, from below upward; twitching in the integument of the occiput, on the right side; violent ringing in both ears; in the evening, sticking in the left palm; tearing in the outer border of the right sole.

(75) *Sixth Proving.*

January 8th. *Fifteen drops of the second dilution* [5 : 95].

Dull confusion of the occiput, ending in a pressing headache which lasted half an hour; sticking on the right side, near the middle portion of the sternum; several stitches coming from the interior of the chest; twitching in the right ear with sticking pains; both ears stopped; tearing in the leg; stitches in the brain, from the occipital foramen upwards; tearing in the right eyeball; sticking pain in the left elbow several times during the day; tearing in the right eyeball, coming from the brain; sticking on the left side, near the scrobiculus, from within outwards; sticking and ringing in the right ear; sticking pain in the right fore-arm near the elbow; tearing in the metacarpal bone of the little finger; frequent tearing in the great toe of the right foot; dull sticking near the middle portion of the sternum on the left side; tearing pain in the metacarpal bone of the index finger; dull sticking in the left frontal region; cutting in the right shoulder-joint; stitches in the right metacarpus and in the left eyeball; cutting from the point of the left scapula through the chest to the edge of the middle portion of the sternum; stitches in the fourth toe of the left foot, in the left sole, and in the right thigh.

9th. Early, after rising, ringing in the ears; sensation of heaviness in the occiput; cutting under the sternum, which embarrasses the respiration; cutting in the right side of the chest, extending from the sternum to the right elbow; very sparing stool, half fluid, with a sensation as if the rectum were very inactive; a feeling in the vertex as if a nail were driven in there; very violent cutting in both loins when walking; ringing in the ears, frequently during the day.

10th. Cutting in the urethra from the perinæum forward; very violent, dull sticking pain in the right testicle; tearing in the left knee; ringing in the ears; evacuation slight, not satisfactory; sticking pain in the pelvic region on the right side near the linea alba; sticking in the splenic region.

11th. Sticking pains in the left testicle, several times during the day; tearing in the right carpus; severe cutting pains in the urethra (perinæal region); dull stitches in the rectum upwards; a stitch from the foramen magnum through the brain to the vertex; dull sticking pain near the lower part of the middle portion of the sternum, on the right side; tearing in the right leg; no evacuation; cutting in the epigastrium, from the spine outward; feeling, when laughing moderately, as though the thorax were strongly compressed, with shortness of breath; dull sticking in the popliteal space impeding the extension of the leg.

12th. Tearing in the right lower leg; sticking in the left knee, early, in bed; several dull stitches near the scrobiculus on the left side; tearing in the metacarpal bones of the right hand; a sticking pain on the left side from the sacrum to the left testicle; tearing in the left lower leg.

13th. In the open air, tearing pains in the region of the heart, and from there into the left scapula; sticking in the left knee; tearing in the left lower leg; roaring in the ears.

14th. Tearing in both legs and in the right thigh.

15th. Tearing in the right thigh; ringing in the ears several times during the day.

16th. Tearing in the right foot.

(76) *Seventh (and last) Proving.*

17th. Ten drops of the first dilution in an ounce of water produced no new symptom. The almost exclusive subjective symptoms which the prover noted from the 17th to the 20th were summarily as follows: *sticking in and on almost every part of the body*—on the vertex, through the brain, in the eyeball, in the sternum, under the nipples, in the ribs, through the chest, from the scapula through the heart, in the groins, in the maxillary bones, shoulder, elbow, and knee-joints, in the ankle and wrist, in the os ilium, in the thigh, in the calf, in the arm and fore-arm, in the metacarpal and metatarsal bones, in the tendo Achillis, in the final joint of the thumb and great toe, at the root of the nails of the thumb and index finger.

Tearing in the concha, the eyeball, the scrobiculus cordis, the shoulder-blade, the shoulder and hip-joints, the thigh, from the ischia to the knee, in the leg, in the arm and fore-arm; *cutting* in the perinæal portion of the urethra; twitching in the flexor of the left thumb, in the right cheek, under the scapula; sensation of dislocation in the knee and hip joints (aggravated by walking in the open air); painful oppression under the sternum (increased by deep inspiration) and in the inguinal region; ringing in the ears for several hours; roaring in the ear (early in bed); increased urgency to urinate; feeling of compression in the testicle; scanty, papescent stool.

U.

Dr. Holleczek also caused three experiments to be made by his sister *Josepha*, a healthy, active girl, seventeen years old. Like those of her brother, they produced for the most part only subjective symptoms.

(77) *First Proving.*

1840, January 6th. Ten drops of the 4th dilution of Thuja in an ounce of water.—During the same day, sensation as though the skin on the temples and forehead were shrunken and hard, continuing two hours; drowsiness; fine sticking in the inner malleolus of the right foot; sticking in the region of the spleen, twice in succession, with consequent soreness there; pressing and fine sticking under the sternum; sensation of weakness in both knees (disappearing in the right in ten minutes, in the left after an hour); sticking in the region of the fifth true rib on the right side; great lassitude and weakness in both arms, with frequent tearing in them; vertigo; superficial headache, as if the skin were rendered tense on all sides; frequent yawning; chills over the whole body; sticking in the left palm, the right axilla, and near the pit of the chin; headache in the forehead, pressing, the whole day; pressing in the eyes; chills in the evening in bed; several stitches in the right axilla and temple.

On the following day, repeated tearing in the forehead and sticking in different parts of the body (elbow, tibia, mammæ, chin, scrobiculus, scapula, shoulder-joints).

(78) *Second Proving.*

January 8th. Fifteen drops of the second dilution.—The same day, *tearing* (in the small of the back, in the nape, over the temple, in the knee-joint, in the tarsi, and some of the finger-joints); *sticking* (in the ear, under-jaw, splenic region, hip-joint, iliac region, in the middle of the thigh and leg, in the tarsus, shoulder-joint, arm and fore-arm, carpus); both these feelings, tearing and sticking, most on the right side; ringing in the ears; heaviness and tension in the back; sensation of soreness in the scrobiculus cordis.

The symptoms developed on the succeeding days, from the 9th to the 16th, are little more than a repetition of those already given.—She had *stickings* and *tearings* sometimes in the same parts, sometimes in others (ear, ear-cartilage, ala of the nose, near the sternum, in the epigastrium, between the shoulder-blades), and sometimes in all the limbs (on the 9th, in the evening in bed). She also complained on the 9th of stoppage of both ears, and on the 10th, of painful soreness in the middle of the back, and pain as if bruised in the right shin-bone.

(79) *Third Proving.*

January 17th. Ten drops of the first dilution in an ounce of water.

The sixty-six symptoms which the prover perceived and noted during the experiment, from the 17th to the 21st of January, consist mostly also of *sticking* and *tearing*, now in this and now in that part of the body—scarcely a spot was intact. The pain seems for the most part to have been transitory. I only find recorded on the 18th, a sticking in the left iliac region "lasting all day." On the 21st she had a tearing in the left fore-arm, shooting from the elbow to the fingers so that they were suddenly flexed. On the 18th she had, besides sticking and tearing, "feeling as if bruised in the back and buzzing in the ears." There is only one objective symptom in addition to the sudden flexion of the fingers just mentioned, "increased secretion of urine" on the day of the dose.*

CHAPTER V.

Symptomatology and Characteristics of the Thuja-Sickness.

The process of determinating the characteristic marks of a remedy, can, from its very nature, be nothing more than that of throwing into natural groups the scattered materials afforded us by the provings, and estimating scientifically the morbid elements thus obtained, in order in this way to obtain its therapeutic indications and raise the drug to the rank of a remedy.

In this difficult task three main points, in our opinion, must be kept in view.

1. The *where* of the morbid manifestations, that is, the organic substratum, the locality, the locus in quo of the sickness.

2. The *how*, that is, in what way and after what fashion the pathogenesis of the drug is developed in subjective and objective symptoms.

3. The discrimination of the drug-symptoms into subjective and objective, idiopathic and sympathetic, essential and accidental, constant and variable, &c., upon the solid foundation of the physiological proving, to the exclusion of all hypotheses and learned refinements.

To this end we will now examine the phenomena presented by the

* The experiments which Dr. Fröhlich instituted with the Thuja upon two rabbits, led, unfortunately, to no result. In order to avoid any possible disturbance from alcohol, he prepared the fresh juice of the arbor vitæ, and for a week several times moistened with it the left eye, the anus, and a bare spot on the skin of one of the rabbits, and administered to the other for the same length of time, at first one, and finally three coffee-spoonfuls of the juice a day. It is to be regretted that Fröhlich, who has already given us several beautiful drug-provings upon animals, was on this occasion, as he himself says, "obliged by divers circumstances to abstain from the prosecution of his experiments with Thuja." In the short period of this trial, there was neither an objective production of the Thuja-sickness, nor were the subjects of it mortally poisoned.—*Mayrhofer.*

action of Thuja in anatomico-physiological order, in order to assist the memory as much as possible.

Nervous System.—The nerves, as the organs for communicating the sensations, are first of all affected by the disturbing forces of drugs, and it is through them that the enormous train of subjective symptoms, manifesting themselves by the different kinds of pains, is developed. Here lies the reason why the nervous symptoms of many drugs frequently so much resemble each other; and on this account it is that they have, as a general rule, but little therapeutic value.

It is only when such manifestations take place in the track of particular nerves and locate themselves in the parts supplied by them, and when there is something peculiar in the mode of their development, that they have any practical import or therapeutic utility.

The operation of Thuja upon the sensory functions of the cerebro-spinal system, is evidenced by the following symptoms: flying stitches through the brain, vertigo, drawing, sticking or boring, screwing, dull, stunning headache, drawing, tearing, sticking in the head, frontal eminences and zygomata, &c. As special nervous affections of the head, we have: *the feeling as though a convex button were pressed upon the head, especially in the neighborhood of the sutures, or a needle or a nail repeatedly thrust in;* hemicrania in the forehead, the pains extending by radiation into the brain. Belonging to the spinal marrow: drawing, tensive, sticking, tearing, creeping, itching, burning, laming, digging, boring pains in the nape, back, sacral region, nates and limbs.

Nor are the motor nerves unaffected by Thuja, as is plain from the frequently recurring, involuntary muscular twitchings. In the ganglionic system the *plexus cœliacus* and *hypogastricus* were the most affected, as appears from the abdominal symptoms of the drug.

We shall treat more fully of all these subjective or nervous symptoms when we come to speak of the particular organs affected.

Sleep and Dreaming.—Under this head, Thuja, like almost every other drug, gives rise to alternate effects; sleeplessness, sleep coming on late, lasting but a little while, restless, and interrupted by dreams; groaning in sleep; unrefreshing dozing with constant terror; uneasy, tormenting, horrible images in dreams, e. g. of the dead; voluptuous, lascivious dreams; quiet, refreshing, deep sleep, &c.

Therapeutic indications cannot be obtained from the symptoms of sleep and dreaming alone, as they are not independent pathological conditions, but only the reflex of organic affections. Thus, sleeplessness, unrefreshing dozing, or restless sleep with dreams, are true accompaniments of fever; tormenting and horrible dreams, with sudden starting and terror, of cerebral and pectoral affections; and lascivious dreams, ending with pollutions, point to an excessive action of the genital system.

The symptoms afforded by the sleep under the action of Thuja, according to their physiological value, are, for the most part, simply signs of febrile action; they frequently indicate the action of the drug upon the genital system, but seldom point to any irritation in the cerebral organs.

Mind and temper.—Thuja exhibits no marked psychical relations. With some of the provers there was little or no disturbance in these functions, and the symptoms that were perceived are again only opposite alternations,* which divide themselves into exaltations and depressions.

The exaltations manifest themselves but seldom; we have disposition to be angry, inclination for intellectual labor, great activity of the mind (with weakness of the body); the depressions, however, are numerous; as, melancholy; discouragement; anxiety; restlessness and lowness of spirits; ill-humor and disgust of life; difficulty in recollecting; difficulty in finding the proper words; slow speech, &c.

From these considerations we must draw the conclusion, that the principal action of the arbor vitæ upon the mind and temper is of *a depressing sort*, and that the signs of the *shackled soul* are the indications that ought to guide us in our selection of it as a remedy.

PERCEIVING FACULTIES.

Visual Organs.—The symptoms which attest the effects of the arbor vitæ upon the organs of sight may be divided into four classes.

1. Subjective: as, *sensation as if the eyes were pressed forward out of the head*, or as though the eyelids were swollen; *drawing, pressing*, sticking or *burning in the eyes;* biting, *burning in the eyelids, canthi* and caruncles; feeling of dryness in the eyes, tension in the interior of the orbits; digging pain in the posterior part of the eyeball, &c.

2. Objective: redness and inflammation of the white of the eye (with pressing and biting); dilatation and contraction of the pupils (alternate effects); watering of the eyes (especially in the open air); obstruction of the eyes with gum; *swelling of the upper lids; twitching of the eyelids;* digging twitching in the eyeball, &c.

3. Symptoms of functional disturbance: short-sightedness; *dimness of the sight; obscuration of the sight as though there were a veil before the eyes:* weak sight; swimming of surrounding objects before the eyes (Wz.); black, self-moving points before the eyes, whether open or shut; *glittering before the eyes, with hovering of numerous dark and bright points before them* (Zl.); *appearance of a bright disk with a dark centre* which follows the movements of the eyes (Dr. Huber); *hovering of clouds and streaks* before the eyes (Lackner).

* The opposite symptoms developed in the psychical sphere by the action of many drugs, depend upon the universal law of dynamic oscillation, and are (and it is the same in health) but striking repetitions of the constant pendulum-swing of psychical life; from sorrow to joy, from grave to gay, from tears to smiles, from hope to fear, from love to hate, from pleasure to pain. But as through all the varying tints of the psychical life of the individual, the temperament and temper, as a sort of ground color still predominate, these exaltations and depressions, viewed as a whole, present a striking picture, and one which is of the highest import as a therapeutic indication in cases of mental disturbances.—*Mayrhofer.*

4. Exanthematous appearances: *red itching eruptions between the eyebrows; suppurating tubercles on the borders of the eyelids, on the eyebrows*, or in the neighborhood of the eyes.

The general character of the sickness produced by Thuja lies at the foundation of the subjective symptoms: suddenly coming and going, irregularly periodical, aggravated by rest, morning and evening, ameliorated in the open air and by movements, especially attacking the left side.

As the symptoms of the eyes never appear independently, but always accompanied by consentaneous affections either of the olfactory and respiratory apparatus, or of the urinary and genital organs, we cannot admit any direct and immediate relation between Thuja and the organs of vision.

In pathological conditions of the eyes, therefore, all the concomitant symptoms are to be considered, and the hints derived from the preceding history of the disease to be weighed, which indicate the choice of Thuja, and assist us in the decision.

Auditory Organs.—These organs, which, in comparison with the other perceptive faculties, are much less often affected, do not escape the action of Thuja.

Subjective symptoms: hammering and tearing in the ear; violent tearing in the concha; penetrating and squeezing in the ear; pressing, obstruction, sticking in the auditory canal; ringing, roaring, and dull vibrations in the ears; thrusting stitches in the right side of the throat, reaching into the ear, with the feeling as though the air pressed through an opening (Eustachian tube) into the ear on opening and shutting the mouth; single, violent stitches in the auditory meatus; feeling of stoppage or as if there were water in the ear; creaking in the ear during empty deglutition, &c.

Objective results: suppurating tubercles; moist warts (Wachtel) in the neighborhood of the ears.

The remarks already made in relation to the eyes will equally apply to the ears. In diseases of these organs, the choice of Thuja must be determined by the character of the ear symptoms, by the accompanying affections, and by the history of the case.

Olfactory Organs.—The symptoms of the nose and its vicinity are again either

1. Subjective: pressure on the root of the nose; tension in the right ala; sensation of dryness in the nose; drawing between the mouth and nose; crawling in the nose; burning in the nose with sensibility of the septum; itching in the nostrils, &c.

2. Objective: frequent sneezing; repeated epistaxis; discharge of blood by blowing; running catarrh; *catarrh suddenly ceasing and returning*, sometimes alone, sometimes accompanied with cough and febrile symptoms, swelling and hardness on the left ala; hard scabs in the nose; itching eruptions or tubercles behind the alæ; vesicles on the septum; a red streak from the nose over the forehead, &c.

These symptoms too must be judged of in connection with the other consentaneous affections, and can very seldom by themselves form therapeutic indications.

Gustatory Organs.—The operation of Thuja upon the organs of taste, to which head we refer all the parts constituting the oral cavity, is evidenced by a variety of symptoms, which may be divided into subjective, objective, and functional.

1. Drawing, tearing, sticking, twitching toothache on entering a warm room; drawing, tearing, sticking in the jaws; burning on the lips, on the tongue and palate; feeling of soreness on the palate and tongue; pressing on the velum palati; rough, scraping feeling on the tongue and in the throat; sore feeling on the point of the tongue; sensitiveness of the gum; soreness and dryness in the throat: violent pain in the masseters as though they were wrenched, &c.

2. White coating upon the tongue; sore tongue; burning vesicles on the tongue; painful, *swollen gums;* inflamed and swollen *tonsils; swelling of the salivary glands; increased secretion of saliva;* saliva mixed with blood; throwing up of a tough, thick mucus; sore palate; *burning, red spots; elevated, itching spots on the lips; quivering of the lips;* creaking of the under jaw when chewing, &c.

3. Sweet, sour, metallic-tasting saliva; sweetish, insipid, sharp, bitter, rancid, resinous taste; taste blunted (food cannot be distinguished by the taste); thirstlessness; thirst; desire for cold drinks, &c.

The subjective symptoms have but little practical value, inasmuch as many other remedies develope them in the same way; the objective, however, are much more important, and highly valuable in a therapeutic point of view, especially when they are manifested in connection with other characteristic symptoms.

SANGUINEOUS SYSTEM.

Fever.—Every medicinal agent in its perfect action excites fever, and thus presents different peculiarities according to the different power of the drug.

The species of fever which is developed in those who have an exceeding susceptibility to the action of Thuja, or which follows in the train of massive doses of the drug, either appears unaccompanied or attended by a catarrhal affection of the olfactory or respiratory organs.

The independent fever, according to the preceding provings, manifests the following peculiarities:

1. It is a well marked *cold fever* (febris algida). Its symptoms all point to a preponderance of the cold stage. The chill commences generally from the spinal marrow, is especially felt in the limbs, more particularly in the feet, at times only on one side or only internally, and, in its highest development, is attended by trembling of the heart, momentary pulselessness and deadness of the fingers; *it either passes immediately over into the sweating stage,* or alternates several times with

heat; nay, the extremities are often still cold after the body has become hot. The hot stage seldom attains much intensity, and is generally first perceived in the face while the rest of the body is still cold.

2. Regularly, it comes on morning and evening, more seldom in the course of the day; *thirst is generally altogether absent* or comes on with the hot stage, and is seldom of any account.

The general weakness and prostration is so remarkable that it by no means corresponds to the degree of the other symptoms.

3. In its course, it shows either a quotidian or tertian type, or an irregular perodicity. The fever that attends the affections of the mucous membranes has the peculiar property of being *as capricious and changeable* as the subjective symptoms of Thuja.

Respiratory Organs.—We come now to the phenomena which the *arbor vitæ* excites in the air passages, larynx, trachea and its ramifications, to which we also add the symptoms of the lungs and pleura.

The very decided action of Thuja upon the mucous membrane of the nasal and buccal cavities, might have already led us to conclude that it would also produce pathological conditions in the lower air passages, and our provings have accordingly shown that it can especially attack the thoracic organs (though only exceptionally).

1. Sensitiveness of the larynx; scraping, sticking in the trachea; dryness and roughness in the fauces; oppression in the chest; pressing immediately under the breast-bone or on one side of the chest; drawing, tearing, sticking on one side of the chest; sensation as though the chest were compressed from without and the corresponding part of the lungs from within; internal sensation of soreness in the chest; pressing in the lower half of the chest; stitches in the left side of the chest, unaffected by inspiration and expiration; dull, interrupted stitches in the chest; violent sticking in the lower part of the lungs, which is aggravated by sneezing, deep breathing and coughing, &c.

2. Hoarseness; short, dry, straining, interrupted cough; troublesome night-cough; raising of thick, tough mucus, like lard; short, constricted, accelerated respiration; moaning and groaning in sleep.

We by no means mean to deny that Thuja possesses the power of affecting the respiratory organs, nor that it can excite in them a congestive or an irritative condition, but we must regard the affections of the lungs and pleura which follow its exhibition as individual exceptions and statistical singularities which are no essential attribute of its operation; in this respect we need only mention *Aconite*, *Bryonia*, *Rhus*, *Tart. Emet.*, to show that it is far surpassed by many other remedies.

On this account we can allow to the chest-symptoms of Thuja but a low and conditional therapeutical value.*

* I cannot entirely coincide in this opinion. The author points out that Thuja acts *first and most especially* upon the uro-genital organs. The intimate physiological and pathological relation between these and the respiratory organs would have made it very probable *a priori* that the latter would be partakers of the effects of Thuja. In effect, not only our own but Hahnemann's experiments show that

Heart, Vessels, and Muscles.—The few symptoms of the heart produced by Thuja, such as palpitation, trembling of the heart, transitory pulselessness, pressure in the scrobiculus with difficult respiration, uneasiness and anxiety (*anxietas præcordialis*), are the attendants of fever, particularly of the cold stage. They point to a repletion of the central organ with blood, and to an impeded circulation. They do not appear, therefore, as direct effects of Thuja upon the heart, and have no special therapeutic value.

Besides the changes in the pulse, the maximum and minimum of which were observed to be over one hundred and under sixty in the minute, there are other symptoms which indicate the action of Thuja upon the venous system; as, swelling of the veins in the neck, temples and hands; turgescence of the hæmorrhoidal vessels; burning in the varices; pressing in the hypochondria.

A peculiar symptom of frequent recurrence is the *twitching* or *jumping* of isolated muscular parts in the legs, calves, toes, arms, hands, and fingers, more seldom in the trunk; also on the lips and chin. This symptom appears in a lower degree as a *subcutaneous vibration* or slight trembling of parts of muscles. The twitching is especially perceived *in the middle, in the body* of the muscles, appears almost exclusively during rest, in short, repeated attacks, and rapidly disappears on movement; *a sudden twitching of the upper part of the body* or of the feet comes on more violently.

We attach therapeutic value to the muscular twitchings of Thuja.

REPRODUCTIVE SYSTEM.

Digestive Organs.—All remedies when taken in sufficient quantity excite morbid affections in the primæ viæ with which they are first brought in contact; and even those which in themselves are innocuous may become injurious if administered in large doses.

Hence it results that many similar phenomena take place in the digestive organs after the exhibition of different drugs, which has led our opponents to assert "that according to the homœopathic materia medica, every drug was good for every disease, and every disease indicated every drug." *

the *mucous membrane of the air passages* (nose, trachea, and bronchi) plays by no means so subordinate and accidental a part in the physiology of the *arbor vitæ* as the author would have us believe. In many of the provings, and especially in those where the uro-genital organs were affected but slightly, or not at all, they form (according to my view) the starting point for a great part of the symptoms detailed. This was the case with *Gross*, *Böhm*, *Lackner*, *Landesmann*, *Liedbeck*, *Reissinger*, *Sterz*, and *Wurmb;* nay, with some of them, for example, with *Maschauer*, with myself, and with that boldest and most persevering of provers, *Prof. Zlatarovich*, the effects upon the respiratory organs, in reference to their independence and therapeutic significance, seem to have carried off the palm from all the other symptoms.—*Ed. Oest. Zeit.*

* This maxim applies perfectly *per inversionem* to the therapeutics of the old school: for a casuistic materia medica can with perfect propriety administer every remedy in every disease, or treat each disease with all remedies.—*Mayrhofer.*

The symptoms of the organs of deglutition are: scraping feeling in the pharynx and throat; pressing when swallowing; feeling of constriction of the pharynx; accumulation of mucus in the throat and pharynx.

Stomach: eructations tasting of the drug; nausea; vomiturition; inflation of the stomach with flatulence; pressing and griping in the region of the stomach; heartburn; cramp.

Bowels: rumbling and rolling, griping and cutting, with inflation of the abdomen; colicky pains; deceptive feeling as though something alive were moving in the abdomen;* flatulence.

The symptoms which indicate an affection of the liver or of its peritoneal envelope, are: pressing in the liver as if from a stone; sticking in the abdomen, rendering walking difficult, &c.

Stool: ineffectual urgency; diminished evacuation; constipation for several days; as an alternative effect, not of frequent occurrence, loose papescent stool or even diarrhœa; while at stool, *sticking pain in the rectum;* after stool, *burning and itching in the anus; biting, itching, and burning at the anus and in the sulcus* without stool; *swelling of the hæmorrhoidal vessels; feeling of swelling at the anus;* a less frequent alternative effect, feeling of emptiness there; *moisture of the anus; sweat on the anus; excretion of bloody slime from the anus, &c.*

The groups of the symptoms of Thuja affecting the anus and rectum are of importance in a therapeutic point of view, because the symptoms exist abundantly in the provings, come on regularly after every dose, and are an integral part of the peculiar condition which that drug excites in the urinary and sexual organs, in connection with which they must be regarded and judged.

Urinary and Sexual Organs.—We come now to the organs toward which Thuja stands in the most intimate relation; the uro-genital apparatus and its connections.

(*a*) *Urinary Organs.*—In order to aid the memory we again divide the phenomena into subjective and objective.

In the first class we have: *burning in the renal region; drawing along the ureter to the bladder; sensation of inflation and fulness in the vesica with urgency to urinate*; *frequent urgency to urinate; pressure on the neck of the bladder;* painful *stitches from the anus to the orifice of the urethra* or in the reverse direction; *stitches in the fossa navicularis; voluptuous itching or tickling in the urethra; cutting in the region of the cervix vesicæ* during urination and at other times; *burning toward the bulbus of the urethra; burning in the urethra and at the orifice during, after, and without urination; itching on the point of the urethra; itching without and also during urination through the whole urethra; drawing and cutting in the urethra and vesica;* deceptive sensation as if a *tenacious fluid were passing forward*

* The sensation as though something alive were moving in the abdomen seems to arise from the stretching of the intestines by the accumulated flatulence.—*Mayrhofer.*

in the urethra, or as if there *were still some drops of urine left after urination, &c.*

To the second class belong: *frequent, copious emissions of limpid*, straw-yellow urine; at times interrupted urine; scanty discharge of dark urine with inflammatory irritation of the urinary organs; red sediment in the urine; *discharge of glutinous mucus from the male urethra;* discharge of *liquor prostaticus* (Hempel); *mucous discharge from the female urethra, &c.*

To these phenomena in the urinary apparatus, correspond the symptoms of the

Sexual Organs. 1. *Subjective symptoms.*

(a) *In the male organs: sticking and itching in the glans: single, flying stitches on the point of the glans; burning itching, sensation of soreness on the glans; great sensibility of the whole glans; painful stitches on the inner surface of the prepuce; tickling, itching, and biting on the glans and prepuce*, alternating with *flying stitches in the anus; twitching pain in the penis; burning stitches in the penis as far as the testicles; drawing, sticking in the testicles and seminal cords; crawling and itching on the hairy parts of the genital parts and the inner side of the thigh; sticking in the perinæum; tension and drawing in the groins.*

(b) *In the female organs: pressing and constriction of the genital parts;* tight pain in the genital parts and perinæum; *pain as if sore; itching in the pudenda; biting and burning in the vagina; sticking in the groins* (extending through the thigh into the knee).

2. *Objective symptoms.*

(a) *In the male organs: swelling of the prepuce; red spots on the glans and prepuce; erosions on the inner surface of the prepuce and on the furrow of the glans*, which become *moist* and purulent; *a red excrescence on the inner surface of the prepuce* (like a condyloma); *a granular, elevated spot on the external surface of the prepuce which suppurates, forms a scab, itches and burns; small elevations on the corona glandis, smooth, red excrescences on the point of attachment of the prepuce; on the glans; a flat, foul, burning ulcer with a red margin on the corona glandis; moistening of the glans; gonorrhœa of the glans; moist eruptions on the scrotum; profuse sweat of the genitals and perinæum; retraction of the testicles toward the inguinal ring; puffing and projection of the perinæal raphé; suppurating tubercles on the perinæum; swelling of the inguinal glands, &c.*

(b) *In the female organs:* swelling of both labia; *leucorrhœa from one period to another*, mild, and leaving greenish yellow spots on the linen.

3. *Functional symptoms.*

(a) *In men*, pointing to an excitement of the sexual system: excessive sexual impulse; frequent erections; pollutions; seminal emission with sensation as if the urethra were too narrow: indicating a lowering of the sexual impulse; *indifference to the other sex; unfrequent desire for coition;* inability to perfect copulation.

(b) *In females: retardation and diminution of the catamenia.*

This formidable host of subjective and objective phenomena, to which Thuja gives rise in the uro-genital system, leaves us no room to doubt that it stands in a near and direct relation to these organs, and in this sense is a urinary and genital remedy.

As however the determination of the therapeutic utility of the recorded results of the provings depends upon the frequency and constancy of their occurrence, as well as upon their agreement with the phenomena of natural diseases, we must subject these numerous symptoms to a scientific arrangement, in order to trace the conditions which indicate the choice of Thuja as a remedy.

The ruling kind of pain produced by Thuja in the urinary organs is *burning.* Its seat for the most part is the *fossa navicularis,* less frequently the *orifice of the urethra,* less frequently the region of the *prostate gland* and *cervix vesicæ,* and seldomest of all the ureters and kidneys. It is manifested especially *during and after urinating,* and without that is often replaced by *voluptuous itching.* The urine generally runs freely *without any delay,* but *urgency to urinate* soon comes on; the stream is seldom interrupted by cramp. By this means Thuja is distinguished from its closely allied drugs, *Cantharides, Sabina, Cannabis, Petroselinum,* and others which hinder the urine more or less. The feeling *as if some drops were still running forward in the urethra* is frequently developed after urination. In quality the urine remains about the same, in quantity it is almost always increased.

There is no special violence in the *irritative condition* which Thuja induces in the urinary organs, as is evident from the fact that the *mucous flow from the urethra* (as an inflammatory product) is mostly wanting or is very slight; in which respect it is far inferior to other remedies, for example hemp. On the other hand, Thuja more frequently excites *inflammation and blennorrhœa of the glans* than other remedies.

In relation to the sexual functions, we find alternating effects, pointing now to excitement and now to depression of the sexual appetite. On taking a general view, however, of all the provings, it becomes evident that the *diminution of the sexual impulse is the more constant, and therefore the reliable therapeutic effect;* and this is especially corroborated by the *deficient catamenia* which Thuja occasions, for deficiency of the menses and weakness of the sexual impulse are as constant companions as excessive menstruation and increased venereal desire.

In this relation, Thuja is connected with *Cannabis,* and stands directly opposed to Sabina, which causes excitement in the sexual system, especially in the female.

The most important peculiarity of Thuja then, is *excitement of the cutaneous system of the sexual parts* and their neighborhood.

Genital sweat, balanorrhœa, suppurating tubercles, swellings and ex-

crescences on the skin, which must be regarded partly as crises, are speaking evidences of this tendency; and in this property Thuja yields to no other remedy.

The symptoms of the testicles and inguinal glands are consensual effects.

We have also the following characteristic marks of the operation of Thuja on the uro-genital system: *burning and itching in the urethra, especially in the fossa navicularis, urgency to urinate, with increased, uninterrupted urine, slight thickish mucous discharge from the urethra, balanorrhœa, cutaneous excrescences, diminution of the catamenia and of the sexual impulse, moderate leucorrhœa.*

Glandular System.—Copious symptoms testify the action of Thuja upon this portion of the organism.

The cervical and salivary glands, the inguinal, and those of the prepuce, swell and become painful; the salivary and sebaceous glands are excited to increased secretion. Irritation lies at the basis of all these symptoms. When we reflect upon the general effect of Thuja upon the totality of the cutaneous surfaces, we could scarcely expect that the glands which stand in organic and vital relations with them should escape its action; though we must regard the glandular affections produced by it rather as sympathetic than idiopathic.

Skin.—The physiological provings of Thuja have shown that it manifests its action by means of eruptions and excrescences on the cutaneous surface. We have already had occasion, when considering the symptomatology of the senses and genital system, to remark this peculiarity, and it now remains to submit to a closer examination the cutaneous symptoms which Thuja produces upon the trunk and limbs.

1. *Subjective: crawling*, itching, biting, burning, pricking and sticking in different spots on the skin; occasionally gurgling and running under the skin, as from single dribbling drops of blood. The most constant and most frequent kind of pain produced by Thuja upon the skin is *itching*, and in a higher degree, *burning:*

2. *Objective.* These are partly inflammations, partly eruptions, partly excrescences, which have been observed under the following forms:

(*a*) *Red smooth spots* (maculæ) which appeared singly, or several at a time, for the most part upon the limbs (those upon the prepuce, glans and lips, were spoken of under these organs); which *itch*, *burn* after being scratched, and in a few hours or during the night disappear as quickly as they come.

(*b*) *Burning vesicles* (papulæ) which were only noticed upon the mucous membrane of the tongue, on the palate and glans.

(*c*) *Moist and suppurating erosions*, which likewise appeared only on the mucous membrane, glans, and prepuce.

(*d*) Tubercles (nodi), of different sizes, which appeared sometimes several together, as on the scalp, sometimes single, in the neighborhood of the parts of generation, on the limbs, on the face, &c., commonly surrounded by a *reddish or brownish base*, *itching* and rapidly passing *into suppuration* on the summit; the smaller appeared like an eruption, the larger resembled chicken pox (varicellæ).

(*e*) Warts (verrucæ), which assumed various shapes; either as *small red excrescences on the genitals*, or as the common *dry warts on the hands*, which are either conical or roundish; in their commencement show a smooth surface, but in the course of their growth become cracked, and resemble mulberries; or as *moist*, *sweating excrescences*, which were observed *at the anus*, *on the perinæum*, *in the furrow between the nates*, *and on one ear*. As indications of cutaneous excrescences, *fulness of the perineal raphé and of the anus* are to be remarked.

These cutaneous symptoms all appeared after a longer use of the Thuja, and on that account we must set them down as among its secondary effects.

The notable peculiarities of Thuja-warts and tubercles are:

1. Their broad conical shape.
2. Their situation in the superficial cutaneous tissues.
3. The splitting and cracking of the superficies in the larger and older warts.
4. The disposition to suppurate or to be moist, especially in the warty tubercles which make their appearance in the neighborhood of the sexual parts.
5. Their chronic course, which with warts may last many weeks and months.

Fibro-serous membranes.—Under this head belong most of those symptoms which we have noticed as Thuja pains under the nervous system, and which have their seat in the muscular sheaths, in the aponeurotic expansions, perhaps even in the muscular tissue itself, and which resemble wandering rheumatic affections. We have already noticed the symptoms of the *mucous membranes* under the separate organs.

Osseous System.—The symptoms which indicate the operation of Thuja upon the osseous system or periosteum are but few. The *gnawing and boring pain* which is characteristic of affections of the bones, seldom appears in the provings. But a sure indication of a periosteal affection is the frequent, painful feeling in the articular extremities of the hollow bones, aggravated by movement, and frequently accompanied by swelling of the painful spot.

General.—The following general characteristics of the Thuja-sickness we derive from the statistics of the provings, and from the discussion of the symptomatology of the *arbor vitæ:* they are identical with the general therapeutic indications.

1. Thuja enjoys a very extended circle of operations; almost every system, province, and organ of the whole body is more or less affected by it; but it stands in the most intimate relation:

(*a*) To the *uro-genital system;* and

(*b*) To the *cutaneous system* in all its ramifications.

In this relation, the arbor vitæ is a *urinary*, *sexual*, *and cutaneous remedy.* In the uro-genital system, the *urinary apparatus is idiopathically* affected, the *sexual organs sympathetically.*

Of the *cutaneous tissues, the fibro-serous and mucous membranes* bear the stamp of *primary effects ; the external skin, of the secondary.*

2. The general character of the pathological condition, which Thuja sets up in the attacked parts, is that of *irritation.*

This *irritation,* which may even increase to inflammation, causes in the secreting organs (mucous membranes, urinary apparatus and glands) an *increased and altered* secretion. In the external skin the irritation is concentrated in single spots, and manifests : *inflammation, suppuration, formation of warts, and excrescences.*

3. The affections of Thuja present the following peculiarities :

(*a*) They attack *only a single organ,* limb, joint, or spot *at a time ; and these local affections usually cease when morbid symptoms arise in a different province.*

(*b*) They come on for the most part in *abrupt paroxysms, begin suddenly,* and *end as though they were snapped off.*

(*c*) They make their appearanee *especially during rest,* and either diminish or disappear by movement ; nay, the pains which appear in circumscribed spots *often instantaneously disappear* on touching the affected spot, and return immediately on quitting the contact. They come on consequently for the most part *in the evening in bed,* and *in the morning* on waking ; they are aggravated, too, by *passing from a cold into a warm temperature,* and are diminished by the opposite. The pains in the joints only are aggravated by movement, and violent affections or febrile symptoms remain the same whether in rest or motion.

(*d*) They more frequently *affect the left side of the body,* though they do not on that account neglect the right.

4. The most constant kinds of pain which Thuja excites in its most extensive sphere of operation in the different organic structures, are : *drawing and tension in the limbs and joints, burning in the urinary organs, itching and crawling on the skin.*

5. The course of the Thuja-sickness is *partly acute, partly chronic.* The symptoms of the *primæ viæ* go off in a short time, but those of the *secundæ viæ* run a very irregular course, and are characterised by *great mutability and caprice.* They return after intervals of *hours, days, weeks,* continue *sometimes shorter and sometimes longer,* and appear *now in this and now in that* part of the body. The *cutaneous excrescences* finally, as the *concluding products of* Thuja, *are as slow* in disappearing as they are in coming, *and remain for months.*

6. The true attendants of a Thuja-fever are *strongly marked, predominant cold,* and *gloomy, depressed state of mind.*

To *express the physiological character of the arbor vitæ in the shortest manner,* it is, "*Exaltation of the cutaneous system, with disposition to dermatic excrescences.*"

CHAPTER VI.

Therapeutics of Thuja.

Physiological drug-provings are so many questions propounded to the living organism; the pathogenetic phenomena thereby developed are the answers returned, and also the material for the foundation of therapeutics; and the accuracy of the therapeutics is determined by the *usus in morbis.*

By the physiological proving of a remedy health is interrogated concerning disease; by the pathological proving sickness is interrogated concerning health; and from the agreeing answers of these two trials of nature results as a whole the science of pharmacodynamics.

By the physiological method, the powers of the drug are discovered; by the pathological, its therapeutic powers are confirmed; these two inseparable parts are related to each other as flower and fruit, as assertion and proof; and confirmed therapeutic indications are the highest flower and fruit of the physio-pathological materia medica. The physiology of a drug without the therapeutics is dead knowledge; its therapeutics without its physiology is blind opinion; sure knowledge is only reached when we obtain the physio-pathology of a remedy blended into one by means of a great general therapeutic principle.

The general therapeutic indications which we have developed by the characteristics of Thuja, have their significance in all the disorders that come under its province, and the particular indications are derived from the physiological effects of the remedy upon the separate systems, provinces and organs.

Before we consider more intimately, and illustrate by cases, the therapeutic indications of the *arbor vitæ* (which are identical with its characteristics) in connection with those special forms of diseases which lead us to its employment, let us for a moment look at the indications laid down by Hahnemann; he expresses himself thus:

"The homœopathic physician will know how to value the clearly observed artificial elements of disease produced by this uncommonly powerful drug as a great addition to our previous stock of remedies, and will not neglect to make therapeutic use of it in some of the most serious diseases of man, for which, until now, no remedy had been discovered. It will appear, for example, from these symptoms that Thuja is a specific for that horrible affection arising from impure cohabitation, condylomata, when it is complicated with no other miasm, and experience shows that it is the only useful remedy for it; it also for the same reason most certainly cures that severe form of gonorrhœa arising from impure connection, provided always it be not complicated with any other miasm."—(*Rein. Arz.* 2 *Aufl.* B. 5. s. 122.)

With how much justice Hahnemann decided upon the remedial

power of Thuja from its provings, let the cures performed by it testify; for blennorrhœas of the sexual organs which have arisen from contagion, and the sycotic condition that so frequently attends them, are especially the therapeutic field in which the *arbor vitæ* has gained its most plenteous as well as its most beautiful laurels.

A.

Diseases of the Urinary and Sexual Organs.

(a) *Blennorrhœas.*—The condition which Thuja excites in the urinary organs, is characterised as irritation of the mucous membrane, with increased and altered secretion.

The special therapeutic indications which insure the selection of Thuja are: contagion from coitus; burning, itching pain in the urethra, generally when urinating, and immediately after, less often without this cause, and which is seated in the fossa navicularis or near the cervix vesicæ; increased, but little altered urine; purulent mucous discharge from the urethra or glans, from the urethra or vagina, sensibility of the glans and penis; swelling of the inguinal glands; tendency to chronicity and to lympathic vascular excrescences.

Hahnemann states that Thuja is indicated by the following symptoms (*Chron. Krank.* B. 1): "Thickish, purulent discharge from the commencement, urination little painful, body of the penis somewhat hard and swollen, or painful on the dorsum and beset with enlarged glands." This agrees with our physiological therapeutic indications.

1. A gonorrhœa of six weeks standing had already been treated with cubebs, camphor, tinctura kalina, and aqua laurocerasi, and had for a short time been subdued. The discharge was copious, rather yellow than white, the urinary secretion natural, tickling in the urethra when urinating, at times cutting in the groin.

Two doses of *Cann.* 2 (one drop), which Dr. Hartlaub administered, with an interval of eight days, produced no impression.

On taking *Thuja* 30 (ten pellets) the discharge became less and white and the pains disappeared. As however some cutting on urination was still perceived at the end of seventeen days the patient again took *Thuja* 30 (five pellets). The discharge at the end of three weeks was white, and only amounted to a couple of drops a day. Hartlaub again administered Thuja (in what dose is not mentioned), and ten days later, when the nocturnal erections were somewhat painful and the discharge continued, but in a less degree, *Capsic.* 9 (ten pellets). After fourteen days the patient was well and had no relapse.*—(*Annalen der homœop. Klinik.* B. 3, s. 214, 215).

The second case of gonorrhœa cured with Thuja by Hartlaub is as follows.

2. A strong young man who had often had gonorrhœa, had suffered from it now for five weeks and had already taken much cubebs. The disease had

* "Perhaps," adds Hartlaub, "I might have saved Thuja, had I waited longer." We rather think that this cure of seventy-eight days might have been somewhat shortened by more frequent doses of Thuja.—*Mayrhofer.*

come on from the commencement with great pain and hæmaturia. The discharge was still very copious and watery, urine natural. When urinating, he felt violent burning, now in the anterior, now in the posterior part of the urethra, the inguinal glands were swollen and somewhat painful.

All these troublesome symptoms disappeared within eighteen days after a dose of *Thuja* 30 (five pellets), and there only remained a very moderate discharge, which so far disappeared after two similar doses, a fortnight apart, that the urethra was only slightly obstructed on waking in the morning. One dose *Cann.* 6 (one drop) caused this also to vanish within a short period.*

3. A man of scrofulous constitution, age 24, contracted a gonorrhœa after a suspicious coitus, and according to his story it first appeared fourteen days afterwards. Before he applied to Dr. Hartlaub he had consulted a quack, and received from him an almond emulsion with camphor, which he had taken for several days. At first he had only discharge from the urethra without any pain; after using the camphor, however, the dischrrge increased and the pains appeared.

Discharge greenish-yellow. When urinating he felt violent burning in the glans, which remained sometime after. When not urinating he had frequently during the day itching pain along the whole urethra, and continual itching on the glans. At night he was driven out of bed by painful erections. Urine reddish, with whitish sediment, bowels sluggish, the right inguinal gland swollen and painful. After the bowels had been regulated by a dose of *Nux Vom.*, no other change in the disease supervening, he took, three days after, *Thuja* 20. In five days the itching on the glans and the painful erections had altogether disappeared; the burning on urination and the gonorrhœa were less, the urine was clearer, but still deposited a sediment. Seven days after the improvement ceased, and for a hasty urgency to urinate, which often appeared, especially when standing still after moving, a dose of *Puls.* 12 was given; in two days after the urgency to urinate disappeared, as did the painful swelling of the inguinal glands, the discharge and burning on urinating were still less, and this last changed into a slight sticking and cutting in the glans. For these symptoms Hartlaub, after a fortnight, gave *Cann.* 2. The pains ceased, but the discharge was unchanged, and was only wholly cured after a second dose of *Thuja*.†—*Annal. der homœop. Klinik.* B. 1. s. 188, 189.

4. Dr. Argenti relates the following case (*Archiv für homœop. Heilk.* B. 18. H. 3. s. 84):

A. D., twenty-four years old, contracted a venereal gonorrhœa. He was advised to take Balsam Copaiba, the more the better; which he faithfully did. After some days violent pressing pains in the testicle and spermatic cord (it is not said of which side) came on, with hard swelling of the testicle, and his nights were sleepless through the pains. After two doses a day of *Pulsatilla*,‡ the trouble in the testicle disappeared after four days,

* Hartlaub observes that *Cannabis* is more useful in acute and *Thuja* in chronic gonorrhœa, which, if taken *cum grano salis*, agrees with our own experience.—*Mayrhofer.*

† We think that Thuja was the homœopathically indicated remedy in this case, and are of the opinion that a few doses of that drug alone would have sufficed to remove the disease.—*Mayrhofer.*

‡ The size of the dose is nowhere mentioned in the history of this case.—*Mayrhofer.*

but in a few days returned, without any perceptible cause, in all its violence, *Puls.* was now of no service, the pains became still more severe; but *Arnica*, taken four times in two days, cured the disorder in the testicle entirely and permanently. The gonorrhœa was first removed by Thuja after a fortnight.*

(b.) *Diseases of the Prostate Gland.*

The affections of the prostate are so often a stumbling block in the way both of the patient and the physician, that we must receive with gratitude a remedy which promises to be useful in lesions of that organ with gonorrhœa.

Our provings have plainly indicated affections of the urethra in its prostatic portion, and if no decided disease of the gland was developed, still we may, at least, infer that that organ was not entirely unaffected. Perhaps experiments of longer duration might develop clearer results than pains in the neck of the bladder and discharge of prostatic fluid (*Hempel*), if they were carried so far as seriously to endanger the health.

We must content ourselves, therefore, with directing the attention of our readers to the fact that Thuja, which corresponds to the chronic and irregular course of a gonorrhœa, may also prove serviceable in lesions of the prostate gland—(*See Editor's note, ante*).

Unfortunately our homœopathic literature, thus far, contains but few communications on the treatment of the prostate.

Dr. Attomyr (*Archiv für hom. Heilk.* B. 18, H. 3. s. 46) states

* Will these four cases stand the test of critical investigation as scientific cures? I doubt it much. The remedial power of Thuja in common (primary, acute, independent) urethral gonorrhœas, is, according to my experience, exceedingly problematical. And our physiological provings give us a sufficient explanation on this subject. This remedy should be more serviceable in gonorrhœa of the glans and prepuce. It affords us, however, certain aid in those secondary (consecutive) sympathetic, chronic, *gonorrhœal discharges* which, as Hahnemann teaches, are derived from (what according to Ricord's able researches is still somewhat apocryphal) condylomatous contagion (a), are accompanied by condylomata (Ricord's mucous tubercles); or which, as Mayrhofer correctly points out (b), are followed by a lesion of the prostate gland (irritation, congestion, inflammation), or, on the other hand, have been excited and maintained by such a lesion. In relation to this last, my learned friend Dr. Böhm informs me, that an extensive experience has taught him that we can count with probability upon a sympathetic affection of the prostate, in all gonorrhœas of regular course, in individuals of a good constitution, which have lasted longer than six or eight weeks, and that the cause of a good half of all chronic gonorrhœas may be sought either in simple hypertrophy, in hyperæmia or infiltration of the prostate, especially of its middle lobe and excretory ducts. It is in such cases as these that Thuja proves especially useful, nay, surpasses every other remedy. He can produce more than twenty cases from his own practice, which, though of long standing, and treated with the most varied remedies, have yet yielded immediately and perfectly to Thuja alone. Nay, so firm is his conviction of the remedial power of this drug upon the prostate, that he administers it even in suppurations of the gland, and when he has not effected a cure he has often by its means obtained a considerable mitigation of the urinary troubles.—*Ed. Oester. Zeit.*

that he has employed Thuja in gonorrhœas with predominant prostatic affection, and has been well satisfied with the result so far as the prostate was concerned. He thus cured in six weeks a considerable and very painful affection of the prostate induced by bad conduct during a gonorrhœa, in the course of which the once corpulent patient had become greatly reduced.

Dr. Hartlaub rapidly cured a painful sensibility when urinating, the remains of a prostatic inflammation, by a single dose of *Thuja* 18. The patient, a young man, suffered from chronic gonorrhœa. The inflammation itself had been cured by *Puls.*—(*Prakt. Mit. &c.* 1837-38.)

(c.) *Condylomata.*

The power of Thuja to produce, besides gonorrhœal affections, cutaneous excrescences on the parts of generation and on other parts of the body, in the form of tubercles and warts, as secondary products, induced Hahnemann to regard it as a specific against the condylomata so frequently attending gonorrhœa. It has also been considered as a powerful remedy in obstinate sycosis, not only by homœopathic physicians, but frequently by those of the old school, sometimes secretly, sometimes openly, but ever without mention of the source from which they derive it.

The special therapeutic indications which point to the employment of Thuja in sycosis, according to the result of the physiological provings and of clinical experience, are the following: gonorrhœa, past or still present, or leucorrhœa, condylomata on a broad base, cracked, mulberry-shaped moist surface, itching and burning in the excrescences, alternate amelioration and aggravation of the affection.

To these positive indications we may add one of a negative character, namely, that mercurial preparations* or caustic, occasionally used against condylomata, remain ineffectual, by which latter means they are driven from their original seat and make their appearance on unusual parts of the body.

Dr. Trinks has written a short treatise on sycosis and its cure (*Annalen der hom. Klinik.* B. 1. § 185).

"This (miasmatic) disease is quite frequent in Dresden, and I have had occasion to observe it in various complications and extent. Like syphilis, it commonly first appears upon those parts that have received the contagion; in man, upon the glans, the folds of the prepuce, the orifice of the urethra; in the other sex, on the labia minora and majora, on the clitoris, &c. If no impediment is put in the way of their growth, they very soon notably increase in circumference and in number upon the original spot; if, on the other hand, they are destroyed by external applications, caustic, amputations, &c.) the disease disappears from that place in order to break out

* Condylomata attendant upon chancres disappear under the use of mercury; those which accompany gonorrhœa do not diminish under that remedy.—*Louvrier's Syphilidologie.*

afresh in another. It then appears in the neighborhood of the anus,* in the axillæ, in the fauces, on the lips, the external surface of the iris; and in women, on the nipple."†

"Their form is likewise various. I have seen them on the penis in the form of many-pointed warts, of cockscombs or cauliflowers, and the same in the fauces. They rest upon a broad base on the lips and breast, on the anus and in the furrow. As to their consistence they are generally soft, seldom hard and horny (when they present the warty appearance). The soft excrescences for the most part distil a stinking moisture; they seldom discharge blood."‡

"I have frequently seen this disease uncomplicated, as small wartlike excrescences upon the glans and prepuce, which gradually increased at the base; all that was necessary for a perfect cure was six weeks, and *one* or at most *two* doses of Thuja."

"Condylomata frequently came, too, complicated with gonorrhœa, the stains of which upon the linen were greenish-yellow, and which was attended with burning pain in the *fossa navicularis* during and after urination. For these cases also, Thuja was a specific; the gonorrhœa commonly disappeared first, then the condylomata."

"More frequently still, I have seen condylomata complicated with primary syphilis; with chancres on the glans, on the frænulum and inner surface of the prepuce, accompanied by simultaneous inflammatory swelling of the prepuce and inguinal glands."

"The cure of this complication is not difficult, if the patient have not taken large doses of the mercurial preparations. Where they had not done so, I began the treatment with a small dose of *Merc. solub.*, allowing it to operate as long as it produced any improvement. In some cases, the syphilis was thoroughly eradicated by this dose alone; but in the majority, a second and even a third were necessary. Then I followed quickly with the arbor vitæ. But if mercury had been previously exhibited in large doses both externally and internally, the difficulty of the cure was much increased. I was then obliged to give first a dose of *Calc. sulph.* or *Acid. nit.* to destroy the excessive effects of the mercury. During the operation of this remedy, the two co-existing diseases frequently took on their original forms."

"Quicksilver given in suitable preparation and dose now completed the cure of the syphilis, and the sycosis soon followed on the exhibition of its proper remedy."

"The exhibition of Thuja is often alone sufficient thoroughly to eradicate

* Condylomata frequently affect the anus, perinæum and thighs, by natural growth in extension.—*Mayrhofer.*

† According to ***Ricord***, who distinguishes the broad condylomata (***condylomata lata, papules muqueuses***) from the pointed, pedunculated excrescences (***condylomata acuminata***) which he calls "***Vegetations***," these growths may also appear in the external auditory meatus, on the nose, tongue, cheeks and tonsils, in the larynx, on the navel and vagina, on the neck of the uterus and between the toes. —*Mayrhofer.*

‡ Condylomata on the nose and commissures of the lips display deep furrows and tend to scab over. Those on the tongue resemble aphthæ, appear singly or in small numbers, and look like little gray, granular prominences, which seem to be covered with false membrane. They frequently return after many years (10 to 15) and not unfrequently withstand every sort of treatment. (See ***Ricord's*** treatise on ***Syphilis***, edited by Dr. Turk, and also ***Ritter's*** Chronic Gonorrhœa).—***Mayrhofer.***

sycosis; in many cases I have found its external application unnecessary, especially to soft condylomata. But wartlike excrescences with horny points on their surface require the external use of equal parts of alcohol and Thuja-juice, and also the subsequent internal administration of nitric acid."

We add in this immediate connection the communication of a follower of the old school upon this same disease, because observations made upon the same subject by men of opposite views, are stringent proof of the truth of those matters wherein they agree.

On the internal and external use of *Tinct. Thujæ* in cases of *condylomata*, by Dr. Warnatz (*Monatschrift für Med. &c.* 1838, B. 1. H. 2).

"Every practising physician must have experienced the intractability and the liability to return, when surgically treated by excision, of condylomata, those lymphatic vascular excrescences in the *rete vasculosum* of the skin, lying near the mucous membrane of the rectum and genital organs, which appear originally as symptoms of secondary syphilis.* The author resided in a district where among a part of the country people secondary syphilis is not unfrequent, and appears pretty often in the shape of condylomata about the anus and genitals. Among these again, those with broad and dry surfaces, were disproportionately more frequent than those with pointed, sore and secreting ones. Such patients often continue to bear the disease for a long time without its apparently exerting any very great influence on their general health, until excoriation, pains, and the extension of the excrescences oblige them to seek the aid of a physician. Then the most minute investigation frequently detects not the slightest trace of syphilis except the condylomata, which in women, however, are commonly accompanied by a suspicious vaginal blennorrhœa, and it is often exceedingly doubtful (especially after a severe mercurial treatment) whether we are to regard the original disease as still present in the cutaneous excrescence or whether it has set up in this shape a new form of disease. We certainly saw many cases cured under the employment of the best known remedies, as under Dzondi's treatment, under the Louvrier-Rust inunction, under red precipitate (without cauterisation of the condylomata). The well known external applications, either purely caustic or such as tend to produce an alteration in the morbid process, were also used, as *Lapis infern.*, *Lap. caust.*, *Cupr. sulph.*, *Liquor hyd. nit.*, *Sol. tart. emet.*, *Acet. saturni*, *Sabina*, Plenck's solution of *Sublimate*, *Camphor and Alcohol*. In many cases, however, the re-action thus excited was too painful and even not without danger; sometimes they could not be employed from domestic and matrimonial considerations; sometimes the knife was finally necessarily resorted to and then the disease returned, especially, according to W.'s observation, in young and plump individuals." †

* It is still a question whether condylomata are forms of primary or secondary syphilis, or whether they may not be both. The thing becomes much simpler to those physicians who recognize the distinction between the gonorrhœal and chancrous sickness.—*Mayrhofer.*

† Condylomata, the result of gonorrhœa, defy the therapeutic triad of the old school, *Mercury*, *Caustic* and the *Knife*.—Nay, Dease has remarked that they did not disappear though the patients were so long salivated that they died of marasmus, thus verifying Hildebrandt's remark, "*Sunt medici qui morbos construunt et aegros destruunt.*"—*Mayrhofer.*

"It is very possible, however that in many cases new and repeated syphilitic infections may have taken place which have been concealed from the physician so long as they were new. Unfortunately, in relation to the moral conduct of such patients, "*quilibet præsumitur malus*" must be the physician's guiding maxim."

"Two years since, the author was especially annoyed by a patient so afflicted with condylomata that none of the usual remedies were of the least avail. On account of the original syphilitic infection, the patient had already been through a course of inunction, but without any result as to the condylomata. W. then recollected that Hufeland, in his "*Journal für pract. Heilk.*," recommended the external application of Thuja to condylomata, and he resolved to try its effect."*

"For four weeks in succession, the warts upon the *scrotum and perinæum* were painted three times a day with the alcoholic tincture of Thuja; the cure which followed is perfect to this day, and no other syphilitic symptom whatever has appeared. W. employed the same remedy in the same way and with similar results with several patients, and finally resolved to try what effects might be expected from its internal use. He administered it internally in several cases of broad condylomata twice, from eight to sixteen drops, and at the same time employed it externally with astonishing success. In several slight cases, a perfect cure followed from the internal exhibition alone. The author relates the following case:

"N. N., a stout country girl, 29 years old, as the result of an impure coitus, had suffered for over a year with *syphilis univ.* (showing itself chiefly in the cutaneous system), and had undergone such a profusion of doctors and doctors' drugs that her pecuniary means, at best but scanty, were pretty much exhausted. On examination he found small chancres (mucous follicles of the vagina in a state of ulceration), a tolerably copious leucorrhœa, with discolored, offensive secretion, and very extensive *condylomata lata.* The anus and posterior portions of the *labia pudenda* were covered with a broad, cauliflower-like excrescence, consisting of broad, slightly reddened, but otherwise almost dry condylomata, so that the anus had precisely the appearance of the external genitals with long, elevated *labia externa.* Besides these, there were, neither in the throat nor any where else, any traces of syphilis to be seen. She was received into the Charity Hospital in Camenz, in Upper Lusatia. The physicians of the establishment, Dr. Roderer, and the author's father, Warnatz, employed various mercurials, and even inunction, without any effect upon the condylomata. The ulceration of the vaginal mucous membrane and the blennorrhœa had indeed almost disappeared, but the condylomata were unaltered."

"Thuja had already been employed externally on the recommendation of the author, but without result. He now advised the internal exhibition of the tincture of Thuja without delay in a dose rising from eight to sixteen drops twice a day. The external use of it upon the condylomata was continued. The case was tedious but the result was striking. After pursuing

* Hufeland could only have recommended Thuja for condylomata upon Hahnemann's authority, for he, as the first prover of Thuja, recognised its specific virtue in sycosis, and employed it for that affection. Our opponents have, ever since the first promulgation of Homœopathy, been in the habit of helping themselves to homœopathic dainties and nicknacks. Their pretended ignorance, evasion, or concealment of the homœopathic source we must decidedly condemn, as a violation of the right of property which Homœopathy is in duty bound to maintain. *Cuique suum.—Mayrhofer.*

this course for three months a perfect cure was obtained, not only of the condylomata but also of the vaginal blennorrhœa.

"Altogether W. has treated 16 cases, fourteen of the broad and two of the pointed condylomata. These latter remained uncured, but rapidly disappeared on exhibiting *Liquor hyd. nitr.* externally, and *sublimate* internally. Eleven of the fourteen cases of broad condylomata were perfectly cured. Of the remaining three cases, one still retained small warty fragments, which the author excised, and in the other two no change was perceived; it ought to be remarked, however, that one of these patients had been cured by Thuja a year before, but when the disease appeared anew no cure was obtained."*

"In eight cases the remedy was applied exclusively internally; in eight both externally and internally. Internally the dose was from six to sixteen drops of the pure drug taken twice a day; externally it was painted on three times a day with a fine brush, until, by and by, burning, excoriation and slight secretion from the condylomata came on. If they were sore and excoriated at the commencement, the application of the remedy occasioned a pretty severe burning pain. Finally, it is not possible, by the closest attention, to observe the *farrago symptomatum* which the Homœopaths pretend to have noticed as effects of this drug.† Patients who took the remedy internally perceived a feeling of burning and warmth in the mouth, throat, and on the tongue, extending into the precordial region, but this soon passed off. No special operation on the digestive organs or bowels was observed; but in several cases nocturnal cutaneous excitement and increased urination seem to have been produced."‡

"A slight itching was the only remarkable feeling in the condylomata, which is, however, rather to be ascribed to the perinæal sweat."§

The patients did not complain at the commencement of the treatment when the Thuja was applied to the dry condylomata; after several days' application, when the skin had become thin and excoriation had commenced, they only felt a little burning. At the same time the warts reddened somewhat, and showed some, though little secretion, which appeared to be the especial agent of cure by the outward application of Thuja. The author, however, has never seen those violent effects from the external use of the drug which Dr. Fricke of Hamburg has observed, in whose practice, though using it in a diluted form, it caused such remarkable irritation that he was obliged to lay it aside. Fricke saw considerable swelling and excoriation of the whole neighbor-

* It is very probable that Sabina, externally and internally applied, would have effected a cure in this case.—*Mayrhofer.*

† The apparent confusion of symptoms in the Hahnemannian system is the greatest stumbling-block to the physicians of the old school. They find it much more convenient to reject the good with the bad than to subject themselves to the trouble of studying the character of a remedy from the physiological proving, or of making experiments with drugs upon their own bodies. As to this case, the few drops of Thuja exhibited produced few primary symptoms, because their powers were exhausted in combating a disease to which the drug was perfectly appropriate. —*Mayrhofer.*

‡ These observations agree perfectly with our provings.—*Mayrhofer.*

§ The sweat on the genitals belongs equally to the operation of Thuja, as our provings testify, and itching and tickling in the condylomata under the use of Thuja have already been observed by Hahnemann.—*Mayrhofer.*

hood where it was applied, follow in every case. Diluted, the remedy produced no results, and only in one case was he able to effect a tedious cure. (*Casper's Wochenschrift*, 1844, N. 24.) The experience of Dr. Köhler of Warsaw is somewhat opposite in character. He never witnessed inflammation, excoriation, or even unfavorable influences or relapses * after the employment of the drug. The same was the experience of Dr. Leo of Warsaw. He constantly associated the internal administration of mercury,† however, with the external use of Thuja. (*Fleker's Annalen*, &c. 1835. H. 3.) The author does not know of any other observations that have been made public.‡ The author does not permit himself to form any opinion upon the pharmacodynamic character of Thuja; since for this, still more extended experiments are necessary, which are to be expected from the heads of great clinical institutions. § He has communicated the little experience he has had, without prepossession and without any sympathy for Homœopathy, ‖ but simply because he conceives it to be the duty of every physician to contribute, according to his ability, to that common good of all, the extension and advancement of science.

* Diversity of effect depends upon the relative irritability of the individual patients. Thus the tincture of Thuja will produce no unpleasant consequences in a torpid patient, while in one who has a well marked susceptibility to this drug, even dilutions will produce violent reaction. The *quantum* of the drug must be taken into consideration in relation to the individual no less than the *qualé*. If Dr. Warnatz is of the opinion that Homœopathy consists in small doses (a notion with which homœopathising allopaths would fain quiet themselves and others) I beg him to know that Hahnemann himself directed the application of the Thuja tincture to condylomata in the oldest and most inveterate cases (*Chron. Krank. Heil. der Sycosis*).—*Mayrhofer.*

† In order to keep up the art of hodge-podge, and to secure the certainty of a doubt as to which remedy effected the good.—*Mayrhofer.*

‡ Because the author had neglected to acquaint himself with the literature of Homœopathy, of which many of the physicians of the old school are still ignorant. All those physicians who neglect the study of Homœopathy richly deserve the reproach of *onesidedness*, and so long as candidates for a degree are not examined on the learning of the new school, so long will our public examinations supply us with only onesided priests of Æsculapius.—*Mayrhofer.*

§ We cherish like hope with the author. But unfortunately, Homœopathy commands as yet no syphilitic clinique, and to all appearance will wait long before she attains so desirable an object.—*Mayrhofer.*

‖ This protest against Homœopathy is a sufficient proof of the prejudice of the author. He who cures condylomata with Thuja is a homœopath, because his treatment is founded on the principle "*similia similibus*," and in truth, he takes part in Homœopathy. Before the world, indeed, he may be an avowed or a secret homœopath, or even a homœopathic smuggler, according as he is honorable enough to acknowledge or weak enough to be silent respecting his faith, or so destitute of principle as to plough with another's heifer and read by another's candle without acknowledging his obligations to the owner. Homœopathy, however, by this time should be well accustomed to the treatment of her rationalist opponents, slapping her in the face with one hand and picking her pocket with the other.—*Mayrhofer.*

1. *Uncomplicated Sycosis.*

Dr. Trinks relates the following case of primary sycosis.

1. A young man was exposed to contagion by a coïtus and eight days after, comblike, horny excrescences appeared upon the inner surface of the prepuce. Trinks diagnosed these excrescences to be condylomata, but the patient, not having confidence in this opinion, consulted another (distinguished) physician of Dresden, who diagnosed Trinks to be an ignoramus (allopathic professional courtesy! M.), and quieted the patient with the assurance that the excrescences were the result of too violent rubbing and erosion of the prepuce (sub coïtu) and that they would soon spontaneously disappear. Thus comforted, the patient departed on a journey, giving no thought to his ailment; but on returning home, at the end of six weeks, he found to his horror that the excrescences had considerably increased both in number and in size.

The formerly incredulous physician now declared them to be condylomata. But the patient declined his treatment and sought aid of Dr. Trinks. The horny condition of the excrescenees led him to the external and internal use of Thuja, which worked a perfect cure in six weeks.—*Annal. der hom. Klin.* 1, s. 177.)

Tietze (surgeon) communicates the following cases (*Op. cit.* s. 369, 370):

2. A man 30 years old, blond, lean, of middle height, had suffered several years from sycosis. He was treated with mercurial remedies, whereupon the condylomata vanished, it is true, but soon came to light again. Driven in again by the local application of quicksilver, the excrescences soon returned. Thus passed several years, the patient keeping constantly by him a pot of mercurial ointment in order to daub over them wherever they broke out next. When he consulted Tietze he complained of vertigo, eructations after eating, grumbling in the abdomen, burning in the urethra, especially morning and noon. There were several warts on the *corona glandis* which became moist during the increase of the moon, and discharged a purulent fluid. He had also cough with discharge of yellow mucus, severe thirst, and twitching of his limbs in sleep, perspired much, and complained of fatigue in his legs. On the 10th of July, 1828, he took a dose of *Thuja* 30: this was repeated at the end of a fortnight, and on August 10th he had three pellets moistened with *Acid. nit.* 24.

In the beginning of September the condylomata had disappeared, and at the end of the month, even the marks on the skin where they had been. The chest trouble was gone. He married, became the father of a sound, hearty child, and experienced nothing more of his tedious complaint.

3. A strong young man had had for a long time two warts upon the prepuce nearly as large as peas, which, however, occasioned him no inconvenience. Dr. Rummel gave him on the 18th of February four doses of Thuja 30. Six days after, no change being perceptible in the condylomata, a considerable swelling made its appearance in the cheek, threatening to end in suppuration. The patient took one dose of *Mercury* 15, whereupon the abcess in the mouth broke and the swelling disappeared. Freed from this interpolated disease, the patient again took advice in respect to the warts, and received two pellets moistened with *Thuja* 30, with the direction to dissolve them in a glass of water and to take a table-spoonful a day. Ten days after, the patient came in consternation to his physician, with the story

that the whole glans was covered with pus. Rummel recommended him to put dry lint between the glans and prepuce, and to do nothing else.

After an interval of two days the genital organs were found entirely freed from warts. No trace of a scar could be discovered and he continued perfectly cured of sycotic affections.—(*Allg. hom. Zeit.* B. 5, s. 102.)

4. A young man, two years before, had contracted a gonorrhœa, and when this was finally suppressed, it was succeeded by condylomata about the anus, which he at first neglected and afterwards bunglingly treated on his own responsibility. When he applied to Dr. Schindler, in January, 1833, the whole perinæum as far as the scrotum and around the anus for a breadth of two inches was beset with large moist condylomata. He complained of violent burning and biting and could scarcely walk. No improvement resulted from a dose of *Thuja* 30; *Acid. nit.* 30, somewhat diminished the burning.

From February 24th to March 16th the patient took every eight days a dose of *Thuja* 30. The warts ceased to be moist, appeared to become smaller, and he could walk better. *Nitric acid* 30, one dose every eight days. The improvement progressed visibly; several small warts disappeared, the large ones became flatter, the burning and biting entirely ceased.

April 28th. The patient again had four doses of *Thuja* 30 to be taken at intervals of eight days; the most of the condylomata disappeared except the larger ones: one pair only was left of those on each side of the anus.

Another four doses of *Thuja* produced no further improvement, and four doses of *Phos. ac.* remained similarly without effect. Dr. Schindler gave now a dose of *Sulph.* against any possible psoric complication; the disease, however, on the 19th of August, was at the point where it had been at the end of April. The patient now took every morning a drop of the pure *Thuja* and also applied lint moistened with *Thuja* externally.

August 27th. Every trace of condylomata had disappeared, the skin was smooth, and the patient perfectly cured.—(*Allg. hom. Zeit.* B. 4, s. 276.)

Dr. Rummel gives the two following cases of sycosis.—(*Archiv für, &c.* B. 8, H. 1, s. 58, 59):

5. In the first case urethral gonorrhœa was also present, and the whole scrotum was beset with hard, only partly moist tubercles. A cure followed the exhibition of one dose of *Merc.* and two doses of *Thuja* (strength not stated) and the external use of the juice.

6. A young man applied to Dr. Rummel by letter, requesting him to remove an ulcer upon his penis consequent upon contagion; from the description, Rummel concluded that it was a chancre, and prescribed *Mer.* 12. No improvement following after a fortnight, and the cure still lingering after *Acid. nit.* 12, he insisted upon seeing the patient. Autopsy showed it to be sycosis. Two condylomata were secreting an offensive purulent mucus, and the patient stated that he had perceived a painful erosion (but decidedly no chancre vesicle) the very next day after the copulation. There was besides in the left axilla a dry, brown elevation, such as Hahnemann has described. On the 24th of December the patient took *Thuja* 30, on which the condylomata perfectly disappeared in three weeks. The brown, herpetic elevation in the axilla, however, remained unaltered, and first vanished after a dose of *Acid. nit.* 18. The exhibition of *Thuja* eradicates condylomata with brown spots under the arms.—(*Allg. hom, Zeit.* B. 1, s. 96.)

7. Dr. Lobethal cured an officer of cuirassiers of an entire circle of condylomata around the anus by the use of *Thuja* 1 (drop doses) alter-

nated with *Acid. nit.* 3 and the external application of the tincture, in some months after the patient had received no benefit from small doses of the same remedy administered by another homœopathic physician.

Dr. Mohnike relates an interesting case of obstinate sycosis cured by Thuja.—(*Hufeland's Journ.* March, 1843. *Extracted into the Oest. Med. Wochenschrift*, 1843, No. 21.)

8. In the autumn of 1839 there applied to Dr. Mohnike a young merchant who some two years before had contracted a violent urethral blennorrhœa from an impure cohabitation. He had never previously had syphilis, and this gonorrhœa even, after a few weeks' use of copaiba, had disappeared. But scarcely two months had elapsed before the warts and excrescences were gradually developed, from which he had now suffered for nearly two years, and against which no remedy seemed to make head. The patient was thus led to believe that his case was incurable, and had made up his mind, as a last resort, to try the water cure at Græfenberg, provided Dr. Mohnike's treatment was ineffectual. The examination of the patient developed the following facts ; the inner surface of the prepuce and the portion of the penis behind the glans were, as it were, sowed over with numerous pointed condylomata. These excrescences of the mucous membrane lay prostrate on the spot whence they had sprouted, but when Dr. Mohnike raised their heads with the forceps, the thin pedicle appeared of nearly a line in length. The exudation of the offensive clammy moisture peculiar to condylomata could only be detected in a very slight degree. The patient had never felt pain or itching in the glans and foreskin. He had had no cohabitation since the appearance of the condylomata. The perinæum was occupied in its whole extent between the scrotum and anus by a large *condylomata latum.* It was certainly half an inch high, and extended on both sides of the raphé. It exuded much, and was covered with a greasy purulent moisture. The patient complained that he could often scarcely endure the torture when walking, and that the inner and upper part of the thigh was often sore and inflamed from the acridity of the discharged fluid.

A similar broad condyloma, but smaller than that in the perinæum, was found on the inner surface of the left thigh. The orifice of the anus, where the skin meets the mucous membrane of the rectum, was surrounded by three large *condylomata lata,* which simulated hæmorrhoidal protuberances. They exuded much, and constantly occasioned a very painful troublesome itching, but intolerable pain when he had a hard stool. Finally, behind the anus and on the coccyx there was an excrescence resembling the others in size and condition. He had never experienced pains in the bones, and the most careful examination of the oral and faucial cavity could detect there no indications of secondary syphilis. He had already taken Zittmann's decoction and Dzondi's corrosive sublimate pills. Besides this, the most varied sorts of caustic had been locally applied to the warts, and even excision and the ligature had been tried. But external and internal treatment was equally unavailing.

Mohnike almost despaired of obtaining a perfect cure. He prescribed internally Berg's formula of *Stib. sulph. nig.* with *Hyd. præc. rub.*, which has often proved serviceable in confirmed lues, especially where the skin and mucous membranes are affected. The patient was ordered to lie abed the greater part of the day, and to promote the cutaneous transpiration by frequent drafts of an infusion of *Spec. Lignor.*, with a spare diet. In addition, Dr. Mohnike used Plenk's solution of sublimate, with which he cautiously touched the warts on the glans and prepuce once a day for a week. The broad condylomata, except those at the anal orifice, he covered with lint, saturated with the same solution. All to no purpose. He now threw aside all caustic applications and waited to see if internal treatment alone would not effect the cure, but with similar result. He then resorted to the use of *tincture of Thuja*, and soon had reason to be amazed at the rapid, scarcely hoped for action of the new remedy,* for already on the third day after the whole condylomata had been several times daily painted with the tincture, they presented an entirely altered appearance; they shrivelled, fell in, and sensibly diminished in circumference. On the fifth day of the treatment all the pointed warts upon the glans and inner surface of the prepuce had disappeared. The smallest remains of the broad perinæal condylomata were visible on the ninth day. The tincture occasioned but little pain, and the sound skin at the base of the warts was neither inflamed nor irritated. The excrescences all disappeared by absorption, and without ulceration or gangrene.

2. *Sycosis with Rhagades.*

A case of this kind is related by Dr. Genzke of Parchim.—(*All. hom. Zeit.* B. 22, s. 22.)

1. A young physician had contracted by contagion a gonorrhœa, which disappeared under the use of Balsam of Copaiba. One year after, violent burning came on in the anus, which became intolerable when walking or at stool, and an offensive moisture distilled which soiled the linen. Examination showed a shining mulberry condyloma, with a broad base close to the anal opening; and on both sides of the anus, in the natural folds of the skin, two deep fissures (rhagades), which, as well as the condyloma, secreted an exceedingly foul fluid. A colored yellowish brown ring two inches broad surrounded the anus. Dr. Genzke prescribed the first dilution of *Thuja*, with directions to take one or two drops a day in the morning, fasting, and to paint the wart and fissures with the tincture. In fourteen days the burning had almost completely disappeared, the condyloma was visibly wrinkled and had lost its polish, the rhagades were smaller, the foul secretion had become less and inodorous, and in short, all the local symptoms progressively diminished. The patient, however, a novice in Homœopathy, mistrusting the small doses, took larger ones than were directed, and experienced *pressing aching in the forehead, restless unrefreshing sleep, and a well-marked balanitis.* The glans was in its entire circumference swollen, inflamed, covered with small pimples, and discharged a tolerably copious purulent secretion.† The Thuja was omitted, and four weeks after the beginning of the treatment the whole train of symptoms, both of the disease and of the remedy, had vanished.

* We must class Dr. Monhike too among the homœopathic freebooters, because he does not state the source whence he obtained his new wisdom. If the remedy was good enough to effect in a few days a cure where the so-styled rational treatment had proved, for years, inefficient, it surely was good enough to have been openly acknowledged as a homœopathic remedy.—*Mayrhofer.*

† *Balanorrhœa* is an effect of Thuja beyond a doubt, as I can substantiate from my own experience.—*Mayrhofer.*

3. *Sycosis co-existent with Syphilis.*

Dr. Schrön gives us an instructive case of Sycosis and Syphilis combined.—(*Allg. hom. Zeit.* B. 5, s. 147.)

1. A girl of sixteen years old had leucorrhœa and bean-shaped warts, especially about the anus. Schrön (then an allopath) subjected her to a course of sublimate pills, and in the meanwhile removed the warts by the knife. She was afterwards treated by another allopath, likewise with mercury; but the warts and leucorrhœa never entirely yielded. In January, 1833, she again applied to Schrön. She had on each side of the nose along the cheeks two chancres of the size of a ducat, which extended into the nostrils and presented elevated red margins and a tallowy bottom.* There lay about the anus a collection of cockscomb-like warts which discharged, and occasioned such a burning that she could not lie in bed at night. The leucorrhœa reddened the thigh. Schrön gave *Merc. viv.* 3 (½ grain), alternating it with *Thuja* 3 (1 drop) every eight days, and applied the undiluted tincture externally upon the condylomata. In six weeks the chancres healed entirely, and, in twelve, warts and leucorrhœa had both disappeared. The burning in the condylomata first diminished, then they ceased to discharge, and finally they shrivelled into mummies and vanished.

2. A peasant girl, 30 years old, had in September, 1844, a soldier on furlough for a lover, and a fortnight after his departure she felt violent burning in the anus and a corrosive leucorrhœa set in. Soon after she remarked little tubercles about the anus which were painful to the touch and when at stool. She consulted a country midwife, who examined her and said she had piles. She went with this opinion to a barber surgeon, who treated her for the piles. But the tubercles becoming constantly larger and more abundant, moist excrescences appearing also upon the genital parts, and an ulcer coming on the right thigh, she consulted an obstetric practitioner, who examined her and prescribed (Nov. 18) fifteen grains of *Merc. solub. Hahnem.*, made into thirty pills with extract of liquorice, of which she was to take every evening.

The ulcer, indeed, healed under the use of the pills, but the excrescences continued to spread. In 1845 (March) the patient came to me. Examination showed a countless number of condylomata. Round the anus was a ring of broad, soft, cracked, moist condylomata. The whole perinæum was crowded with a host of warts, which had become confluent, and so formed one great *condyloma latum.* Between the *labia externa* and the thighs a double row of condylomata ran up on both sides to the *mons veneris.* The *labia majora* were inflamed, much swollen, and covered internally and externally with warts of all sizes. Finally, there were solitary condylomata down the inner side of the thigh almost to its middle. It was, in truth, a disgusting sight, for the number of warts must have been over a hundred. The vaginal blennorrhœa corroded the thigh. She felt burning in the condylomata; the catamenia had ceased during the disease.

I gave twenty drops of *Thuja* 2 in six ounces of water, with directions to take a table-spoonful three times a day. On the 7th of April the patient returned with the news that she was much improved. The burning was much diminished; the condylomata discharged less and looked shrivelled and perishing; the swelling of the labia and the leucorrhœa were less. On

* Were these chancres the consequence of the original infection, or had a new contagion taken place in the mean time?—*Mayrhofer.*

the 13th the patient had another vial of *Thuja* 2, upon which the amelioration proceeded and the menses appeared. I now gave her the tincture, one drop three times a day, internally, and directed her to moisten the condylomata with it morning and evening. By the end of May over half of them were gone, and as the cure seemed to be at a stand I gave her *Acid. nit.* for a week (a few drops in six ounces of water, one spoonful morning and evening).

The *arbor vitæ* operated with renewed energy after the administration of the nitric acid, which last produced but little alteration in the disease. The solitary warts vanished completely in June, and the complex ones were reduced in size one-half. All the other troubles were much lessened.

In July the girl fell from the thatch of the cottage upon which she was spreading hemp to dry, and injured herself so severely that she was necessarily treated for the consequences of the fall for a month after. In August I made an experiment with the tincture of *Sabina*, and had the condylomata painted with it daily, in order to see if in this neglected condition the savine would not hasten the cure. This was not the case. I was obliged to have recourse again to *Thuja*, under the persevering use of which all the morbid symptoms ceased, and the condylomata disappeared, except a small spot on each side of the anus, toward the perinæum, where the colony formerly existed.

In October the patient took no more Thuja, and I cannot say whether these last traces of the condylomata finally disappeared or not; we may, however, judging from the rapidity of the cure up to that time, almost certainly conclude that they did.

I may also remark that the patient, who entirely despaired of a cure in the commencement, exhilarated by her progress, may have taken the doses stronger than they were directed; in the second month of the treatment she exhibited, as signs of the operation of Thuja, single *large vesicles* upon the thighs and arms, which were surrounded *by a red areola* and passed *into suppuration.*

4. *Sycosis after the cure of Syphilis.*

Dr. Portalius relates a case in which condylomata succeeded to the cure of syphilis.—(*Arch. für hom. Heilk.* B. 19, H. 3, s. 80 et seq.)

1. Mr. M. had two large genuine syphilitic ulcers on the prepuce. No signs of sycotic affection were to be perceived on a daily examination. Both chancres healed in eight days (from the 13th to the 22d January), during which time the patient took daily one dose of *Merc. nig.* 12., kept strict diet and lay abed (two absolutely indispensable conditions, if syphilitic affections are to be rapidly and permanently cured). Five days after the perfect healing of both chancres, condylomata sprouted luxuriantly upon the *frænulum præputii*, which were cured by Thuja. (It is not stated what dose was given nor in what time the cure was effected.—*Mayrhofer.*)

Tietze relates an analogous case.

2. A stout girl had suffered from a very copious leucorrhœa since her delivery a year before; it was accompanied by violent itching on the genitals. On inspection, the *labia majora* were found considerably swollen, and numerous ulcers with pale, tallowy bottoms, from the size of a lentil to

that of a groschen, covered not only the external organs of generation but also stretched deep into the vagina. Their syphilitic character was undeniable. She took daily *Merc. nig.* 12. After a fortnight a considerable improvement appeared, and the patient took from the 10th of August to the 18th September, six doses of Sulphur 30, which not only removed the leucorrhœa, but perfectly healed the remains of the ulcers.

Fourteen days after, however, such a profusion of condylomata had appeared that the whole presented a most shocking sight. Even on the right corner of the mouth there was a wart. She took externally *Thuja* (tincture) and internally *Thuja* 30, every day. The treatment was interrupted by many accidents, but resulted in a perfect cure at the end of three months.

5. *Masked Sycosis.* (Radetzky's case.)

1. An illustrious personage, seventy years of age, had frequently suffered for many years from a cough, which since 1836 increased in autumn to an inflammatory catarrhal fever, and yet no pulmonary lesion could be detected. In that year he broke two ribs by a fall; the accident was followed by a very violent pneumonia which ceased after purulent and offensive sputa. During the two following years he was not seriously sick; he had at times, as he had had before, attacks of headache in the forehead, sour eructations, and diarrhœa, which however were soon cured. In July and August, 1839, cephalic congestions with violent vertigo often distressed him, and to these were soon added pressure in the forehead and in the right eye, with inflammation of the eyelids, watering and protrusion of the eye. By appropriate remedies the affection was indeed diminished, but the under lid still remained inflamed. On the 9th of October, 1840, the patient (a distinguished military officer) sat on horseback five hours in the sun; in the evening he was attacked with violent fever accompanied by intolerable pain in the forehead over the right eye. This latter was much inflamed and protruded somewhat from the orbit. The fever soon disappeared; the trouble in the eye too was somewhat lulled, but there still remained inflammation of the lower lid, watering of the eye, and a swelling at the external canthus back in the orbit, which was not painful nor did it interfere with vision.

Toward the end of October, the patient went on a journey and only returned after an absence of six weeks. During this time, there had arisen in the eye a vegetation of the size of a bean, which, commencing in the internal canthus, extended along the under lid. The tumor already existing in the external canthus had enlarged, and the eye was considerably protruded from its socket. Occasional headache in the forehead and violent congestions were also present. The domestic physician of the illustrious patient, Dr. Hartung, considered the case as a critical one, for it was his opinion that a fungus had formed in the orbit, the development of which he dreaded.

The homœopathic treatment now commenced had no special issue; the general strength was preserved by the various remedies employed, but the growth of the fungus could not be stopped. The tumor over the external canthus had now a purplish color, and both it and that in the internal canthus had increased, and there appeared between the ball of the eye and the under eyelid a fungous, elastic, pale, red, painless, spurious growth, which pressed the ball out of the normal axis of vision. The pupil was directed upwards and outwards, and the free motion of the eye impeded, but the power of vision was as yet unimpaired.

An oculist, called into consultation on the 6th of January, 1841, confirmed the diagnosis of the ordinary physician, and gave a very unfavorable prognosis, declaring "that there was nothing to be done in the case, and that no method whatever could effect a cure." At Hartung's solicitation that he would at least recommend something, he prescribed corrosive sublimate (a quarter of a grain daily), at the same time remarking "that it would do no good, but he knew nothing better." Dr. Hartung acquiesced in the prescription, but from caution administered only one-twelfth of a grain (whether only once or oftener is not stated), but was immediately obliged to give an antidote on account of the violent cephalic congestions that came on.

On the 26th January, 1841, Hartung describes the state of the disease as follows.—(*Allg. hom. Zeit.* B. 20, s. 145 et seq.)

A hard grayish blue tumor filled almost the whole orbit and displaced the ball of the eye outwards; on the under lid it was clearly fungous, it was painful under strong pressure, and bled easily; the ball was pushed against the external canthus and immovable. The patient perceived various pains in the fungus, sticking, tearing, burning and itching. The eye itself gave him no pain, but the visual power was so affected that every object opposite the external canthus appeared black. The eyelids were also stretched and swollen, black and blue, and immovable. The conjunctiva, especially that of the lids, the *plica semilunaris*, and the *caruncula lachrymalis* were loosened, of a dirty red, and covered by a thick tissue of varicose vessels.

In the morning the crevice between the lids was filled with a white, viscous, purulent mucus; the eye watered in the daytime; in the evening it was hot, dry and painful. In other respects the patient was free from febrile symptoms, and his strength and the vital functions of the organism were as favorable as could be desired.*

The case now fell wholly to the charge of Dr. Hartung, as the patient emphatically declared "that he would have no treatment but the homœopathic." Dr. Hartung employed at first, *Ars.*, *Psorin* and *Herpetin* (all three of the 30th dilution), but without result. The bleedings ceased after *Carb. anim.* 30, and the fungus ceased to grow, but no amelioration followed. Hartung now gave one drop of *Thuja* 30 in three ounces of distilled water, a table-spoonful three times a day. On the first day appeared some reminiscences of the previous morbid condition, as, aching on the right side of the forehead, nocturnal cough, slight diarrhœa, renal pains and itching on the

* The communications of the consulting physicians do not agree in relation to the special diagnosis. The ordinary, in his account (*loc. cit.*) speaks constantly of a *fungous excrescence.* Another physician, who was called in consultation, says "that he had satisfied himself, by the presence of all the commonly reputed characteristics of that disease, of the existence of a scirrhous metamorphosis," and a third physician calls the affection, "*Ophthalmiam syphiliticam ex schirro orbitæ syphilitico oriundam.*"

Since we too have a right to express an opinion on the subject we take the liberty of saying, that we consider the spurious growth in question as a sycotic excrescence, and upon the following grounds: 1. because the pathognomonic signs of the disease point that way with the greatest probability (notwithstanding that the veil that conceals the previous history of the case is not removed); 2, because the *mercury* administered produced no amelioration; and 3, because *Thuja did* prove the specific—according to the allowed rule of probabilities, "*ex juvantibus et non jus vantibus judicium sumendum est.*"—*Mayrhofer.*

inside of the thigh with a miliary eruption.* These symptoms diminished on the second day and vanished on the third. The local symptoms were, itching in the inner canthus of the diseased eye, and secretion of a creamy fluid about the whole circumference of the fungus. This result induced Hartung to apply Thuja also externally. He caused the fungus to be moistened every two hours with warm water (four ounces) containing six drops of the tincture. On the fourth day after the exhibition of Thuja, the pain in the eye had ceased, the secretion of the milky fluid had increased, and the fungus was notably diminished, especially at the upper orbital border. The amelioration steadily proceeded under the employment of Thuja through the fifth, six and seventh days, and, to the astonishment of all who had seen the disease earlier, the fungus in the internal canthus and under eyelid disappeared. On the evening of the eighth and the morning of the ninth days, the patient had a dose of *Carb. anim.* 30. The fungus was also painted every morning for eight days with the twelfth dilution of *Carb. anim*, and the Thuja baths were continued.

These two remedies (Thuja and animal charcoal) were now employed, externally and internally, in eight day alternations.†

The result was so beyond all expectation successful, that within six weeks the fungus, progressively diminishing, disappeared, the eye regained its normal power of vision, the ball returned into its socket possessed of its former mobility, and in short, a complete cure was effected.

Dr. Bärtl relates a similar case of a fungous excrescence cured by Thuja, which he had occasion to observe when physician to the Syphilitic Hospital at Palermo.

2. "A man was attacked with a panaritium upon the thumb after having been cured of a balanitis by mercury. The inflammation terminated in suppuration, the abscess was opened, and a simple bandage recommended with lukewarm ablutions. The wound not only did not heal, but became redder and more sensitive, and burning pains came on in it.

"The remedies theretofore used, *Puls.* and *Sulph.*, produced no result; the pains increased, especially at night, and a red, fungous, cauliflower excrescence began to show itself from the wound; it felt hardish at the base, was very sensitive to the touch, and bled slightly.

"Under the idea that it might be an excrescence depending upon caries, I examined with a probe, but found the bone covered and sound.

"Touching with *Lapis infern.* was of no service; after twenty-four hours, the fungus was again there, and increased even more luxuriantly than before; the same result followed with burnt alum." This fruitless treatment, the previous disease, the form of the spurious growth, and also its accompanying symptoms, finally led Dr. Bärtl to the well-grounded conjecture that the fungus arose from a sycotic source, and induced him to employ *Thuja*, internally at first, afterwards externally also. The result was, that within a short time "*violent inflammatory irritation aud suppuration was excited in the morbid growth*," by means of which the fungus, then of the

* Do not these symptoms still more indicate *Thuja?—Mayrhofer.*

† We cannot gather with certainty from Hartung's account whether the drugs *Thuja* and *Carb. anim.* were given separately in eight day alternations, or whether the external use of Thuja was continued also during the week of the charcoal, so that the fungus was only once painted with the Carb. in the morning and then frequently through the day with the Thuja, which is most probable.—*Mayrhofer.*

size of a hazelnut, melted away, and the man was discharged perfectly cured.*

Dr. Bärtl takes occasion to make the following remarks on the use of Thuja: I have found Thuja a very effective remedy in many forms of disease founded on pure sycosis. I have especially cured with it, condylomata which appeared on the inner surface of the prepuce or on the glans in the form of cauliflower, after urethral gonorrhœa or balanorrhœa, were pale red, itched, and bled easily on being touched. I employed it in high dilutions and repeated doses until signs of increased pain (in sensitive persons) and partial decay of the excrescence appeared, which commonly manifested itself by gray or blackish points on the surface; I then caused the whole growth to be painted once a day with the tincture. The condylomata dissolved in a short time by the *suppurating process* and a perfect cure resulted.

6. *Chancre Warts.*

There are chancres which instead of eating into the depth of the tissues, increase upward, and are cured either not at all or with great difficulty by mercury, which shows their sycotic character.

Dr. Attomyr gives us two cases of this sort.

1. A man 31 years old had had a small, flat, tallowy ulcer for three days on the inner surface of the prepuce. He took three doses of *Merc. sol. Hahn.* 4 to be taken every other day. The suppuration became greater, the ulcer larger, and showed now a red bottom. He had four similar doses to be taken in the same way. The chancre now rose above the surface of the prepuce—it continued to rise more and more after two doses of *Acid. nit.* 3, taken every other day, but rapidly healed after three doses of *Thuja* taken at intervals of two days. The whole treatment lasted 27 days.—*Archiv für homœop. Heilk.* B. 18, H. 3, s. 141.

2. A perfectly healthy young man contracted a chancre on the inner surface of the prepuce as the consequence of an impure connection. It disappeared on the use of external and internal remedies, but, from time to time, little aphthous ulcers appeared upon the glans and foreskin, which vanished spontaneously after from five to eight days.

At first, three such erosions appeared on the spot where the chancre had been; then by degrees came six more which were half on the furrow of the glans, half on the prepuce. A new ulcer constantly appeared near the still visible spot left by the one just healed. Once a spontaneous ulcer appeared upon the external surface of the prepuce, and healed likewise of itself after it had been covered with a loose crust.

These symptoms induced the patient to submit himself to a rigid mercu-

* Dr. Ritter, in his essay on the essential difference between chancre and gonorrhœa (p. 224), relates a case in which a violent inflammation of the testicle (*Epididymitis gonorrhoica*) supervened on suppressed gonorrhœa in the case of an officer; the inflammation left the testicle hard and swollen. Nine months after inflammation and suppuration came on with increase of the pains, and a fungous excrescence grew from the testicles which soon reached the size of a goose-egg. All the remedies administered were of no avail, and the fungus was removed by ligature.—*Mayrhofer.*

rial after-treatment, but notwithstanding this, the occasional ulcers did not cease to appear. Three years after he exposed himself to a second contagion and was treated by Attomyr. In the beginning, five very flat, confluent ulcers were to be distinguished. A week later there where ten chancres, which appeared, remarkably enough, upon the identical spots where the spontaneous eruptions had been. In the fifth week of the treatment, a chancre appeared on the external surface of the prepuce, which became covered as before with a slight loose crust. The whole eleven became raised instead of becoming deeper, and suppurated so profusely for full seven weeks that the patient wasted.

At first Attomyr prescribed one drop *Merc. sol. Hahn.* 4 each day, and because of the upward growth of the chancres, one dose of *Acid. nit.* 4 daily, for three weeks. As the suppuration did not diminish, however, though the ulcers looked very clean, the patient had *Thuja* 3 one drop, at first twice a day, then once a day, and finally every other day: the ulcers now healed perfectly. The whole treatment lasted nine weeks.—(*Archiv für hom. Heilk.* B. 29, H. 2, s. 162 et seq.)

B.

Verrucae, Warts.

Thuja creates warts in those constitutions which are disposed to cutaneous excrescences, and must, therefore, under the proper conditions, possess the power of curing them. The therapeutic indications and conditions in this relation are: broad base, conical form, superficial seat in the skin, cracked, mulberry-like surface, simultaneous presence of other symptoms indicating Thuja. Warts, which appear after chronic gonorrhœa, in the most diverse parts of the body, yield without a struggle under the curative power of Thuja.

1. Dr. Frank of Osterode, who, fourteen years ago, was troubled with many warts on both hands, which were rubbed with antimonial soap, has had for some years on the left nostril a broad-seated, somewhat movable excrescence, which he often caused to bleed by pulling, upon which an unpedicled wart was developed which reached the size of a large pea. Frank rubbed this a couple of times daily with the tincture of Thuja.

After some days the wart became black, and developed many furrows on its surface. Frank now removed with a knife the chapped surface and left the excrescence alone. This increased again, which Frank had noticed when he first applied the Thuja; but the surface remained smooth, shining, horny and uncracked.

He now again applied the Thuja externally in the manner already stated, and on the very next day the same change took place in the form and color of the excrescence as on the first occasion. He now proceeded less rapidly, moistened the wart several days with Thuja, and then again ceased for a while. The wart became smaller, and in four weeks (including the pauses) the process of destruction was complete and the wart gone.

Dr. Huber* of Linz has observed two cases in which warts have been cured by Thuja.

* Dr. Huber communicates these two cases as *provings*. They are, however, *cures* with excessive action of the remedy, which had been administered in large doses, with an eye to the proving.—*Mayrhofer.*

2. A boy 14 years old, of scrophulous habits, had numerous (30 to 40) warts on his hands, and especially upon the back of his hands. Their size was various, from that of a millet seed to that of a pea. The surface of the smaller was smooth and almost translucent; of the larger roughly marked and cauliflower-like. Their consistence was not hard.

The boy had Thuja 1 on the 6th of October, 1844, with directions to take five drops every evening, and at the same time to wash the warts daily with the tincture of Thuja somewhat diluted. Although he used the remedy with great irregularity, yet on the 17th of November not the slightest trace of a wart was to be seen; the place where they had been, even, was not to be detected by any change in the skin. But during the treatment symptoms arose which we must set down to the account of Thuja: a very severe, twitching, sticking toothache, which came on several days in bed, in the evening, and disappeared every time in a quarter of an hour after a dose of *Cham.* 1; also a dark-red tubercle on the edge of the upper eyelid close to the internal canthus of the right eye. On the 13th of October it was soft, became harder by degrees, on the 18th attained the size of a sweet pea, after some days passed into suppuration, spontaneously separated, discharged much pus, and healed without the aid of art.

3. A girl fourteen years old, with dark hair and eyes, and who had not yet menstruated, had numerous warts on her right hand (20 to 25) which were partly horny like corns, partly less hard and rough upon the surface, partly smooth and small. She had besides on the back of the right forearm near the wrist, a pale-red herpes of the size of a copper Kreuzer, covered with little epidermic scales. She had Thuja internally and externally, at the same time and in the same way as the boy. When she had taken over thirty drops of *Thuja* 1, without experiencing any effect, she omitted the internal employment of the remedy, but used it externally for five weeks. The result was not so gratifying as in the case of the boy. Half of the warts, indeed, disappeared, and those that were left became flatter and less prominent, but they did not entirely disappear.* The cure took place in a twofold manner; in the case of three horny warts the subcutaneous reticular tissue became inflamed, an abscess formed, and on its bursting the skin and wart departed together. The small, smooth and soft warts became by degrees flatter, and entirely disappeared by desquamation of the two concentric cutaneous strata, without leaving a trace of their existence.

Dr. Huber afterwards made a second experiment of a week with the same girl, using internally the first dilution and the tincture. On taking five and eight drops of the tincture on the two last days, the most striking symptom was a tearing *digging pain in the nape*, aggravated by moving the head; in its greatest violence it became furious, and she shrank from pursuing the experiment. This confirmed Dr. Huber in the idea that the pain in the neck which had troubled him during his proving, was truly caused by the drug.

We have no account of any further changes in the warts, nor of the condition of the tetter upon the arm.

4. Dr. Blödau gave *Thuja* 30 against warts in great numbers, succeeded

* Doubtless the horny warts would likewise have entirely disappeared under the continued external and internal use of Thuja. Five weeks were not sufficient to complete the cure.—*Mayrhofer.*

by violent aggravation. A week after he gave a pellet moistened with *Thuja* 30, and four weeks afterwards the warts had all fallen off.—(*Archiv für hom. Heilk.* B. 14, H. 2, s. 107.)

Dr. Gross relates a remarkable case of warts, with an accompanying herpetic eruption.—(*Archiv, &c.* B. 15, H. 3, s. 37 et seq.)

5. A young man of about thirty years old, gave the following account of himself in writing: "I am laboring under an herpetic eruption, which spreads over my whole face. It shows itself, especially after being heated, as red spots, which then throw off white scales, and is accompanied by sticking, burning, and itching. Sometimes the eyelids are entirely covered with it. I have, besides, weakness of the stomach, with acidity and eructation, inflation of the abdomen with flatulence, constipation, with burning itching at the anus, palpitation of the heart, and occasionally pains in the back. When a child I had an eruption on my head, and at fourteen and twenty-one, on my face. At seventeen I perceived little elevations of the skin of my hands, similar to warts, which increased from year to year in size and number. At twenty-five I used some external remedy for them, after which they disappeared; after ten or twelve days, however, re-appeared in this facial herpes, of which, to this day, I cannot get rid. I have already taken tea for purifying the blood, sulphur, graphite, and mercury, but without success. After six weeks' treatment in Carlsbad the tetters disappeared for several months, but have now for a long time been re-instated."

Dr. Gross sent the patient eight doses of *Ars.* 30, with directions to take one every fourth day. After taking these powders, the patient wrote that there was no change in his condition, except that several warts had made their appearance on his hands, but the tetter had not gone. Gross now made choice of *Thuja* (dilution not stated), of which he sent six doses to be taken at intervals of four days. The warts and tetter disappeared together in consequence.

C.

Swellings and Excrescences on the Eyelids.

The general physiological character of Thuja is to create dermatic growth and excrescences, by stimulating the cutaneous system; these may exist upon any part of the body. It also excites pains, irritation, and swelling of the eyelids, suppurating tubercles on the eyelids and brows. Those morbid affections of the eyelids which in ophthalmic medicine are named from their varying forms *Hordeolum, Milium, Chalazium, Verruca,* and *Condyloma*, become proper objects for the action of Thuja, when their special symptoms, or the fundamental sickness of which they are local manifestations, indicate its exhibition.

1. Dr. Bleifuss of Ochsenfurth treated a young lady who had scattered *Hordeola* upon the eyelids.* The conjunctiva was sympathetically affected, and her digestion was disturbed. She sought aid from every quarter, but in vain. *Iodium* even produced no effect, and she began to think of extirpation. Dr. Bleifuss accidentally (! M.) read the symptoms of Thuja recorded by Hahnemann, applied the tincture externally, and beheld, with astonishment, a rapid decrease of the disease. He now exhibited it internally (ten drops several times a day) and effected a perfect cure.

* They appear to have been *Milia* or *Chalazia.*—*Mayrhofer.*

From that time Dr. Bleifuss learned to value Thuja, and subsequently wrought with it other wonderful cures.

"Let us pick," says he, "the grains of wheat out of this homœopathic chaff! they are of excellent service to our therapeutics, as I have frequently had occasion to be convinced." *

D.

Pains in the Limbs.

The arthritic pains which Thuja excites, especially in the limbs, are among the most frequent and most constant of the symptoms during the provings; they never entirely failed to appear in the most unsusceptible and least productive provers.

The special curative indications are, drawing, tensive, tearing, twitching pains, appearing suddenly, confined to one spot or limb, or wandering, aggravation in rest and warmth, amelioration by movement and in the open air, and in feverish conditions, predominant cold with numbness (deadness) of the affected limbs and desponding frame of mind.

Homœopathic literature is still very poor in vouchers for the therapeutic virtues of Thuja in corresponding arthritic affections.

Dr. Mschk relates a single case (*Annal. der hom. Klin.* B. 1. s. 216).

A woman came crying and weeping to him, and begged him to cure her of the violent pain from which she had suffered for a fortnight. The pain was tearing, and extended from the right shoulder to the points of the fingers. She also felt twitching in the muscles, now here, now there, from the top of the shoulder to the middle of the arm: the forearm and index finger were, as it were, dead, the other fingers numb. The pain was most severe on letting the arm hang down; in warmth, especially in bed at night, the tearing and twitching were aggravated, but were better in the cold and on motion. Perspiration produced an amelioration. Chills, with yawning, came on after midnight, and sleep appeared late, and was disturbed by horrible dreams. The patient frequently had tenesmus. She had an evacuation with difficulty every two or three days only, and it was sometimes mixed with blood. To these symptoms were added nocturnal thirst with sensation of cold in the arms, palpitation, and depressed spirits.

The patient had a dose of Thuja 27, with directions to return; which she

* We thank our allopathic colleague for the honorable frankness with which he has announced the source of his new knowledge; he has thus nobly distinguished himself from those physicians of the old school, who, as we have had frequent occasion to remark, secretly appropriate the useful grain from the homœopathic field and openly denounce its whole produce as chaff, or who, dressed in borrowed feathers, go cackling about as though themselves had laid the egg The daily spread of homœopathic dilettantism among allopathic physicians is indeed a most striking indication, on the one hand, of the pharmacological poverty of the old school, and on the other of the therapeutic wealth of the new; for what says the proverb? "The robber is in need, but the robbed has plenty." But we must most solemnly protest against any amalgamation of the physiological pharmacodynamics of the new school with the casuistic pathological materia medica of theold —*Mayrhofer.*

did not do. Her physician accidentally met her, and she excused herself for her neglect by saying, that soon after taking the dose, her pains entirely disappeared, and the other troubles so far vanished that she only felt some weakness in the arm and fingers.

E.

Intermittent Fever.

We have seen that Thuja, in its perfect effects, develops a fever characterised by the predominance of the cold stage, to which sweat immediately succeeds (*Febris algida imperfecta*), coming on mostly in the tvening, seldom in the morning, commonly without thirst, seldom ateended with severe thirst, and manifesting a quotidian or tertian type.

Dr. Herrmann states in his treatise on the homœopathic treatment of intermittents (*Annal. der hom. Klin.* B. 2, s. 398) that in the year 1830, when, by the command of the Emperor Nicholas, he made some homœopathic experiments in a division of the Garde-Central Hospital at Tulzyn in Podolia, the intermittents (which are very prevalent there, as an endemic, and commonly exhibit a very capricious character) during one season of hot and dry weather assumed a very similar type. Thus, the attacks began with cold shiverings, with external and internal chill, in some cases with thirst, were immediately followed, without the intervention of a hot stage, by general perspiration.

In intermittents thus constituted, Thuja (the dose is not stated) effected a rapid cure; but somewhat later, after rain had set in, this remedy proved no longer serviceable.

These are the only cases which we have in relation to the employment of Thuja in intermittent fevers, and judging from the physiological provings, it can but seldom be a specific in that disease.

Besides the cases already enumerated, Thuja promises to be useful in the following affections:

1. In left-sided hemicrania of the fifth pair, especially of the frontal branch, and in cerebral nervous affections, with the sensation as though a nail were driven in, or a convex button pressed upon a particular spot on the head (*clavus hystericus*).
2. In stiffness of the neck, with the feeling as though the muscles were too short, especially if there be present any other symptoms which point to Thuja.
3. In *Varicellæ acuminatæ, verrucosæ*, during the period of suppuration.
4. In muscular twitchings of a rheumatic origin, especially in the limbs, which come on suddenly when at rest, and cease on motion.
5. In amblyopia with mists and flakes before the eyes, when it is attended by symptoms which indicate Thuja.*

* May not Thuja be also specially indicated in chronic catarrh, in ozœna after precipitate cures of gonorrhœa and condylomata, and in obstinate bronchial catarrhs. —*Ed. Oest. Zeit.*

Those physicians who, with Lobethal and others, consider condylomata as constantly and without exception a result of secondary syphilis, and do not allow that they ever appear independently, must, consequently, consider Thuja as one of the remedies for syphilis.

It cannot indeed be denied that the symptoms which Thuja develops in the sexual, glandular, and cutaneous systems present similarities to the phenomena of secondary syphilis; but this drug has not produced in a single prover ulcerative sickness and peculiar sores, as mercury excites them. We cannot, then, attribute to Thuja any special therapeutic power in primary syphilis, and homœopathic literature has as yet no cases to show of chancre cured by its means.

F.

Cures in cases of Animals.

Homœopathy proves itself true, not only in the cure of men, but also in that of animals; and she receives great commendation both from cattle doctors and cattle owners, for the three virtues of *simplicity*, *effectiveness*, and *cheapness*.

Physiological provings of Thuja on animals, are as yet wholly wanting; still this admirable remedy, from its property of exciting warts and cutaneous excrescences, has been used in analogous diseases in veterinary medicine.

1. *Horses.*—The tincture of the *arbor vitæ* has been used by veterinary physicians with the best results in grease, which is related to sycosis in this, that if the disease be neglected, warty excrescences form in the fetlock, which bleed easily, and, like condylomata, secrete an offensive fluid (*Dr. Elwert*, *Hygea*, B. 19, s. 415).

Thuja has also testified its power in the cure of warts in horses, which arise in various spots, especially in the neighborhood of the ears, eyes and nose, if these excrescences exhibit a rough, split, cauliflower-like surface, and, like condylomata, bleed easily, are moist and suppurating.

Oberamtmann Kleeman cured a horse, within three weeks, of warts, which he had had for several years on the head and chaps, with a few doses of Thuja 2 and 15 (*Archiv für. hom. Heilk.* B. 14, H. 2, s. 108).

2. *Cattle.*—Warty excrescences often appear in great numbers, and of various sizes, upon the udders of cows.

Thuja has been exhibited in case of these warts with success, when it was indicated by their character.

According to Dr. Schindler, Thuja perfectly cured five very similar cases of warts in cows, whose udders were entirely covered with the excrescences (*Archiv für hom. Heilk.* B. 14, H. 2, s. 108).

3. *Dogs.*—Dogs are not unfrequently affected with mulberry-like, moist, easily bleeding warts, which sometimes cover the whole naked

inner surface of the ears, in the form of a cauliflower, or arise in the cavity of the mouth, and greatly resemble condylomata.

Dr. Wachtel observed the following case: a little, two months old, male pup (wolf dog) got, without any known cause, near the anterior border of the tongue, a fleshy excrescence of the size and shape of a hemp-seed, which, in eight weeks increased to the size and form of a mulberry. On the inner surface of the mouth also, fleshy cauliflower-like excrescences were visible, thickly sowed on both sides. He was sprightly, and well, but took food and drink with difficulty.

From the striking similarity of these excrescences to condylomata, Wachtel attempted to cure them with Thuja, and caused the whole of the warts to be painted twice a day with the tincture.

During the first eight days no change could be perceived in the excrescences, except that they grew no more. On the twelfth day, little cracks showed themselves on their surfaces, which occasionally bled. From the sixteenth day on, small pieces separated by degrees, dried, and fell off. At the end of four weeks, his mouth was clean and every trace of an excrescence was gone.

CHAPTER VII.

Essay toward a theory of the operation of Thuja.

Dr. Huber is the only one of the provers of Thuja who has communicated his views on the subject. They are *verbatim* as follows.

"The head, muscles of the nape, and the genitals were the points upon which the force of Thuja was especially expended in me. It seems equally to affect the systemic solids and fluids. It seems to create in the blood a peculiar condition whereby it, through increased innervation, acquires the disposition to excite the vitality of the reticular tissue (especially the subcutaneous and intermuscular) in the form of increased warmth, congestion, and swelling (*inflammatio*), and to form there products which appear in the provings partly as excrescences (tubercles) and partly as suppurating exsudations. Among the solids, it is the sensitive portion of the nervous system the activity of which is increased by Thuja. The *plexus cœliacus and hypogastricus* of the ganglionic system receive the first impression, which by means of the sympathetic is reflected on one hand, upon the *trigeminus*, and on the other, upon the sensitive nerves of the spinal marrow, especially upon those of the neck and sexual organs (*nervus pudendus communis*). But since these nerves are for the most part distributed to and ramify in the subcutaneous and intermuscular reticular tissue, their increased activity can only be considered as heightening the vitality of that portion of the organism. The sanguineous condition produced by Thuja seems to bear the same proportion to the increased nervous influence as the disposition does to the noxious cause (*causa occasionalis*). If then Thuja possesses the power not only of changing the blood but also of increasing the vitality of the nervous and reticular systems, why should it not be endowed with the faculty of curing excrescences of various kinds, such as warts, condylomata, and other spurious growths* which are plainly founded upon conditions such as those we have stated. The fundamental operation of Thuja therefore *appears to depend upon a peculiar condition of the blood, and on an excitement of the vitality of the sensitive, nervous, and reticular systems.*"

We may be allowed to remark that a theory founded upon the results of a single proving must necessarily be one-sided. It is only by means of an association of provers that the whole sphere of operation of a remedy, in all its breadth and depth, can be developed, and the theory of the operation of drugs must stand upon a statistical foundation. The single prover develops only isolated portions of the full operative sphere of the remedy.

The effects upon the sanguineous and nervous systems together, are exhibited by every drug in common with Thuja, and you may have as many "conditions of the blood" as you have drugs; for every intoxication passes into the blood.

Our own view of the matter is this, that *the general physiological effect of Thuja is irritation of, and increase of, vitality in the system of the tissues;* causing, in *fibro-serous* membranes, *wandering arthritic* pains; in *mucous* membranes (uro-genital apparatus and air passages, *Ed.*), increased and altered secretion, and upon the *external skin*, warty excrescences. The *trigeminus*, the *plexus cervicalis* and *pudendo-hæmorrhoidalis* are especially attacked; hence the most important specific symptoms of Thuja are developed in those provinces and organs which are supplied by these nerves and their ramifications.

CHAPTER VIII.

Dose, Duration of Action, Allied Remedies, and Antidote.

Dose.—On this subject Hahnemann has recommended the 30th dilution as the highest dynamic potence, and the undiluted tincture as the lowest material dose, so that here we have the most refined dynamism and the grossest materialism standing in conjunction. The employment of the high potencies is declared to be sufficient in simple cases of recent origin, and that of the mother tincture to be necessary in severe ones of long standing (though only in external applications). In this extensive therapeutic scale we have, on the one hand, the proof that Hahnemann had departed from his decreed normal dose of the decillionth (of which fact many examples are to be found in the second edition of the *Materia Medica Pura*), and on the other, the information for those opponents of Homœopathy who in some incomprehensible manner, place its essence in the smallness of the doses instead of in the principle of similarity, that cures performed with the tincture of a specific remedy are still homœopathically wrought.

* Thuja cures warts, condylomata, and such spurious growths, for the simple reason that it actually creates *similar* excrescences.—*Mayrhofer.*

We repeat here what we have heretofore said in relation to posology (*Hygea* B. 19, s. 215): "The relation between irritability, and the size of the dose, is different in different individuals, and in different diseases, and the sliding scale of doses must go parallel with this varying standard."

The individualisation of the *quale* and *quantum* of a drug must be reciprocally regulated, and the practising physician must be permitted the discretion of ascending or descending the therapeutic ladder, according to the exigency of the special case in hand.

For the practical man, the sole effective cure of disease lies neither in the seventh heaven of the high potencies,* nor in the lowest hell of the mother tinctures, but the maxim, "*medium tenuere beati*," has its full value here also.

According to our own experience, the first dilution of Thuja, (10: 90.) corresponds to the larger part of patients and diseases; still there are subjects who manifest so much sensibility to the action of Thuja that they tolerate only high and infrequent doses, while with torpid individuals and in neglected cases, the external and internal employment of the tincture is frequently necessary for a considerable length of time.

Duration of Action.—The course of the Thuja sickness like that of all other drug diseases, is partly of an acute and partly of a chronic sort.

Many of the symptoms, especially those of the *primæ viæ*, which come on immediately after the dose, disappear again in a short time. The nervous affections and pains of Thuja extend over a longer period, on account of their frequently recurring at irregular intervals of hours, days, and weeks, and the objective products run a chronic course, sometimes of weeks and months, as the provings have shown. In this relation we must rank Thuja rather among the chronic remedies.

As to the repetition of the dose, we may here also rely upon the maxim that, regularly, in acute diseases stronger and more frequent doses are required, (repeated in from two to three hours,) and that in chronic cases, higher and less frequent doses will answer (at intervals of one, two or three days). Torpid subjects bear strong and repeated doses, while erethic constitutions need but little medication.

Allied remedies.—The nearest neighbors of Thuja in reference to the urinary organs are, *Cannabis*, *Petroselinum*, *Copaiba-balsam*, *Cantharides*, *Pulsatilla*, and *Mercury*. *Hemp* is useful in acute gonorrhœas, with a thin, very copious discharge, and very painful urination. *Par-*

* Without wishing to dispute the possible efficaciousness of the so-called high potencies, I wish merely to suggest the following doubts:

1. The high potencies appear to possess virtue, only when they are freshly prepared.

2. Their preservation must be watched over with the greatest caution and fear of depotentising (two very uncertain particulars both for doctor and patient).

3. The high potencies carry the materia medica into the metaphysical region of the world of shadows and of spirits, a most dangerous circumstance not only in reference to our opponents, who believe nothing without proof from physics, but also in reference to the science itself which has a solid foundation.—***Mayrhofer.***

sley is only serviceable in slight cases, with constant urgency to urinate, and *Copaiba* corresponds to blennorrhœas, whose chronic course is attended by torpidity of the mucous membrane. *Cantharides* are indicated in cases of decided inflammation of the urinary organs and hæmaturia. *Pulsatilla* is indicated in gonorrhœas characterised by the passage of urine in drops, or by affections of the testicles. These remedies are effective and curative, especially in irritation of the urinary apparatus, arising from rheumatic, mechanical, and chemical causes. Our choice falls upon *Mercury*, when gonorrhœa is combined with chancre.

Farther removed we have *Acid. nit.*, *Alum.*, *Capsic.*, *Cubebs.*, *Nat. mur.*, *Petrol.*, *Sab.*, *Sepia.*, *Sulph.*, which are especially indicated in those gonorrhœas which have become chronic or complicated with dyscrasic and drug diseases, and must be selected according to the peculiarities of the accompanying symptoms.

In blennorrhœas, however, arising from contagion and accompanied by condylomata, *Thuja* is, and remains the master remedy, as *Mercury* is in urethral chancres. In sycotic conditions, *Sabina* and *Lycopodium* come next to Thuja; Sabina frequently effects the cure of condylomata alone, often completes it after Thuja, and these two remedies seem even to take higher rank than Thuja, in cases of solitary, dry, whitish and pedunculated condylomata. For the employment of *Acid. nit.*, which Hahnemann recommends in alternation with Thuja, in condylomata of long standing, two grounds may be stated: 1, its physiological relation to the urinary organs, and 2, its antidotal power to Mercury in gonorrhœas and condylomata, which have been treated and maltreated with Mercury in allopathic doses. Nitric acid is also, according to our experience, a very valuable remedy in urethral strictures, which are manifested by spasmodic urination and vesical blennorrhœa. In the common warts which appear upon the hand, the nearest allied remedies are *Rhus* and *Dulcamara*. Further removed, *Caust.* in those which are inflamed and painful, *Lycop.* in those which are pedunculated, and *Calc.* and *Sulph.* in those which are accompanied by chronic eruptions.

Antidote.—Hahnemann gives *Camph.* as the antidote to Thuja, which, with *Coffee*, stand, though not in antidotal yet in palliative relation to the most of the vegetable remedies.

We know of no cases of poisoning by Thuja, and none happened in the course of our provings, although some of the provers went great lengths, among whom Prof. Zlatarovich stands distinguished as the boldest Thujophagite. They would be mitigated by drinking warm milk or mild oil.

To isolated manifestations of the Thuja sickness, several remedies are antidotal. *Cham.* removes the nocturnal twitching toothache; *Cocc.* appears to be serviceable in the acute fever of Thuja,* and *Merc.* to alleviate the affections which appear at night.

* See Zlatarovich's provings of Thuja upon an adult female.

The best antidote, however, is the administration of higher and less frequent doses of the remedy, when it has excited excessive effects in constitutions susceptible to the action of the drug.

APPENDIX.

Are Gonorrhœa and Chancre results of the same disease?

Since the discovery of syphilis, more than three hundred years ago, two thousand works have been written by physicians on these sin-born scourges of the human race, and it might be thought that in this superabundant wealth of the literature of syphilis all important questions in relation to the subject treated of, would have been exhausted. But it is not so. Not only is the veil which covers the origin of the disease still unremoved, but the very weighty question whether gonorrhœa and chancre are identical or different morbid processes, is as yet unsettled.

A few physicians and authors, as *Bell*, *Autenrieth*, *Ritter*, *Haase*, and others, distinguished gonorrhœa from chancre as independent forms of disease, which were, however, capable of existing together; but the greater number of the Æsculapian priesthood consider them as only two varieties of the same disorder, syphilis. This floating controversy was blown into a flame anew by Hahnemann's categorical assertion, that syphilis and sycosis are two entirely different miasmatic diseases; and that spirit of contradiction which leads the old school, in order to affirm its own existence, to deny everything that Hahnemann has said, fell also with grim violence upon this tenet of the therapeutic reformer.

The old school, as the universally generalising system, holds to the view that the blennorrhagic process of gonorrhœa and the ulcerative process of chancre are only modifications of one and the same fundamental disease, syphilis; while the new school, as the individualising method, cannot agree to the identification of the two maladies.

The advocates of the identity theory found their belief upon the following grounds:

1. Gonorrhœa and chancre are communicated by means of a fixed contagium.
2. They both frequently appear in the same subject and at the same time.
3. According to Hunter and Harrison's experiments in inoculation, the gonorrhœal discharge excites chancre, and chancrous pus produces gonorrhœa.
4. Gonorrhœa and chancre differ only because of the different organisation of the tissue attacked. If the contagion falls upon the mucous membrane of the Urethra, *blennorrhœa virulenta* (*syphilitica*) appears, but if it fall upon the sexual parts, it is succeeded by *ulceratio syphilitica.*

5. Gonorhœa is the milder, chancre the more virulent form of syphilis.

6. Constitutional symptoms may follow simple gonorrhœa as well as chancre.

7. Among several persons who have received the contagion from one and the same individual, some will have gonorrhœa, and some chancre.

The defenders of the essential distinction between gonorrhœa and chancre rely upon historic, nosographic, and therapeutic grounds.

1. On the first appearance of syphilis in Italy, in 1494, contagious gonorrhœa (*blennorrhœa virulenta*) was still entirely unknown. The writers on syphilis during the first decennia do not describe the urethral discharge; even Vigo, who had spent ten years on his work upon syphilis, was not then acquainted with gonorrhœa. *Blennorrhœa urethræ virulenta* was first observed and described by the physician *Antonius Musa Brassavolus*, thirty-nine years after the eruption of chancre, and his pupil *Gabriel Follopius* affirms, in his work (*De morbo Gal. Patavii*, 1563), that the urethral discharge was a more recent disease than syphilis, and had been entirely unknown before it was observed and described by his master.

2. Hahnemann states (Chron. Krank. 2. Auf. B. 1, s. 104) that sycosis, under which appellation he includes not only condylomata with and without gonorrhœa, but also the contagious, virulent, urethral discharge without the so-called excrescences, has only raged from time to time, and was extensively disseminated as an epidemic, especially during the French war from 1809 to 1814; since which, however, it has continued to manifest itself less and less frequently.

3. Hunter and Harrison's trivial experiments have not only not been confirmed on a more careful repetition, but have been wholly refuted by the numerous and standard experiments of Ricord in inoculating with pus from gonorrhœa and from chancre. No chancre pustule is excited by inoculation with gonorrhœal pus either on the external skin nor on the mucous membrane; while chancre causes chancre both upon the external skin and mucous membrane. Inoculation was so performed upon a patient who had both gonorrhœal and primary chancre, that one thigh received the gonorrhœal virus and the other the chancrous; the last only developed a chancre pustule, the other did not.—(*See Ricord.*)

4. If chancrous matter could develop gonorrhœa, and gonorrhacel virus, chancre, gonorrhœa and chancre should almost always appear together, for in *blennorrhœa virulenta* the glans and prepuce (the common situations of chancre in man) must necessarily be fouled with the discharge, and in the same manner the pus from a chancre must inevitably be brought in contact with the mucous membrane, especially in women. Besides, from pretended observations that gonorrhœa has caused chancre by infection, and chancre in another subject gonorrhœa, we cannot exclude the possibility of deception: because urethral chancre may

be easily mistaken for gonorrhœa, and give rise to false observations, while in fact the chancre has only given rise to its like.

5. Chancre and gonorrhœa depend upon pathological conditions which are altogether diverse. Chancre is an ulcerative process, healing with loss of substance; gonorrhœa is a blennorrhagic process, heeling without destruction or loss of organic matter.

6. Both the acute and chronic sequelæ of gonorrhœa and chancre are different—The suppression of acute gonorrhœa excites again acute forms; as, *epididymitis, cystitis gonorrhoica, ophthalmia blennorrhoica*, and, according to Ritter, *synocha cum deliriis furibundis.* But on the premature destruction of the primary chancre the symptoms of secondary syphilis make their appearance.

7. Syphilis affects exclusively the human race, while sycosis under various forms appears likewise in animals.

8. The most effectual though not sole specific against chancre is mercury, while in gonorrhœa it is far surpassed in efficiency by other remedies, which fact does not agree with Hufeland's view (*Enchiridion Aufl.* 5, s. 495), who lays it down that the gonorrhœal and chancrous virus are products of the one syphilitic contagion, but that the blennorrhagic infection is the milder of the two; for we cannot understand how a remedy, which is powerful enough to subdue the more deadly virus, should be too weak for the milder form of the same poison. That distinguished authority upon syphilis, Louvrier, states as follows, in his monograph on that disease (page 51), "Mercurial remedies, in whatever form they may be administered, are useless and injurious in simple gonorrhœa; useless, because gonorrhœa is not a (general) venereal disease, and experience has shown that that disease, when combined with gonorrhœa, has been cured with mercury, but that the gonorrhœa still continued after the cure; injurious, because by the administration of mercury increased disease of the affected parts, in the form of renewed inflammation and interruption of the gonorrhœal discharge, is not unfrequently produced."

"As to condylomata, which have appeared after gonorrhœa, the patient may be salivated into marasmus, and there they will remain unchanged; but should they have succeeded to chancre, they readily vanish under the ordinary mercurial treatment. This is a truth, of which every physician, experienced in the treatment of this disease, is well aware, and which I have a hundred times found confirmed in my practice. We should therefore minutely inquire whether gonorrhœa or chancre has been the predecessor of the condylomata." *

9. The chronic sequelæ of gonorrhœa are essentially different from the symptoms of secondary syphilis.

Ritter describes them under the name of lingering gonorrhœa, and divides it into three degrees or stages.

* This categorical opinion of Louvrier leaves no room for doubt but that two different diseases may lie at the foundation of condylomata.—*Mayrhofer.*

First Stage.—This is characterised by itching on the hairy portions of the genitals, which, by degrees, becomes intolerable, is most violent in the evening and night, is increased by warmth and covering, and irresistibly compels the patient to scratch. As the itching diminishes, an itching sticking comes on in isolated circumscribed spots on the genitals, and after scratching, numerous moist points appear about the roots of the hair, which change in from twelve to twenty-four hours into dark brown or black scabs and easily fall off. This scene is re-enacted almost every day. Similar points even appear on the border of the navel with itching; later they make their appearance also on the perinæum and on the thighs, in the neighborhood of the sexual organs. In the female sex, the pain of the tormenting itching is greater and the discharge of lymph more considerable. The hairs themselves are not painful either upon the head or upon the genitals, and the alopecia peculiar to chancre never follows.

At the same time or later pear-shaped warts appear on the female patients, which occasionally itch, and when excised immediately return. Men most commonly do not exhibit these warts; but yellowish-white shining grains of the size of fine barley appear upon the scrotum, which do not itch, but disappear again unnoticed.

After some weeks or months an elastic tubercle appears upon the inner side of the inner lip exactly over the labial artery, under which the artery pulsates briskly every evening. Sometimes a spot appears on the under lip which looks inflamed, burns somewhat, and shows the bluish white epithelium in some cracks; this scales off in three or four days, and is immediately replaced by another. This symptom is frequently repeated at intervals of weeks or months, always in the same way. The urethra, so far as the eye can reach, is affected with whitish spots, which are but little painful, have here and there a depression, feel somewhat callous, and show the mucous membrane still unaffected. Similar spots appear in the female sex in various parts of the internal sexual organs.

Second Stage.—After a certain time, pressing in one or more of the articular extremities of different bones comes on in the evening, until the patient goes to sleep, which may be absent again for days, weeks, and months. The bones most frequently attacked are the sternal extremities of the clavicles, the end of the radius, the ribs, and the tibia. The periosteum is inflamed, and the painful spots are swollen; but the pains never appear in the middle of the hollow bones. Copious, deep-seated, hardish tubercles are perceptible to the touch on the inner surface of the lips and cheeks, and afterward in the soft palate. A particularly painful spot appears from time to time in the concha of one of the ears, or a slight inflammation is developed in the external ear. Permanent little erosions of a whitish blue tint form upon the lips or cheeks, sometimes on the tongue and palate, and the epidermis repeatedly scales off from various spots on the scalp. Cracks and fissures (*Rhagades*) arise in the soles of the feet, oftener in the palms of the hands, which are for the most part dry, less frequently moist, and a transverse crack of an inch in length frequently forms in the neck opposite the atlantic articulation, which discharges, and commonly closes spontaneously. Isolated, dark red, inflammatory spots, of the size of a pea, hard to the touch, come to light upon the breast, back, shoulders, arms, and thighs, and occasionally in the conchæ; they suppurate at the point, and leave behind elevated dark-red nodosities upon the skin which only disappear after months. Small reddish-brown spots appear likewise upon the elbow-joint, remain a few days, then suddenly disappear, and frequently return in the course of the disease. During this time the spots already alluded to in the urethra become gradually larger, their callosity increases, the depressions enlarge by the circumference, and erosions appear, which however result in very slight loss of substance. In fact, pus or offensive fluid is not secreted from these points; they are most frequently dry, or covered with a moisture which rather resembles healthy mucus than a morbid secretion.

These superficial erosions have been improperly called primary gonorrhœal ulcers. Sensibility is rather diminished than increased in these affected spots; urination is neither difficult nor painful; only toward evening or after coitus a very unpleasant pressing manifests itself in the urethra. At the same time or later than these mostly chronic erosions in the urethra, similar, entirely painless erosions are observed upon the lips and cheeks, seldom in the nostrils, the color of which borders rather upon blue than white. These may last a long while without sensibly increasing in size, and they never corrode deeply with any material loss of substance.

A periodical itching of the scalp, obliging the patient to scratch, is also often perceived, and a thick moisture exudes and forms little crusts, which after a few days fall off. The herpetic eruptions which are added, though not always, to the already described symptoms, are more considerable and more troublesome; they may appear on various parts of the body, but principally affect the dorsa of the hands. This herpes surpasses all the other symptoms of this disease in obstinacy, and in spite of every remedy has been observed in a patient for thirty years. It is almost always dry, seldom causes violent itching, frequently removes the epidermis and never forms scales.

The general health is still but little affected, all the vital functions are normally performed, and the glandular system is not perceptibly sympathetically affected.

The chronic gonorrhœa now under consideration never appears without erosions in the urethra, and the urethral callosities, strictures, caruncles and fistulas, which frequently arise as sequelæ of chronic, neglected or maltreated gonorrhœa, only so far belong to the lingering gonorrhœa as they are accompanied by its other symptoms. The eyes and lungs are occasionally affected in the subsequent course of the disease. The symptoms of the eyes are commonly like those of a chronic rheumatic ophthalmia, and the affection of the lungs resembles a neglected catarrh.

Sometimes the knee swells and becomes stiff and painful.* All these symptoms may continue for years, and creep on with a scarcely observable progress for the worse until the disease in a few cases reaches its highest development.

Third Stage.—This is distinguished by the formation of spurious products, preceded in the commencement by pains which indicate a mechanical compression in the abdomen. These spurious growths are tallowy concretions, whitish or yellowish in color, sometimes of a harder, sometimes of a softer jelly-like consistence, are enveloped in membranes, and when they lie superficially, sometimes pass into suppuration. They are sometimes situated externally on the neck or chest, sometimes internally, where they may appear in any of the intestines, e. g., in the omentum and mesentery, in the liver and pancreas, in the lungs and kidneys, &c., and in the female sex frequently in the ovaries. Occasionally only isolated or a few large growths are found in the abdomen or in the neighborhood of the clavicles.

The grouped parasites which are frequently arranged like a rosary, are from the size of a pea, to that of an egg, when they resemble a potato tubercle. The solitary ones may attain an enormous size. In the female sex, a round elastic swelling sometimes appears in the uterine region, which finally bursts (by a violent commotion) and discharges its purulent contents through the vagina, but fills again by degrees, and again, at the proper time, discharges.† The menstrual function is irregularly performed, and a mild, moderate leucorrhœa appears from time to time.

With the appearance of the tallowy concretions (Steatomata), the patient becomes ill-humored and indifferent to every thing which had formerly given him pleasure; he seeks solitude; his face assumes a hectic appearance; his sleep departs, and lingering fever, dreadful prostration, and death, close the scene. Less frequently the disease simulates the form of an *angina pectoris.* The patient at first feels oppression of the chest, then attacks of pain when walking, and cramps in the chest at midnight, which end with syncope. All the functions fall into disorder, and he dies in one of the nocturnal asthmatic attacks, and the autopsy shows the spurious growth already described.

Such are the essential characteristic marks attributed by Ritter to the chronic gonorrhœa, which he made the object of his especial researches for five and thirty years. They led him to the painful conclusion that this disease, considered identical with syphilis, was incurable, and that

* This elastic swelling of the knee is called by the English "*white swelling.*" Many physicians consider this articular rheumatism as a consequence of the administration of balsam of copaiba for gonorrhœa, but Cumano (*Syphilid.* B. 5, s. 461) considers it as a metastasis entirely analogous to a gonorrhœal ophthalmia.—*Mayrhofer.*

† I have known a similar case myself.—*Mayrhofer.*

its course, though long and lingering, was not to be stayed.* (See Ritter's exposition of the apparent similarity, and essential difference, between chancre and gonorrhœa, Leipz. 1819.)

We annex to this lengthened description of Ritter's, the short and comprehensive account of Hahnemann.

Sycosis, which lately, especially during the French war, from 1809 to 1814, was widely spread, but has since showed itself continually on the decrease, was almost always fruitlessly and injuriously treated, by the internal use of mercury (because it was thought to be identical with the venereal chancre); the excrescences on the genital parts, on the contrary, which commonly, though not always, appear several days, or perhaps some and even many weeks, after contagion received by coitus, under a discharge of a sort of gonorrhœa from the urethra, seldom dry and warty, more frequently soft, fungous, and distilling a peculiar, sweetish moisture almost as offensive as herring pickle, bleeding easily, having the shape of a cockscomb or cauliflower, in man upon the glans, or on or under the prepuce, but in woman occupying the neighborhood of the pudenda, and even the pudenda themselves in great number, have been, until now, destroyed by allopathic physicians, by the most violent external treatment, by cauterising, burning, excising, or the ligature. The natural consequence of this was, that they generally returned, or if they suffered themselves to be thus annihilated, the sycotic affection being deprived of the vicarious local symptom of the internal evil, now appeared after another and worse manner, in secondary affections. Thus neither by the external destruction of the excrescences, nor by the internal use of a remedy not indicated, mercury, was the miasm in the least diminished in its control over the whole organism. Besides the undermining of the general health by means of the noxious use of mercury, generally administered in the largest doses, and in the most virulent preparations, similar excrescences break out on other parts of the body, either whitish fungous, sensitive, flat elevations in the cavity of the mouth, on the tongue, palate, and lips, or large, elevated, brown, dry tubercles in the axillæ, external neck, scalp, etc.,—or, otherwise, other bodily sufferings come on, of which I will only mention, the contraction of the flexor tendons, especially of the fingers. (*Chron. Krank.*, 2. *Aufl.* B. 1, s. 104, 105.)

* We give this descriptive portrait of gonorrhœa, with the remark that the copious symptoms are brought together from the observation of many different cases, and that in individual patients only individual parts of the description will be applicable—according to the proverb, "*non omnia adsunt in omnibus.*" Single cases of the form of disease here described with such accuracy, have undoubtedly occurred to every practitioner, and we recommend to the further examination and impartial investigation of our colleagues, this, in our opinion, most important matter. We ourselves, in fault of sufficiently extensive experience, can form no decided opinion whether the chronic disease, described by Ritter, is the natural and necessary consequence of an uncured gonorrhœa, or a variety of blennorrhœa, caused by a vitiated state of the blood, or, still further, a combination of sycosis and hydrargyrosis, consequent upon mercurial treatment.—*Mayrhofer.*

We add now, to complete the triad, Autenrieth's communication on scrofulous gonorrhœa (*Tubingen Blätter* B. I. H. 2, s. 187, *et seq.*), which confirms Ritter's observations on the spurious growths standing in causal connection with gonorrhœa.

Autenrieth describes with accuracy the spurious organisations referred to, without its having been possible for him to have known of Ritter's experience, and his remarks upon the sequelæ of gonorrhœa agree with Ritter's description.

"Gonorrhœa has the peculiar property of producing only *one* local disease at a time; if this cease, immediately another local affection appears in another place. In men, sarcocele often appears; in women, degeneration of the ovaries. Gonorrhœa is nearer allied to lepra than to syphilis. The peculiar superficial ulcers of gonorrhœa, with a cancerous appearance, secrete only a watery fluid; and the gonorrhœal poison is in itself incurable, and can only be excreted by nature as long as it is a local disease.*

We have thus extracted and brought together the points of agreement and difference between gonorrhœa and chancre from competent authorities, without expressing a decided opinion upon the question ourselves, in consequence of a deficiency in our private experience. As things stand at present, however we by no means hold the controversy as ripe for judgment, but are convinced that this weighty question will only then receive its scientific solution, to the relief of suffering humanity, through the individualising therapeutics of Homœopathy, in connection with the revelations of pathological anatomy, when opportunity shall be afforded to emancipated Homœopathy to make decisive investigations on the subject by the aid of syphilitic cliniques.

In reference to the treatment of gonorrhœa, we can neither admit the absolute incurableness of the malady with Autenrieth and Ritter (allopathically), nor its absolute curability with Hahnemann (homœopathically).

In choosing a specific remedy, two considerations must be borne in mind; 1, the most accurate estimation of the entire symptoms of the disease; 2, the minutest examination of the history of the disease in reference to the origin of the affection, its previous treatment, and the at present existing dyscrasic complications.

Thuja is the chief remedy in sycotic cases, in alternation with nitric acid, where mercurial treatment has been resorted to. Obstinate tetters indicate *Nat. mur.* and *Lycop;* if itch have preceded, *Sulph.* and *Hepar.;* disgust of life points to *Aur.;* scrotal herpes to *Rhus.* and *Arsen.* A radical cure, in fine, is only to be obtained from a so-called antipsoric treatment, conducted with the closest individualisation of the malady of the patient and of the remedies prescribed.

* Compare, on this subject, the ideas of *Eisenmann, Schönlein, Timon* and *Jahn* in the *Versuch. für die prakt. Heilk.* (*Eisen.* 1835, s. 84–107.) "*Bemerkungen über die Tripperseuche*" *of the latter.—Ed. Œst. Zeit.*

2.—ÆTHUSA-CYNAPIUM.

ÆTHUS. Fool's parsley. *Fr.* Petite cigüe, faux persil, cigüe des marais. *Ger.* Hundspetersilie.

1. *Description and Preparation.*

This remedy belongs to the order *Umbelliferæ.* It is a little annual plant, growing in this country in waste places and by roadsides, from one to two feet high, and much resembling common parsley. Many dangerous accidents have been caused by the similarity. From a taper, whitish root arises an erect branching stem generally stained with purple near the ground, but free from the spots of the *Conium*, and covered with finely cut leaves of a deep glossy green. The whole plant emits a nauseous odor and is very poisonous. The leaves are bi-triternately compound; the ultimate lobes or segments linear-lanceolate; umbels terminal and opposite the leaves, rays very unequal; leaflets of the involucels linear, all on one side; fruit very prominently ribbed and keeled.

The expressed juice of the fresh plant at the time of flowering is used in medicine.

2. *Prior knowledge of its effects.*

Dr. Roth makes the following notes on this subject.

The old school has never made use of this plant as a remedy; it figures only in toxicology, and the accounts given of its effects previous to the eighteenth century are of no service, as it was frequently confounded with *conium-maculatum* and *cicuta-virosa.* For this reason I have made no use of Gmelin's citations (*Hist. venenor. vegetab. Sueviæ indig. Nova acta physico-medic.* 6, 259). The cases related by the following authorities contain nothing of interest: BOERHAAVE (*Acta reg. Loc. hafn. med.* 1, 54); BLAIR (*Pharmacobotanologia*, Lond. 1, 725, p. 122); SCHREBER (*Sammt. versch. Schrift.* 4, 273). Except *Kallenbach's* note cited among the authorities subsequently, no other account of the use of the plant has been published. My own unpublished case is the cure of a scrophulous ophthalmia in a young girl of eighteen. The symptoms are incorporated in the symptomatology. Kallenbach used the sixth dilution. I used the same in a hundred and twenty grammes of vehicle, a spoonful every day for six weeks, without the intervention of any other remedy.

3. *Digest of the Symptoms.*

The following symptomatology is taken from Dr. Roth's *Materia Medic.* 1, 169. He cites the following

AUTHORITIES. **1.** Muller, *Ephemerid. natur. curios.* cent. 10, observ. 52, p. 369. **2.** Trew, *Commerc. littérar. norimberg.* 1731, p. 178. **3.** Rivière, *Hist. de l'Acad. roy. des Sciences de Montpellier*, 1766, 1, 170. **4.** M. V. *Bullet. de Pharm.* 6 année, no 8, p. 339. **5.** Rust, *Magazin für die gesammte Heilk.* 21, 248. **6.** Hartlaub, *Praktische Mittheil.*, 1828, p. 13. **7.** Nenning, ibid. **8.** Wittke, *Hufel. Journ.* 69, 122. **9.** Mayer, *Neue Bresslauer Samml.* 1, 178. **10.** Lallé, *Bulletin de Ferrusac*, 21, 308. **11.** Pétroz, *Bull. de la Soc. hom. de Paris*, 4, 337. **12.** Trinks, *Annal. der hom. Klin.*, 4, 112. **13.** Kallenbach, *Gaz. hom. de Paris*, 1850, no. 9. **14.** Griesselich, *Hygea*, 23, 255. **15.** Roth, *Unpublished Cases.*

The pathogenetic symptoms are in roman letters; the toxicological in *italics*, the curative are denoted by a cypher (°), and the other figures in parentheses refer to the above names.

MIND. **Moral.** Great flow of spirits (6). Flow of spirits, loquacity, facetiousness (11). Gay, in a good humor, in the forenoon; sad and anxious in the afternoon (7). Excess of moral susceptibility (11). **5.** *Very great nervous susceptibility lasting a long while* (4). Sadness when alone (11). The disposition becomes retiring, weeping as in nostalgia (11) Cross and ill-tempered in the afternoon (7). Disposition to impetuousness (11). **10.** Uneasiness, discontent even to grief. **Mental.** Difficulty in fixing his attention (11). Slowness or instability of his ideas, even to absence of thought (11). °Hallucinations. *Delirium; he thinks he sees dogs and cats* (2). **15.** *Delirium; he jumps out of the window* (1). *Stupor* (5). Loss of consciousness or a kind of stupefaction as though something intervened between the organs of sense and exterior objects (11). *Stretched out without consciousness* (8, 9).

HEAD. **Headache.** *Cephalalgia* (3, 5). **20.** *Pains in the head and stupefaction* (3). Throbbing in the head (11). Lancinations and throbbing in the whole head (7). Sensation in the head, as if it were broken (7). Tearing pain in the head (11). **25.** Confusion in the head as though the brain were compressed (7). Confused head during the coryza (11). *Stupefaction; he cannot remain up* (3). Feeling of tension in the head (11). *Vertigo* (5), **30.** Vertigo in the open air (11). Vertigo when seated; increased by making an effort to quit the seat (11). The vertigo comes on more especially towards the middle of the day (11). The head pains are periodic, often co-exist with paleness of the face, trembling in the jaws, pains in the præcordial region (11). The head pains are especially felt on waking; they are readily renewed by a chill; they are diminished by the emission of flatus and cease on going to sleep (11). **Hemicrania.** **35.** Tearings and throbbings in the right half of the head, then lancinations in the left (7). Very painful lancinations and drawings in the left side of the head (7). Twitching in the left half of the head, then lancinations below the left nipple (in a woman), especially painful during an inspiration (7). **Frontal.** *Pains in the sinciput* (9). Violent pains in the sinciput as though it were forcibly compressed at the same time behind and on the vertex (12). **40.** Lancinations in the forehead when turning the head to the right (7). Tension above the root of the nose (11). Tearing pain across the eyes (11). Pain in the eyebrows (11). **Parietal.** Lancinations and throbbings in the right parietal bone (7). **Vertex. 45.** Pain in the vertex (11). Dull pain in the vertex (7). Lancinations and painful throbbings in the vertex, which disappear by rubbing (7). **Temporal.** A rapid tearing thrust in the right temple (7). Lancinations, then throbbings, in the upper part of the left temporal region (7). **50.** Lancinations and violent throbbings in the left temple, disappearing on pressure, but returning as soon as the pressure is removed (7). A lancinating blow in the left temple, then drawings towards the sinciput (7). **Occipital.** Lancinations and throbbings in the upper part of the right occipital bone (7). Rheumatic (tearing) lancination from the occiput forwards (7). A tearing shock which passes across the whole head from the left side of the occiput to the right side of the head (7). **Scalp. 55.** Feeling of contraction of the hairy scalp (11). Inclination of the head to fall backwards (11).

EYES. Lancinations around the eyes and in the orbits (11). Excoriating pain around the eyes (11). Excoriating pain in the eyelids (11) **60.** Uncomfortable sensation around the lids (11). Swelling of the Meibomian glands; gum in the eyes (11) °Scrofulous ophthalmia (15). °Swelling of the Meibomian glands (15). °Chronic inflammation of the edges of the lids (11). **65.** °The edges of the lids are glued together in the morning by a dried matter, which must be softened to prevent its tearing out the lashes (15). Itching in the corners of the eyes (11). Pressure on the eyes (11). Spasm of the eyes (11). Distension of the eyes (11). **70.** *Brilliant injected eyes* (9). °Pustule upon the cornea (11). Pupils much dilated and insensible to light (8). °Incipient amaurosis (11) *Pupils dilated, but sensible to light* (9). **75.** Things look larger and sometimes double (11). *Fixed look* (8, 9). °Chronic photophobia (15) The symptoms of the eyes come on mostly on waking and in the open air (11).

EARS Lancinating pain behind the ears (11) **80.** Sensation of heat escaping from the ear (11). Dryness of the ear; deficiency of cerumen (11). Puriform discharge from the ear (11). °Yellowish discharge from the right ear (14). Troublesome hissing in the ears (11). **85.** Lancinating pain in the ears, from within outwards (11). Lancinations in the right ear from without inwards (6). Lancinations in the right ear disappearing on introducing the finger into the meatus (7). Lancinations in the left ear, with feeling as if something warm were issuing; these lancinations alternate with an analogous lancinating pain in the left costal region (7). Lancinations in the left ear, followed by a slight tearing around the ear extending to the vertex (7). **90.** Pain, at times lancinating, at times tearing in the right ear, which is only slightly relieved by rubbing (7). Touch and pressure ameliorate many of the symptoms of the ear (11).

NOSE. Feeling of pressure on the nose (11). Lancinations on the left side of the nose, then burning pricking on the right side; afterwards, pricking as if from a hot needle on the exterior of the scrobiculus (7). °Herpetic eruption on the end of the nose (11). **95.** Lancination and drawing in the left zygoma; then titillation in the left upper teeth; afterwards violent lancination in the left ear (7). Insipid taste of coryza (11).

FACE. Drawing, tearing pains in the face (11). Transient heat in the face (11). Cold sweat on the face (11). **100.** Sweat on the face (11). *Pale face* (8). *Wan, red face* (9). The countenance looks fatigued (11). Expression of anguish on the countenance (11). **105.** *The features express great anguish and acute pains* (9). Puffing of the face during the menses (11). *The face periodically puffed and spotted with red* (5). °Puffed face, speckled with red spots (15). Little vesicles on the skin of the face (11).

MOUTH. **Lips. 110.** Yellowish spot on the upper lip (11). Crack in the upper lip (11). Tearing in the lower lip extending into the corresponding tooth (which?) (7). Twitching of the muscles around the mouth (11). Sensation of cold on the chin and at the commissure of the lips (11). **Jaws. 115.** Tearings in the lower jaw when standing up (7). Pain in the submaxillary glands (11). **Teeth.** Gnawing sensation in the lower teeth (11). Sort of shocks in the lower teeth (11). **Cavity.** *Buccal cavity dry* (9). **120.** Aphthæ in the mouth (11). **Saliva.** *Flow, of saliva as copious as though she had been mercurialised; it lasted fourteen days* (4). **Tongue.** Feeling as if the tongue were too long (11). *Moist tongue* (9). **Palate and throat.** Lancinating pain in the arch of the palate (11). *Aphthæ and pustules in the throat, which render the state of the patient almost desperate* (11). **125.** Itching in the throat, scraping (11). Redness of the throat (11). Redness and swelling of the velum palati and the neighboring parts; inconvenience so as to threaten suffocation (11). *Heat in the throat* (11).

APPETITE. *Bitter taste* (9). **130.** Taste of cheese in the mouth (11). Salt taste of food (11). Oniony taste (11). Taste difficult to define; it exists before as well as after a meal (11). Want of appetite although the tongue is clean (11). Want of appetite in the evening (11). Want of appetite (5). Burning thirst (4, 9).

STOMACH. **Eructations.** Nausea with depression (11). Eructations of air (7). **140.** Regurgitations which have the taste of the ingesta (7, 11). °Regurgitation of food an hour after the meal (15). Eructations after having drunk (11). Difficult eructations (11). The eructations are ameliorated on lying down (11). **Vomiting. 145.** *Violent vomitings of frothy matter, as white as milk* (8). *Vomiting after the administration of milk* (8). °Intolerance of milk; children return the milk almost as soon as it reaches the stomach, coagulated or not, in the course of ten or fifteen minutes, by a sudden and violent fit of vomiting; they then sink for some minutes, in consequence of weakness, into a drowsy state (13). Vomiting of greenish matter (11). *Copious greenish vomiting* (5). **150.** *Vomitings and diarrhœa* (3). *Vomiting and diarrhœa of greenish mucosity* (9). *Vomiting and diarrhœa of mucosity tinged with blood* (9). *Vomiting and fever* (3). *Vomiting with chill, sweat and weakness* (11). **Stomach. 155.** Painful sensitiveness of the epigastric region (11). *Very violent pains in the stomach* (2). Painful contraction in the stomach (11). Sensation in the stomach as if something were inverted; then feeling of burning which ascends into the chest (7). *Tearing pains in the stomach extending into the œsophagus* (9).

ABDOMEN. **160.** Throbbing in the abdomen (11). Sensation of digging in the abdomen (11). *Abdomen tight and tense* (4). *Abdomen inflated, sensitive, especially in the region of the liver* (9). *Swelling of the abdomen* (2). **165.** °Abdomen large, inflated (15). *Colic pains and diarrhœa* (9). **Hypochondria.** Painful sensitiveness of the hypochondria (11). Lancinations in the right hypochondria and then in the right ear (7). A lancinating thrust in the left hypochondrium, behind; then lancinations in the depth of the left mamma (7). **170.** Continual lancinations in the left hypochondrium with burning, only disappearing, except for a little while, by rubbing (7). Lancinations in the region of the left hypochondrium, which frequently return and are persistent (7). **Umbilicus.** Bubbling as of boiling water in the umbilical region, followed by gripings in the stomach (7). Colic pains about the navel, followed by two soft stools in the morning after having risen (7).

ANUS AND STOOLS. **Anus.** Contraction of the rectum (11). **175.** Sensation of dryness at the anus (11). Feeling of excoriation in the piles (11). Swelling of the hemorrhoids (11). Bleeding hemorrhoids (11). **Stool.** Constipation (11). **180.** °Constipation (14). Stools, consisting of matters imperfectly digested, a short time after a meal or at night (11). Normal stool in the afternoon (7).

URINARY ORGANS. Cutting pain in the bladder (11). **Urine.** Frequent call to urinate (11). **185.** Frequent call to urinate in the night (11). Copious discharge of urine (11). Urine red, discharged with difficulty (11). The urine deposits a white sediment (11).

GENITAL. Lancinating pains in the (female) sexual parts (11). **190.** Itching in the (female) sexual parts (11). Eruption of pimples upon the (female) sexual parts (11). The menstrual blood is watery (11).

RESPIRATORY ORGANS. **Nasal Passages.** Coryza in the morning (11). Coryza in the open air (11). **195.** Coryza, secretion viscid (11). °Nose stopped by very thick mucus (15). Abortive desire of sneezing (11). A single sneeze in the afternoon (!?) (7). Speech almost prevented (11). **200.** Slow speech (11). **Respiration.** Hoarse respiration (11). Hissing respiration (11). Hoarse and hissing respiration, especially when lying on the back (11). *Unobstructed respiration* (9). **205.** *Painful, anxious respiration* (5). *Very difficult respiration* (1). *The respiration is very painful and short* (2). *Great oppression; she breathes with difficulty* (4). **Cough.** Slight cough (11). **210.** Several paroxysms of dry cough in the afternoon (7). Cough with sensation of tickling in the throat (11). Cough with tearing pain in the chest (11). Cough with stunning pain in the head (11). Cough increased when lying down (11). **215.** Cough followed by mucous expectoration (11). Cough with paleness of the face (11). Cough with sweetish taste in the throat (11).

CHEST. Feeling of pressure as though the chest were encircled by a band (11). *Lancinations in the left side of the chest* (5). **220.** A lancinating thrust on the right costal region (7). An acute lancinating thrust in the middle of the chest; then burning in the same spot, so violent that she thinks she shall die, disappearing on external pressure, and returning after (7). **Heart.** *Violent palpitations of the heart* (4). Palpitations which are felt in the head (11). Palpitations with vertigo, headache, agitation (11.) **Breasts.** **225.** Swelling of the mammary glands (11). Isolated pain in the mammary glands (14). *Acute, smarting pain with heat and redness of the breast,* (from external application); *a multitude of phlyctenæ, vesicles filled with lymph, appear on the breasts the next day and discharge a good deal of serous fluid on removing the covering* (4).

BACK. **Neck.** °Swelling of the lymphatic glands of the neck in the form of a string of beads (15). Swelling of the cervical glands (11). **Nape.** **230.** Lancinating stitches in the nape (7). An acute lancinating thrust in the left cervical muscles; then throbbing over the whole body, but particularly on the right side and behind, with feeling of weight (7). **Dorsal.** An acute, lancinating thrust between the scapulæ (7). Feeling of weakness in the back (11). Drawing in the back (11). **235.** Sensation of heat in the back (7). **Lumbar.** Burning as though from a hot needle, first in the left lumbar region, then in the right hypochondrium (7). Lancinations, like pricks, first in the right, then in the left lumbar region (7). A lancinating thrust in the right lumbar region, then sensation of slight pressure (7). Drawings in the left lumbar region when walking, disappearing when seated (7). **Sacrum.** **240.** Burning on the exterior of the sacrum, disappearing on rubbing (7). Feeling of weakness as if paralytic in the sacrum when rising from or turning in the bed, during the motion (11). Stinging as if from a flea on the sacrum (7). Sensation of constriction as though from a screw in the sacrum (7). **Hips.** Griping on the exterior of the right hip (7). **245.** Tension in the right hip, then tearing lancinations in the right ear (7). Lancinations and drawings, extending from the left hip into the thigh (7.)

EXTREMITIES. Cold extremities (3, 8).

UPPER EXTREMITIES. Pains in the sub-axillary glands (11). °Swelling of the axillary glands (11). Arthritic stiffness of the elbow joint(11). Heaviness of the forearm (11). Swelling of the forearm

(11). Lancinating drawing in the middle of the forearm to the carpal joint (7). A lancinating thrust in the inferior extremity of the left ulna (7). **255.** Cramp in the hand (11). Twitchings in the left thumb (7). Formication in the fingers (11). Contraction of the fingers (11). Swelling of the fingers (11).

INFERIOR EXTREMITIES. **260.** Boring pain in the inferior extremities (11). Lancinating tearing pain in the inferior extremities (11). Lancinating and paralytic pain in the inferior extremities (11). Formication, which seems to be in the bones of the lower extremities (11). Lancinations in the upper part of the thigh (7). **265.** Lancinations in the right knee, when standing up (7). Tearing pain deep in the tarsi (7). Lancination in the right heel (7).

SKIN. Burning heat in the skin (11). °Eruptions, itching from heat (11). **270.** Dryness of the skin (11). °Dryness of the skin (11). °Eruption around the joints (11). °Nodosities of the skin (11). Itching from heat (11). **275.** Crawling itching (11). Itching in the parts of the skin most slightly affected; they become swollen (11). A herpetic eruption became very itching from heat, especially in the evening (11). °Tetters bleeding easily (11). *The whole body is blackish blue* (2). **280.** °Anasarca (11).

SLEEP. Sleep without yawnings in the afternoon (7). Sleep disturbed by frequent wakings (11). Sleep hindered by pains in the limbs (11). Sleeps exceedingly well, the first night (7). **285.** Rolling of the eyes during sleep (11). Slight convulsive movements during sleep (11). Frequent waking produced by a sensation of cold (11). Waking followed by several hours of sleeplessness (11). Unquiet dreams (11). **290.** Wearisome dreams, in the morning (11).

FEVER. **Cold.** Chill in the room (11). Chill after having walked in the open air (11). Chill more frequent in the afternoon (11). General coldness during sleep (11). **295.** General coldness (11). Internal coldness (11). Internal coldness sensible to the touch, so violent that he cannot succeed in warming himself, accompanied by somnolence during the whole day (6). Coldness embracing the whole body and which is even perceptible to external touch, without thirst, for two days (6). Redness of the face during the coldness (11). **300.** Horripilation in the open air (11). Horripilation with heat extending over the whole body (11). Painful lassitude, hot breath and jactitation during the horripilation (11). **Heat.** *General heat* (5). General heat (11). **305.** *Heat notably increased* (9). *Complete absence of thirst, notwithstanding the great general heat* (5). Great suffering during the heat (11). **Sweat.** General sweat (11). Sweat on going to sleep (11). **310.** He cannot bear to be uncovered during the sweat (11). **Pulse.** Small, frequent irregular pulse (11). *Rapid, hard, small pulse* (9). *Irregular pulse* (9). *Full, accelerated pulse* (5). **315.** *Imperceptible pulse* (3). *Small and frequent pulse* (3). The febrile symptoms manifest themselves, more especially in the morning, with very great malaise and disposition to delirium, which go off during the sweat (11).

GENERAL. *General malaise* (5). *Great agitation* (3). **320.** *Præcordial anxiety* (1). *Anxiety and depression* (9). *Agitation and very painful distress* (4). Anxiety characterised by a sensation of weight upon the chest (11). Cries of anguish (2). **325.** *Great general weakness* (5). °General weakness of children (13). °Remarkable emaciation of children (13). *Want of power to hold up the head and stand up* (5). *Epileptiform convulsions; thumbs bent inwards, face red, eyes turned downwards, pupils dilated and immovable, milky froth before the mouth, teeth set, pulse compressed, small, hard and frequent, temperature of the skin natural* (8). **330.** *Very violent convulsions followed by death* (9). °Great liability to excoriate the thighs in walking (15). °Great disposition to perspiration on the slightest physical effort (13).

POST-MORTEM APPEARANCES. 1. A blackish serum was found in the stomach; the liver was hard and yellow, the spleen livid, the mouth black; but the abdomen was not inflamed (3).

2. *Case of two children.* One of the bodies exhaled a very strong smell; the other very little. The scalp adhered very closely to the skull, face a little puffed, eyes half closed, pupils a little dilated, jaws set. The tongue was not swollen, but covered with a whitish coat. Upper extremities moveable; inferior stiff; back, chest and extremities covered with a great number of large blotches. The abdomen of one was very much swollen; it was less so in the other, but was green. The vessel of the dura mater contained but little blood; those of the pia mater were engorged. All the sinuses were distended with a black fluid blood. The brain was soft, with red points; lungs normal; right ventricle of the heart filled with black fluid blood. Stomach reddish; upper orifice contracted; that of one of the children still contained milk and fibres of the root, that of the other, only a yellowish mucus. The one only displayed a few red spots; the other very many. There was no proper inflammation in the mouth, palate, œsophagus or stomach. The small intestines were all a little red and filled with gas, the large contained only a little excrement, and were no more inflamed. The liver and spleen were gorged with blood. The duodenum exhibited several spots of a clear yellow, as did the anterior biliary edge, a part of the colon and of the epiploon. The gall bladder was filled with clear, greenish brown bile. The kidneys full of blood, the rapid cooling of the bodies, the slightly advanced stage of putrefaction and the setting of the jaws, which according to some authors are characteristic of paralysis, did not accord with the other results of the autopsy. The author regards the bright yellow color of the parts adjacent to the gall bladder as characteristic of poisoning by *æthusa-cynapium;* he considers that it is not identical with the common discoloration of that region, inasmuch as the bile contained in its natural reservoir was of a brownish green (9).

3. Extensive ecchymoses over the whole surface of the body; inflammation of the stomach and peritonæum; engorgement of the spleen, plethoric state of the lungs and heart. The brain not examined (10).

4. The individual had previously suffered from a chronic gastritis. Extreme emaciation, inflammation of the peritonæum and bowels. Suppuration of the exterior membrane of the stomach; sloughing spots at various points on the small intestines; scirrhous places in the epiploon (10).

---

3. ALCOHOL-SULPHURIS.

ALO-SULPH. Liquor Lampadii; carburet of sulphur; bisulphuret of carbon.

1. *History, Description and Preparation.*

Lampadius, in 1796, while distilling a mixture of pyrites and charcoal, procured a clear liquid in the receiver, which he named *Alcohol-sulphuris*, the alcohol of sulphur. It was at first regarded as a compound of carbon, hydrogen and sulphur, until a more accurate analysis by modern chemists showed that its component parts were one equivalent of carbon and two of sulphur, CS^2. (*Ann. de Chim.*, vols. 42 & 84. *Phil. Trans.*, 1813.)

It is a transparent, colorless, volatile, and inflammable liquid, having a specific gravity (1.272) greater than that of water, but less than that of chloroform, and boiling at 160° Fahr. It has a very pungent taste and a peculiar odor, somewhat ethereal, and yet partaking of that of sulphuretted hydrogen. It is insoluble in water, and being exceedingly volatile, is preserved under the surface of that liquid; it is soluble in alcohol and ether, and in the oils generally. Its solvent powers are somewhat remarkable, as it dissolves rapidly and in considerable quantity, those two rather refractory bodies, sulphur and phosphorus. It produces a great degree of cold by its evaporation, a thermometer having the bulb kept moist by it and placed in an exhausted receiver marking as low as—80° Fahr.

It is prepared by placing small fragments of charcoal in a porcelain tube, bringing it to high red heat, and then slowly passing the vapor of sulphur through the incandescent mass, and conducting the product by means of a glass tube to the bottom of a vessel containing ice-cold water. The liquid is sometimes yellow from excess of sulphur, from which it is to be freed by careful re-distillation at a low temperature. It may be also prepared in Lampadius's method by distilling six parts of yellow iron pyrites with one of charcoal. The vapor, instead of being conducted into water, may be passed through a Liebig's condenser into a receiver, kept at a temperature below freezing by a mixture of ice and salt. (GOMELIN, *Handbuch ;* MITSCHERLICH, *Lehrbuch*)

Its equivalent, according to the hydrogen scale, may be taken as 6+32 = 38.

2. *Prior knowledge of its effects.*

Very little can be gathered from medical writers concerning the use of this remedy. Dr. Roth has collected the following observations.

1. LAMPADIUS, its discoverer, published several clinical experiments undertaken by Dr. Kappe in 1804 (*Ueber den Schwefel-alcohol.* Freyberg, 1832, 2d ed., p. 54), but they are valueless to us, being badly reported, and the drug having always been administered in combination with camphor, volatile liniment or cologne water.

2. DR. WITTICH (*De alcohole sulphuris,* Gættengæ) recommends it against chronic rheumatism, but mixes it with an ammoniacal liniment.

3. DR. SPIELMAN's memoir (*De alcoholis sulphuris virtutibus chimicis et salutaribus,* Marburgi, 1828) has not been examined.

4. DR. KRIMER, of Aix-la-Chapelle (*Hufeland's Journal* 79, p. 32), has used it in asphyxia produced by the vapor of charcoal, in doses of twenty drops every ten minutes. His cure of a white swelling by the internal use of the bisulphuret is not so satisfactory, inasmuch as *conium* was administered at the same time, and baths of wood-ashes employed twice a week. He thinks highly of the remedy dropped slowly on to an incarcerated hernia—it was very speedily rendered capable of reduction.

5. DR. MANSFELD (*Dresdener Zeitschrift* 5, p. 454) recommends it as an emmenagogue, and is followed by others in so doing, but on examining his experiments we find that he used it containing iodine in solution.

6. DR. OTT (*Casper's Wochenschrift,* 1838, No. 13) is also a great admirer of this remedy as efficient against rheumatism; but on reading his cases, the cessation of an articular rheumatism after every sort of treatment for six months, ending with the employment of the bisulphuret of carbon in conjunction with Russian vapor-baths, gives us no great reason to expect very great wonders of the remedy.

7. In addition to the authorities collected by Dr. Roth we may add the following:

"It may not be out of place here to state that I have employed, with great success, the *bisulphuret of carbon* to enlarged, indurated, lymphatic glands. In the first instance I rubbed equal quantities of the bisulphuret and alcohol upon the parts affected, but without any effect upon the glands. But as its effects were so great when its vapor was confined to the eye, I was led to employ it in the form of vapor and by means of glass bottles. By these means I excluded the action of the medicine from the external air, and thereby prevented its speedy evaporation.

When it had been applied about one minute the patient felt the part very cold, but immediately after, a gradual heat, accompanied with great prickling—the heat increasing the longer the medicine was kept in contact with the part, until it could no longer be endured. On removing the glass, the part was red to an extent two or three times greater than the part enclosed. In a few days the change in the size of the glands was very great, and by its daily repetition a complete and speedy removal of the disease was effected. I also find that its action upon diseased glands is more decided if the surface of the skin is well moistened with water previous to the application of the bottle to the part." —(*Mr. Turnbull, in Pharm. Journal*, vol. 2, p. 352.)

3. *Digest of the Symptoms.*

The following symptomatology is translated from Dr. ROTH's *Materia Medica*, vol. 1, p. 441. He cites the following

AUTHORITIES. **1.** KNAF, *Dissert. inaug. med. de liquidi Lampadii virtute medica.* Pragæ, 1835. **2.** BUCHNER, *Augsburg Journal*, 1850, p. 65. **3.** MAD. H., ibid. 67. **4.** HELD, ibid. 69. **5.** ANNA GASBERGER, ibid. 71. **6.** KONINGSHOFER, ibid. 73. **7.** MAD. KONINGSHOFER, ibid. 75. **8.** M. M., ibid. 77. **9.** PRIMBS, ibid. 78. **10.** PEMERL, ibid. 81. **11.** MOSER, ibid. 90. **12.** QUAGLIO, ibid. 92. **13.** VEHSEMAYER, *Leipsig Journal* 6, p. 269.

The pathogenetic symptoms are in roman letters, the toxicological in *italics*, the curative are distinguished by a cypher before them.°

MIND. **Mental.** **1.** Excitement of the intellectual faculties (1). Vivacity of intellect (1). Head confused, difficulty in thinking with acceleration of the pulse (3). Distraction and difficulty of understanding what one is reading (10). **5.** Unfitness for every kind of exertion; somnolence when at work and pressure on the eyes (11). **Moral.** Bad humor, irritability (3). Sad frame of mind, obstinacy (4). Moroseness and disposition to violent anger (4). Transport of passion, rage (10).

HEAD. **Headache in general.** **10.** Slight headache, lasting only two hours (4). Headache when reading (7). Pressive headache (7, 9). Heat in the head and face (9). ° Tearings in the head (5). **15.** Embarrassment of the head (11)—with distraction (10)—as though from spirituous liquors (4). Head confused (1, 6, 7, 9). *Confusion of the head* (5). **20.** Heaviness of the head (1). Vertigo (2). Sudden vertigo (4). Frequent attacks of vertigo when sitting (4). The headache is increased after drinking wine (2). **25.** The morning headache, which had disappeared in the afternoon, returns in the evening (9). **Frontal region.** Slight frontal headache (9). Slight, transitory, frontal pain which gradually approaches the temporal regions (9). Slight pain in the forehead, drawing towards the left parietal and remaining there two hours (9). Sensation of heat and moderate pressure in the forehead, and necessity to wipe it continually with the hand (9). **30.** Embarrassment of the head, lancinations and twitching pain in the forehead (11). Tearing pain in the frontal region lasting several hours and disappearing in the direction of the temples (4). Embarrassment and vertigo in the sinciput (2). Embarrassment and pressure in the sinciput (7). Frontal region confused (3). **35.** *Heat of the forehead* (5). Sensation of pressure in the sinciput (1). Slight pressive frontal headache (9). Embarrassment of the head, slight aching and digging in the forehead (11). Pressure and dull but transitory pain in the forehead all day (11). **40.** Pressive pain in the frontal region stretching towards the temples and some tearings in the same direction (9). Pressive pain in the frontal region, with feeling of heat, lasting two hours (9). Malaise and pressive frontal headache (6). On waking in the morning, slight pressive frontal headache, which soon vanishes (9). Pressive frontal headache, with few interruptions during the whole day, accompanied by transitory attacks of pain in the temples (6). **45.** Dull pressive pain in the forehead, all day (6). Dull pressure in the forehead and temples, with desire to sleep (6). Pressive frontal headache, increased by stooping and reading (7). Drawing and tearing pain stretching from the forehead to the temples, lasting all day, more severe in the room and during rest; ameliorated by walking in the open air (3). Dull pain in the frontal region, with pressure on the eyes (7). **50.** Dull pain in the frontal region, with nausea and heaviness in the whole head (3). Vertigo in the sinciput, which almost makes him fall forwards (2). **Parietal region.** Pressure in the right parietal bone (9). Pressure at the origin of the temporal muscle (4). **Temporal region.** Thumping pain on the two temples, lasting a long while, caused and aggravated by moving the head and by stamping on the ground (6). **55.** Tearing pains in paroxysms in the left temporal region (7). When stooping, transitory tearing in the right temporal region (7). Lancinations in the left temporal region, which stretch into the occiput (9). Pressive pain in the temples (9). Violently pressive pain in the right temple with malaise, desire to vomit, borborygmi, without colic (6). **60.** Pressure on the two temples from without inwards, subsequently extending also to the vertex (2). Dull pain in the temporal and frontal regions (6). Drawing pain in the left temple (6). Drawing pain in the temples (6). **Scalp.** Itching of the scalp (3). **65.** Little pimples on the scalp, which cause a smarting pain (10).

EYES. Sensation of pressure in the orbits (1). Burning in the edges of the eyelids (7)—which are red (7). Itching of the right lower lid (7). **70.** Itching of the lids, as well as of the skin of the back and two thighs, lasting two days (4). A little pustule, which itches a good deal, forms on the upper lid, accompanied by a sensation of acute burning (4). Pustule lasts four days (4). Heaviness of the lids (7). Pressure on the eyes; he is obliged to close the lids (11). **75.** Pressure on the eyes (9, 11). Pressure and itching in the eyes (4). Pressure on the globe of the left eye and feeling of heat in the interior (9). Dull lancinations in the right eye when reading (10). Single lancinations in the right eye (10). **80.** Transitory dilatation of the pupils (3). Transitory dilatation of the pupils and accelerated pulse (3). *Dilated pupils* (5). Disturbed and veiled sight (3, 10). *Eyes fixed* (5). **85.** Abundant secretion of whitish, yellowish mucus in the eyes (4). Lachrymation of the eyes when reading (9). Paroxysms of lancinating and twitching pain alternately in the different muscles of the eye (10). Smarting in the orbicular muscle of the right eye towards its internal angle, especially during movement of the lids (10). Twitching lancinations in the superior rectus (10). **90.** Trembling of the eyelids (6).

EARS. Sharp, isolated stitches in the ear (10). Lancinations in the right ear (9). Lancinations in the left ear (7). Sharp lancinations in the right ear (10). **95.** Single stitches in the right ear after the noon meal, renewed every quarter of an hour (9). The lancinations in the ear increase towards evening; they last a quarter of an hour (9). Paroxysms of pressive pain in the right ear, as though some one were striking upon the tympanum with a dull instrument (9). Boring in the right ear (10). Tinkling before the ears, lasting four days (4).

NOSE. **100.** Obstruction of the nose (3, 4). The nose is somewhat stopped on blowing it (10). Creeping in the end of the nose like a desire to sneeze (10). Sneezing (10). Sneezing with traces of blood in the nasal mucus (10).

FACE. *Face red and puffed* (5). **105.** Heat of the face and hands, especially of the palms (1). Heat of the face, especially of the cheeks, in the afternoon (7). Heat of the cheek for three quarters of an hour, confusion in the sinciput and sensation of compression of the cerebral hemispheres (2). °Lancinations and tearings in the right cheek, stretching into the temporal region; they had lasted two months (5). Disagreeble sensation in both cheeks during the abdominal pains (10).

MOUTH. **Lips. 110.** Lips dry (4). Burning of the lips and tongue (12). *Twitching of the corners of the mouth* (5). **Jaws.** Drawing pain in the right inferior maxillary (9). **Cavity of the mouth.** Burning in the cavity, breath hot, oppression of respiration and pressure on the sternum (2). **115.** Irritation of the cavity and of the isthmus of the pharynx, followed by a sensation of contraction of the larynx, cough, even to vomiting, and accelerated respiration (2). **Teeth.** Odontalgia in the evening and night; the pains are burning, and aggravated by the heat of the bed (5). Teeth on edge (1). Throbbing and burning pain in the last molar on the left side, not very violent, but lasting all night (4). The toothache in the posterior molar increases; a swelling of the gum forms around the tooth which extends towards the palate, occasions tension and itching, but no pain, and renders mastication difficult (4). **120.** The swelling of the gums does not disappear until the fourth day (4). The toothache comes on in the afternoon, is tearing and drawing; aggravated in the evening; diminishing towards midnight; the cold open air makes it more endurable. Slight shooting in a carious upper tooth (10). Shootings from the crown to the root of a perfectly sound right inferior molar (10). Shooting pain in paroxysms in the carious tooth (10). **125.** Dull drawing and shooting toothache in an upper carious molar and in the corresponding lower tooth, in the morning on waking; it persists in the upper tooth until after he has got up (10). **Taste.** Pasty, disagreeable taste in the mouth (10). Pasty taste, want of appetite and frequent yawnings (11). Foul taste of the pharyngeal mucus which he raises (10). Metallic taste (9). **130.** Metallic, sulphurous taste (1). Bitter, sharp taste in the morning (4). Very repulsive, acrid taste (4). Sweetish, putrid taste (3). Blunted taste during the whole day (2). **Tongue. 135.** Burning on the point of the tongue and in the pharynx (9). Transitory burning, as if from pepper on the point of the tongue and in the pharynx (6). Burning on the tongue and in the pharynx (12). Shooting burning on the tongue (2). Sensation of pricking on the tip of the tongue (9). **140.** Sensation of cold on the tongue, followed by a lancinating burning, and this succeeded by a feeling as though he had taken pepper (at once) (1). **Saliva.** Accumulation of saliva in the mouth with sweetish taste, during the whole day (6). Malaise and accumulation of saliva in the mouth (6, 10). Accumulation of saliva in the mouth (10). Increased salivary secretion (9). **145.** *Increased salivary secretion* (5). Very frequent spitting (1). Saliva viscid with desire for drink (2). **Palate.** Burning in the velum palati (2). °Swelling of the uvula and velum, which are pale red (5).

APPETITE. **150.** Increased appetite (1). Appetite somewhat increased (4). Appetite and salivary secretion increased (1). Hunger, accompanied by rumbling in the belly (2). The appetite continues, notwithstanding the great constrictive pain in the stomach (9). **155.** Hunger, and yet repugnance to food (10). Diminution of appetite (10). Decrease of appetite at noon and in the evening (18). Complete absence of appetite (1). Rapid satiety in eating (11). **Thirst. 160.** Very violent thirst; beer is pleasanter than anything (4).

PHARYNX. Burning in the throat, extending into the stomach (3). Violent burning in the pharynx, with malaise (9). Burning pain in the pharynx (9). Burning in the pharynx and œsophagus (4). **165.** Burning and scraping in the pharynx and œsophagus (9). *Burning and scraping the whole extent of the pharynx* (5). *Very violent burning in the pharynx and stomach* (5). Feeling of acridity in the pharynx (on swallowing the drug) (1). Scraping in the throat (10). **170.** Scraping in the throat for a whole day, as though a cold were about to set in (7). Sensation as though there were a hair in the throat (3). *Difficult deglutition* (5).

STOMACH. **Eructations.** Empty eructations (6). Unsatisfactory eructations (10). **175.** Frequent eructations, with the smell and taste of the drug (1, 6). Flatulent eructations smelling of black radish (10). Eructations and inclination to vomit, especially when he changes from the open air to a room or *vice versa* (11). Acrid and burning eructations twice (10). Very abundant eructations (2). **180.**

Regurgitations. Escape of inodorous flatulence, with burning at the scrobiculus (10). Sour, burning, acrid regurgitations (pyrosis) one or two hours after eating (10). Regurgitations (2). Regurgitations of air (7). Nauseating regurgitations (1). **185.** Regurgitations and discharge of wind downwards (12). Regurgitations and desire to vomit (9). Regurgitations and malaise (9). *Continual acid regurgitations, but without vomiting* (5). °Frequent sour regurgitations (5). **190.** Regurgitations of something sour (3). Acid regurgitations (3). **Vomiting.** Desire to vomit (3, 12). Desire to vomit with embarrassment of the head (2). Desire to vomit, and pressure in the stomach, but very transitory (6). **195.** Vomiting of a small quantity of bitter water (7). **Epigastric Region.** Sensation of burning in the stomach, aggravated by external pressure (9). *Burning in the scrobiculus and in the stomach* (5). Burning in the stomach and hepatic region, increased by external pressure (9). Heat in the epigastric region, which ascends and occupies the whole chest (1). **200.** Agreeable heat in the whole stomach (1). Violent heat ascending from the stomach to the head, and descending to the umbilical region (1). Pain in the stomach, especially on taking a deep inspiration, after breakfast (7). *Lancinations in the stomach* (5). Transitory lancination in the epigastric region (6). **205.** Feeling of malaise in the stomach (7). Malaise and sensation of emptiness in the stomach (11). Malaise in the stomach, nausea, regurgitations of air having the taste and smell of the drug (11). Fulness in the stomach (9). Sensation of fulness of the stomach, with eructations, yawnings and desire to vomit (2). **210.** Sensation of fulness in the whole epigastric region, accompanied by slight vertigo (2). Sensation of fulness at the stomach, which is sensitive to the touch (9). Supper dispels the fulness of the stomach and the vertigo (2). Pasty taste, pressure at the stomach and lancinations in different parts of the hypogastrium (11). Slight pressure at the stomach (1, 7). **215.** Pressive pain in the stomach (9). Pressure and sensation of cold at the stomach (3). Pressive pain in the epigastric region and very abundant emission of flatus (6).

ABDOMEN. Abdomen inflated (2). Inflation of the abdomen, after eating (11). **220.** Inflation of the abdomen, with sensation of excoriation (9). Borborygmi (6, 10). *Great noise in the intestines*, (3). *Borborygmi and tearing colic in the abdomen* (5). Borborygmi and sensation of dryness in the throat (7). **225.** Borborygmi, escape of flatus and desire to urinate (1). Indefinable colic pains after the noon meal (3). Malaise in the abdomen, followed by a soft fæculent stool (10). Malaise in the hypogastrium increased by stooping and by movement (10). Abdomen full and distended, soft stool (2). **230.** Frequent slight colics (1). Slight intestinal colic from time to time, and desire to urinate (1). Slight colic (9). Slight colic pains after eating (10). Slight colic pains followed by a liquid, unsatisfactory evacuation (10). Colic and borborygmi, as if a diarrhœa were about to come on (8). Colic such as follows the exhibition of a purgative (8). Colic here and there with emission of flatus (10). Colic, emission of flatus, stools and remission of the pain (7). Colic pains which disappear on going to stool (6). **240.** Colic and regurgitation of the milk taken, without malaise and without vomiting (7). Violent colic in the evening after having eaten a little salad, followed by a stool of globular substances (10). Colic, with movements of wind in the abdomen on waking at 4, A. M.; on inspiration and by external pressure the pains become lancinating and become permanently located for an hour nearly in the region of the cæcum (10). Malaise in the hypogastrium, abundant expectoration and desire to vomit after having drunk coffee (10). Itching on the abdomen and right shoulder after rising and washing the body with cold water. (10) **245.** Sensation of excoriation in the abdominal integuments (9). Painful sensitiveness of the abdomen to external pressure (7). **Umbilical region.** Colic in the umbilical region with a stool (6). Cuttings in the umbilical region and slight attack of malaise an hour after having dined (10). Attacks of pinching twitching in a little spot two inches from the navel towards the right, lasting a half minute (10). **250.** Slight lancinating and pruritous pain on the right side below the navel, followed by an almost liquid stool (10). Single, very acute stitches on the right of the umbilical region, extending towards the bladder (10). Colic in the small intestines, with emission of much flatulence (6). **Hypochondria.** Lancinating and twitching pain, first in the right then in the left hypochondrium, remaining in both sides for several minutes, and not increased either by pressure or movement (10). Paroxysm of lancinating pain in the right inferior costal region, two inches from the scrobiculus, at five o'clock, P. M. (10). **255.** Paroxysm of disagreeable but indefinable pain in the region of the left lobe of the liver (10). Lancinating twitching in the left hypochondrium (10). Two pappy stools at 11, A. M.; preceded by pains in the region of the left lobe of the liver, and followed by pains in the cæcal region (10). **Hypogastrium.** Dull shootings when bearing upon the hypogastrium (6). Cuttings in the hypogastrium, followed by a moderately soft stool (10). **260.** Slight cuttings in the hypogastrium; contact is disagreeable, and seems to excite them after they have ceased; stooping causes feelings of malaise (10). Slight colic pains in the hypogastrium as though diarrhœa were about to set in (10). **Cæcal region.** Lancinating and twitching pain in the region of the cæcum (10). Lancinations, pinchings in the region of the cæcum (10). The lancinating pain in the region of the cæcum is not relieved by the discharge of flatus. Turning from one side to another, or doubling up the body, aggravates the pain or excites it afresh when almost relieved (10). **265.** Dull shootings in the region of the cæcum, with discharge of flatulence in the morning on waking (10). Lancinating, dull, itching pain in the region of the cæcum, lasting one or two minutes (10).—Isolated lancinations here and there in the left side of the abdomen and in the right eye when reading (10). Lancinating, nipping pains in the right side, frequently during the day (10).—He discharges, during the day, a great deal of flatulence, having the smell of the drug (11). **270.** Discharge of very fetid wind (12). Discharge of flatus, with sensation of itching in the rectum (3).

STOOL. Desire to go to stool (9). Pressing desire for stool at noon (2). Two stools in succession without any pain (7). **275.** Hard, insufficient stool, with slight tenesmus towards evening (10). Constipation (10). Evacuation drier than common (10). Hard stool at first, then soft, with rumbling in the abdomen as though a stool were about to follow (10). Stool at first hard, then soft, with burning at the anus, followed three hours afterwards by a second fæculent evacuation likewise accompanied by burning at the anus (10). **280.** Difficult stool, soft and scanty, as though from inactivity of the rectum (10). Pappy stool preceded by cuttings, shortly after breakfast (10). Two liquid stools (9). Liquid stool having the odor of the drug (11). Stool liquid, as if after a purge (10). **285.** Slimy diarrhœa (9). Watery diarrhœa (9). Liquid diarrhœa and violent pain above the sternum, twice repeated (9). Sudden diarrhœa, after having dined with great satisfaction, recurring twice in the afternoon accompanied by colic (9). *Violent diarrhœa; evacuations of a sour smell and accompanied by tenesmus* (5). **290.** °Chronic diarrhœa, appearing every month or six weeks, lasting one or two days with colic, especially in the umbilical region, which is drawn in, with liquid, yellowish, frothy evacuations of a sour smell and accompanied by tenesmus (3).

ANUS AND RECTUM. Transitory lancinations in the rectum (6). Itching and burning at the anus (9).

URINE. Desire to urinate (1). Increased but not altered secretion of urine (1).

GENITAL ORGANS. **295.** Flaccidity of the genital parts, a constant symptom during the whole proving (2). Transitory irritation in the navicular fossa at night, without desire or need to urinate (4). Erections (9). Very restless night; erections and pollutions (9). Lancinating and twitching pain in the left testicle lasting two minutes (10). **300.** Menses five days before the time without any pain (3).

LARYNX. Heat and irritation of the larynx, temperature of the expired air, higher (2). Hoarseness, irritation of the larynx, especially of its posterior surface, manifesting itself by a continual desire to hawk, but rarely by a cough, for thirty-six hours (2). Hoarseness for two hours (9). Voice a little veiled without any other catarrhal symptom (10). **305.** Veiled voice (10). Rough veiled voice (10). Sensation of scraping and transitory lancinations in the neck (6). Sensation of scraping in the larynx provoking cough (6). Irritation in the neck provoking a cough (12). **310.** Desire to cough provoked by a tickling at the bifurcation of the bronchi (2). Slight, dry cough (6).

CHEST. *Sensation of heat in the chest* (5). Congestion in the superior portion of the lungs manifested by accelerated respiration (2). Oppression of the chest aggravated by going up stairs (2). **315.** The oppression of the chest is aggravated in a room the air of which is not renewed, and is accompanied by anxiety (2). Fulness of the chest and embarrassment of respiration, arising in the anterior portion of the diaphragm (2). Sensitiveness of the anterior portion of the thorax when sneezing (2). Dull, pressive pain in the right side of the chest (6). Pain in the left half of the chest and beneath the sternum from time to time (9). **320.** Attack of stitches in the left half of the chest without cough (9). Transitory and isolated stitches in the chest and below the left false ribs (10). Dull stitches in the inferior part of the right chest (10). Pressure beneath the sternum (9). Transitory stitches near the sternum on the left side after having drunk coffee (10). **325.** Itching stitches in the nipples (male) (10).

BACK. **Cervical.** °Stiffness in the muscles of the right side of the neck (5). Drawing pain in the right sterno-mastoid muscle (6). Itching stitches in the right sterno-mastoid (10). Painful scraping as though from a foreign body in the left side of the neck at 9 A. M., extending into the left ear when swallowing, lasting one or two minutes (10). **Loins. 330.** Lancinating and twitching pain in the right lumbar region lasting a minute or two (10). **Sacrum.** Tension in the sacrum with some shocks towards the coxo-femoral articulation (2). Tearing and pressure in the sacrum (9). Drawings in the sacrum in the afternoon (9). **Shoulders.** Lancinating and twitching pain in the right scapulo-humeral articulation (10). **335.** Very slight lancinating pains extending from the shoulder-joint to the carpus, in the morning (3). Jerking lancinations in the arm and shoulder joint (10). Attacks of lancinating and itching pain in the left deltoid (10).

SUPERIOR EXTREMITIES. Slight formication along the whole right arm with feeling as though the arm were about to become numb (3). Numbness of the left arm with pain and feeling of fatigue (9). **340.** Pressive pain in the right arm from time to time (9). Itching on the anterior surface of the right arm and fore-arm, in the bend of the left elbow and on the thighs (10). Paroxysm of lancinating and dull pains on the internal side of the arm and thigh (spasmodic contraction of small isolated muscular fasciculi) (10). **Elbow.** Transitory tearing pains in the right elbow and left shoulder (8). Twitching in the region of the olecranon (10). **Fore-arm. 345.** Attack of lancinating pain at the insertion of the biceps on the fore-arm during the whole evening and succeeding night (10). Slight lancination extending from the left olecranon along the extensor muscles into the carpus, several times during the day (3). Formication extending from the olecranon to the end of the fingers, excepting the thumb (3). Formication in the fore-arms, alternating with slight shootings (3). Pressive pain in the left fore-arm aggravated by touching and by resting on the fore-arm (9). **350.** Trembling of the left fore-arm, with lancinations especially about the right joint (9). A spot on the right fore-arm (urticaria) which itches a good deal and forces him to scratch (10). Several isolated papules on the right fore-arm which itch when touched (10). Itching in a small spot on the right fore-arm, inclining one to scratch, and followed by an eruption of small pimples (10). **Carpus.** Pain in the carpal joints (9). **355.** Lancinations in the left carpal region (9). **Metacarpus.** Slight, twitching pain in the joints of the hand for several weeks, sometimes in the right, at others in the left, several times a day, but only lasting a few seconds (11). Lancinations by jerks in the metacarpo-phalangeal articulation of the index and in the fleshy part of the right great toe (10). Dull shooting in the metacarpo-phalangeal articulation of the left index (10). **Fingers.** Lancinating and twitching pain in the first phalanx of the fourth finger of the left hand, frequently renewed (10). **360.** Lancinations in several of the finger-joints (10).

INFERIOR EXTREMITIES. **Hips.** Violent itching, forcing him to scratch in the region of the right hip (10). Drawing from the left hip-joint to the knee-joint, with feeling of a sprain in the knee (4). **Nates.** Violent pain in the ischiatic tuberosity and along the posterior surface of the lower extremity, in the afternoon, while riding in a carriage (10). The lancinating and itching pains often appear in different parts of the body, especially in the region of the right ischiatic tuberosity and at the insertion of the gracilis and sartorius (10). **Thighs. 365.** Shootings in the middle of the right thigh (10). Occasional shootings in the muscles of the thighs and in the toes (10). Shooting pain in paroxysms along the middle of the thigh like a neuralgia, after the noon meal; it lasts half an hour, is very painful and is repeated the next day before noon. In the afternoon the same pain is perceived between the tibia and the fibula (2). Itching on the two thighs, on the right side of the back as far as the renal region, and right fore-arm, forcing him to scratch in the morning on waking (10). Little colorless pimples on the thighs, on the right side of the back and arm, the itching of which is aggravated by scratching; they become red and form an eruption analogous to scabies (10). **370.** Drawing pain in the left thigh when walking (7). **Knees.** Pain and drawing in the knee-joints (12). Tearing pain in the knee-joints and tarsal-joints, in the afternoon (9). Lancinating pains in the internal side of the left knee extending into the great toe (4). Tensive pain in the right ham when walking and extending the foot (6). **375.** Lancinating and twitching pains, sometimes in the hollow of the right ham, sometimes in the hypogastrium, spermatic cord, lasting until after dinner (10). **Legs.** Itching in the calves and legs (10). Itching of the legs, in the evening when going to bed (10). **Feet.** Frequent transitory pains, in paroxysms, in the joints of the feet (11). Pain resembling the result of fatigue after a prolonged walk in the joints of the feet (11). **380.** Tearing pains in the left foot, especially in the tarsal bones, transitory (6). Twitching lancinations at the insertion of the tendo-Achillis into the calcaneum (10). Pain in the point of insertion of the tendo-Achillis into the calcaneum when going up stairs (10). Dull aching in the left heel (6). Transitory twitching pains in the dorsum of the right foot and in the right carpal region, equally transitory (6). **385.** Violent cramp in the sole of the right foot, removed by pressing the foot firmly upon the ground (10). Several lancinations in the fleshy part of the great toe (10).

SLEEP. Somnolence (4). Great somnolence during the whole day (11). Somnolence during the whole day and agitated sleep at night; head heavy; he is obliged to change his position every instant (11). **390.** Somnolence at 2 P. M. (3). Somnolence at 3 P. M., and at night she cannot sleep (3). Somnolence after noon and in the evening she goes to sleep with equal ease (3). Very great somnolence in the evening, in company (6). Great somnolence and wavering in the head, in the evening (11). **395.** Very great somnolence with heaviness of the upper eyelids which close involuntarily (7). Sleeplessness on account of dryness of the skin and a general unpleasant heat; he is obliged to rise and moisten his skin with cold water in order to produce a perspiration, but without result (11). *The pains in the head prevent him from sleeping* (5). She goes to sleep very late (3). Late and very restless sleep (4). **400.** Deep and refreshing morning sleep (3). Restless sleep and heavy head for several nights in succession (11). Very restless night, alternate unquiet dreams and wakings (9). Very restless nights with erections and burning in the urethra (9). Sleep interrupted after midnight, full of disagreeable dreams (2). **405.** Sleep troubled by many disagreeable disquieting dreams accompanied by tears (7). Restless sleep disturbed by dreams (4). Restless sleep, disturbed by confused dreams (3). Sleep disturbed by dreams (7). Much dreaming towards morning (10).

SKIN. **410.** Skin hot and in many places burning as though he had touched nettles (11). Sharp, itching stinging in different parts of the skin (10). Itching lancinations in different parts of the integuments (10). Itching in various parts of the skin, in the morning in bed, not very violent if it is not aggravated by scratching (10). Bleeding and burning of the scabious eruption from scratching (10). °Impetigo on the backs of the hands, three cases, little vesicles on a red, inflamed, swollen base, sometimes nearer, at others more separated, containing a yellowish cloudy serum which discharges and forms thick yellowish crusts, which sometimes irritate the neighboring parts and torment the patient with the violent itching to which they give rise. Three globules (dilution?) were administered; shortly afterwards the hand swelled considerably with violent smarting. At the end of eight or twelve hours the pain and swelling began to diminish and the impetigo disappeared in from three to eight days (13).

FEVER. **Cold.** General coldness (3). Sensation of cold and desire to go to stool (9). Sensation of general internal heat and coldness of the feet (7). **Heat.** General heat, slight headache, strong pulse, cramps in the calves and toes, without thirst. The heat lasts two hours and leaves great weariness behind (8). **420.** Coldness of the feet and general heat of the upper part of the body (2). **Perspiration.** Cutaneous perspiration suppressed (11). Skin dry, perspiration suppressed, appetite diminished for several weeks (11). **Pulse.** Arterial pulse more frequent (1). Pulse accelerated for ten minutes only; it rises from seventy-six to ninety-two (3). **425.** Acceleration of the pulse (4). *Pulse ninety to ninety-five* (5).

GENERAL. Great weariness and depression (11). Extraordinary fatigue after a long walk; respiration a little embarrassed (6). General weakness, especially in the left arm, in the morning, disappearing towards noon (9). **430.** Transitory physical excitement (4). *She lies down,* *weeps and groans* (5). Transitory attacks of malaise (10). Transitory attacks of malaise as though he were going to faint (11). Uncomfortable all the afternoon (10). **435.** The malaise returns in fits, even after having been to stool (10). The attacks of malaise are especially brought on by the compression of the abdomen in the sitting position; the open air seems to mitigate them (10). Lancinations in paroxysms in different parts of the body (10). Twitching lancinations in different parts of the body, especially in the muscles of the right eye (10). Twitching (jerking) pains, sometimes in the forehead, at others in the joints of the feet, and again in the joints of the arm (11). **440.** °Great liability to rheumatic pains (5). °Rheumatic pains in different parts of the body. The symptoms are diminished after eating and by motion in the open air (10). The drug does not seem to act for more than twelve or eighteen hours (6).

---

4. AMPHISBÆNA-VERMICULARIS.

AMPH. Amphisbæna.

1. *Description and Preparation.*

This genus of serpents belongs to Brazil and other parts of South America, and derives its name from the fact that its head is so small and its tail so thick and short, that they are with difficulty distinguished from each other, while, at the same time, it has the habit of proceeding either backwards or forwards as occasion may require. It is said to be destitute of fangs and to be perfectly harmless and inoffensive, living for the most part upon ants and other insects. Mure, from whose *Pathogénésie Brésilienne* the following proving is taken, gives the following description of the species used. "Its body is cylindrical, from fifty to eighty centimetres long, terminated by a very obtuse tail. It is destitute of proper scales, but its skin is divided into quadrilateral compartments disposed in rings around the body, two hundred and twenty-eight on the body and twenty-six on the tail. The lip of the cloaca is divided into six long and narrow plates; the head is small, a little pointed, protected by scutella and confounded with the neck. The eyes are very small; the jaws not dilatable, the teeth conical, bent, unequal and distinct from each other; the nostrils lateral and pierced in a single naso-rostral plate. Its color is brownish above and a slightly pinkish white beneath.

"We procured the poison by cutting off a portion of the jaw from the living animal and immediately triturating it." If the Amphisbæna is destitute of fangs and harmless, according to the opinion of the naturalists, this poison will be somewhat apocryphal.

2. *Prior use.*

The dried and powdered flesh of the Amphisbæna is said to be administered by the natives of Brazil as a specific in dislocations, sprains, and bruises.

3. *Digest of the Symptoms.*

AUTHORITIES. MURE, *Pathogénésie Brésilienne*, p. 261.

GENERAL. Debility. Sadness and great lassitude in the morning, removed when walking. Tender sadness tending to mildness. Great pain in the whole vertebral column, aggravated by walking, moving the arms and stooping. **5.** Depression. Ennui. Impatience.

HEAD. Heaviness in the forehead and parietal regions. Heaviness in the forehead. **10.** Great confusion and vertigo with swinging sensation, which seems to tend to one side by a series of successive impulses, and then to the other by a similar operation. Repeated strokes in the right side of the forehead as though he were struck by hail. Sweat on the head. Disturbance of the sensations; he experiences dreadful headaches and would believe his feet were in his brain. Confusion as if from intoxication, when turning the head.

EYES. **15.** Pain as from a stye in the internal canthus of the right eye. Continual trembling of the right upper lid, and especially of the left. Constriction of the right eye; it feels as if it were tied. Pain and lancinations in the external canthus of the left eye. Feeling of a grain of sand in the right eye. **20.** Fatigue of the eyes in the evening; pain and pricking when looking at the light. Lachrymation and constriction of the left eye.

EARS. Pain in the meatus as if from the introduction of air.

FACE. Little prickings and heat over the cheekbone of the right side. Dull pains on the right side of the inferior maxillary bone. **25.** Pains and lancinations attacking the whole right side of the head. Pains in the right lower jaw and some swelling, aggravated by the air and moisture. Swelling of the right lower jaw, aggravated by the air. Very large and painful pimple on the left side of the upper lip, ending in suppuration.

MOUTH AND THROAT. The teeth feel prolonged and are set on edge, especially the right inferior molars, and in the interior of the mouth. **30.** The toothache is worse in the afternoon and evening. He cannot chew without pain, but the impression of liquids is not painful. Swelling of the tonsils. Difficult deglutition; he cannot swallow his saliva.

ABDOMEN. Protrusion of an umbilical hernia. **35.** Coldness and pains in the epigastrium. Tearing pain in the navel all day. Suppuration of an inguinal hernia. The hernia is painful, and pent-up air is perceived in it. Lancination like a dagger-stroke in the navel.

STOOL. **40.** Constipation.

EXTREMITIES. Very painful swelling of the arm, (15th day). Cramp in the left leg. Painless retraction of the legs. Cramps in the left leg; it drags in walking as though paralysed.

SLEEP. **45.** He wakes precisely at midnight for ten days in succession. Interrupted sleep.

SKIN. Red miliary eruption (dry itch cured) in extensive plates of an elliptic form; furfuraceous desquamation takes place in every spot when the eruption is healed. The spots of miliary eruption of little red pimples extend over the whole chest, neck and back, with itching, more violent in the morning and diminishing until evening. A white vesicle forms by degrees on every papule and discharges a clear lymph, after which the eruption dries up on the fifth day. **50.** Miliary eruption of little pimples, especially on the forearm.

5.—ANAGALLIS-ARVENSIS.

ANAG. Scarlet Pimpernel. Red Chickweed. Poor Man's Weather-glass. *Fr.* Anagallis mâle. Mouron rouge.

1. *Description and Preparation.*

This plant belongs to the order of *Primulaceæ* in the natural system; Pentandria, monogynia, *Linn.* Calyx and corolla, five-parted; stamens, five; capsule globose, opening horizontally all round. A square, procumbent stem, with opposite branches, and ovate, sessile, opposite leaves, dotted underneath, about half an inch long. The flowers are borne on solitary axillary peduncles longer than the leaves; the corolla scarlet, with a purple centre. It is found near New York, and on Long Island, and Staten Island, and is said to be the European species introduced. It flowers from June to October.

The expressed juice of the whole plant is used.

2. *Prior Knowledge of its Effects.*

Dr. Roth has collected the following instances of its use.

1. HIPPOCRATES used the plant mixed with alum as an application to foul ulcers. (*Opera omnia*, Genev, 1657. *De ulceribus*, 879).

2. Dioscorides (lib. 2, cap. 174) says "that the *Anagallis* has the power of mitigating and arresting inflammations. It draws foreign substances out of the body and represses corrosive ulcers. Its juice evacuates the brain of phlegm, if used as a gargle and discharged by the nose. It relieves toothache if inserted into the ear of the opposite side. Used with Attic honey it cures spots on the eyes and disorders of the sight. Infused in wine it is good for those who have been bitten by serpents, and for those having diseased kidneys or liver. The plant with the blue flower is said to cause the prolapsed rectum to return, while that with the red is said to cause its descent by rubbing."

3. Serapion (*de simplicibus ex plantis*, 1497, p. 119, CLV.) endeavors to prove that the Arabian physicians used the remedy. "*Virtus ejus est quod calefacit partes et desiccat sine mordicatione. Et secunda est quod abstergit et attrahit. Et tertia est quod extrahit sagittas et spinas et alia infixa corpori. Et succus ejus injectus in nares purgat cerebrum ab humoribus qui sunt in eo et incarnat ulcera et confert corruptionibus membrorum.*"

4. Chomel (*Histoire des plantes usuelles*, Paris, 1782, p. 276) says "that it is useful in mania and epilepsy."

5. Hartmann, Mynsicht, Willis and others, also consider it useful in the frenzy which comes on in continued fevers. It is employed by the handful in the drinks and decoctions prescribed for hypochondriacs; water distilled from it has the same virtue. The alcoholic tincture of the flowers, and the extract of the whole plant, especially if mingled with the flowers of *Hypericum*, are remedies not to be despised in epilepsy.

6. Tragus asserts that a glass of wine, which has been slightly boiled with a handful of pimpernel, is a good remedy against the plague; the patient must keep himself well covered up in bed, the object being to sweat him. He considers the juice good against dropsy, and renal and hepatic obstructions.

7. Simon Pauli (*Quadripartitum Botanicum*, p. 196) mentions a poultice of pimpernel boiled in urine as a popular remedy in his country applied to the hands and feet of gouty subjects.

8. Suadicani (Hufeland Jour. 44, p. 84), among others, has recommended this plant against hydrophobia in a long memoir, which may be referred to as above. It is a copious exposition of its efficacy against hydrophobia, from the most ancient times to the present, and maintains that the anagallis is as certain a therapeutic agent in canine madness, as quinine in intermittents, or mercury in syphilis.

In addition to the authorities cited by Dr. Roth, we may add that—

9. Orfila found three drachms of the extract sufficient to destroy a dog, with marks of inflammation of the bowels. The plant with blue flowers referred to above is described by Linnæus as *A. cœrulea*, a mere variety of the *A. arvensis*.

3. *Digest of the Symptoms.*

AUTHORITIES. DR. ROTH (*Matière Medicale* 1, 251) cites SCHRETER, *Arch. hom.*, vol. 23, p. 174.

MIND. **Moral.** Great flow of spirits for several days; everything causes him pleasure. Hilarity; more lively than usual; he attends to business with great pleasure and is very well satisfied with himself. **Mental.** He is constantly thinking, his mind is very active.

HEAD. **Forehead.** Pressive aching in the sinciput from a current of cold air. **Temples. 5.** Spasmodic lancinations in the temples; from there they extend into the eyes, in the centre of which there is a feeling of pressure.

EARS. Obstruction in the right ear, preceded by pressure upon the eyes.

THROAT. Sensation of dryness and scraping in the throat.

STOOL. Desire to go to stool. Well digested stool· **Rectum. 10.** Itching in the rectum and pressure on the sacrum as if from piles.

URINE. **Urethra.** Burning pain in the urethra when urinating, especially in the morning; the meatus seems stopped up; he experiences a strong pressure when the urine issues, and the stream divides into two, three, or more jets. Tickling itching along the urethra, and especially at the meatus, which is not very painful nor very disagreeable, and which incites him to coitus.

GENITAL ORGANS. **Coitus.** Desire for coitus. Burning pain in the urethra before coitus, and during the erection, which ceases during the copulative act.

CHEST. **15.** A sort of restlessness in the chest. Sensation in the interior of the chest as if it were pricked by a great number of needles. **Heart.** Violent trembling of the heart, with general trembling and coldness, preceded and accompanied by a dull pain in a carious tooth, and agitation in the chest.

BACK AND EXTEMITIES. **Shoulder.** Tensive drawing which ascends from the left shoulder into the nape, and recommences after it had ceased, whenever he raises and extends his arm. **Metacarpus.** Dull drawing, sometimes tearing pain in the right metacarpus; oftenest on the right side, sometimes on the left, and returning at irregular intervals. **Finger. 20.** Sensation resembling cramp in the right thenar, when cutting with scissors, changing into a dull drawing; when it ceases on the right side it reappears in the same part on the left.

SLEEP. Bad, agitated night's rest; he goes to sleep late, wakes early, and desires to sleep still more in the morning.

FEVER. **Heat.** Heat rises into his head, and he experiences a slight sweat on his forehead, followed by a pressive lancination in the globes of the eyes, and a tickling formication in the urethra exciting him to copulation. **Cold.** Trembling and chills.

6.—APIS-MELLIFICA.

APIS. The common honey-bee.

We are principally indebted for the proving of this very admirable remedy, to the indefatigable zeal and perseverance of our colleague, Dr. F. Humphreys, of Utica. Having been experimented upon by him, he proposed it for trial to the Central Homœopathic Society of New-York, upon which a committee was appointed to prove the drug and report upon it. Drs. Bishop and Munger were joined to Dr. Humphreys, and the result was a report to the Central Society which is incorporated in the following article.

1. *Description and Preparation.*

This useful insect is too well known and too widely diffused to need a particular description. It and its products, honey and wax, have apparently been familiar to man from the very earliest ages.

The preparation with which the following provings were made was procured by placing the living working bees, taken in the month of August, in a large open-mouthed vial, and pouring alcohol over them when in a state of excitement. The tincture is suffered to stand awhile, and is then decanted clear for use.

Dr. Hering suggests that a better mode of procuring the pure virus of the insect, would be to seize the bee by the head and with a little forceps extract the sting and poison bag together, which may then be triturated with sugar of milk.

A preparation has also been obtained by placing the living bees in a closed vessel until they were suffocated and dried, and then pulverising them with milk-sugar.

2. *Prior Knowledge of its effects.*

That the bee possessed a powerful weapon of offence in its sting, and that the effects arising from its delicate puncture were sometimes formidable, has always been known, but from the want of a true therapeutic guide, this knowledge could never be made serviceable in the cure of the sick.

1. Deseret relates that a workman fifty years old was stung by a bee over the right eyelid; he immediately fell to the ground and in a few moments died. His face was inflamed, and after death there was a copious discharge of blood from the nose.

2. Zacutus saw, after a sting in the eyebrow, an inflammation, violent pain and gangrene of the part follow.

3. In a Munich Journal, a case is related where a man was overtaken by a swarm of bees and so stung in the hands and face, that he soon died from the pain, inflammation and swelling of the affected parts.

4. "The *poison-apparatus* is found in the females and neuters only. It consists of two thin convoluted secreting organs, opening into a pyriform receptacle, from which a small duct passes to a sting which consists of two portions, placed side by side, barbed at the extremity and contained in a sheath. The poison is said to be hot and acrid to the taste. The consequences produced by the sting of a bee are pain, redness, swelling and hardness of the part; and might prove fatal if a swarm were to attack an individual." (*Pereira*).

5. Mr. Lawrence mentions the case of a French gentleman, who was so severely stung by bees about the upper part of the chest that he died in fifteen minutes, with all the symptoms of mortal collapse usually produced by the bite of venomous serpents. (*Med. Gaz.* 5, 582.)

6. Dr. Marcy (*Theory and Practice,* 547) states that the first trituration of the honey-bee has proved successful in his hands in *ascites* and *hydrothorax.* "In large doses, it causes a sense of fulness, constriction, or of suffocation in the thorax; difficult and anxious respiration; pain and tenderness of the abdomen, increased by pressure or contact, symptoms worse in the horizontal posture; great secretion of urine, which is pale or of a straw color, and deposits a reddish or brick-colored sediment; frequent desire to urinate, and strangury." After citing a case of *ascites*, which will be found under the clinical remarks, he adds: "We have witnessed the effects of this remedy in two other cases of ascites, in one case of protracted general dropsy, and in one case of hydrothorax, and with the same favorable results. The powder of dried honey-bees has long been used as a remedy in dropsies by the aborigines of our country."

7. A lady, aged 65, had been in the habit of attending and taking care of honey-bees for forty-five years, had been frequently stung, and always with but slight inconvenience. In September, 1849, her attention was directed to some apples, which were drying, among which some bees were present, when one of them stung her on the chin. She hurried into the house, remarking that a bee had just stung her, and that she "felt strangely," which were her last words. In less than fifteen minutes all signs of life had disappeared.—*Amer. Magazine.*

3. *Digest of the Symptoms.*

AUTHORITIES. **1.** Dr. Barker. **2.** Dr. Bigelow. **3.** Dr. Bishop. **4.** F. D. **5.** Dr. Greene. **6.** Dr. Hays. **7.** Dr. Humphreys. **8.** Dr. Kellogg. **9.** Dr. Munger. **10.** Dr. Robinson. **11.** Dr. Wells.

The figures at the end of the symptoms refer to the authority; the ordinary type indicates the pathogenetic effects; the symptoms which have disappeared under the use of the drug are distinguished by a cypher (°), and those which have been confirmed by cures are preceded by an asterisk (*).

MIND. Irritable disposition the eighth day; nothing appeared to satisfy him, all out of place (7.) Unfitness for mental exertion (7, 11). Dread of death, or sensation as if he should not be able to breathe again (2).

SENSORIUM. Confused vertigo for several days, at times very violent, worse when sitting than when walking, and extreme when lying down and on closing the eyes, from several doses of the 30th (7). **5.** Head is dull and slightly confused (7). °*Crazy, wild, blind staggers in horses* (old observation) 7. Furious mania? (7).

HEAD. Weight and fulness in the upper part of the head (2 Heaviness and pressure in the head, continued three or four days, commenced one hour after taking one drop of the 3d att. (11). °Great sensation of rush of blood to the head (3). **10.** *Headache over the eyes*, which is dull, heavy, tensive, with pain through the orbits, lasting but a short time; this headache has occurred in three provings ( ). °Semilateral headache over and in one eye and in the whole left side of the head, with redness and puffy swelling of the cheek, nausea and vomiting (6th dil.) (4). °Headache on the right side, involving the eye and side of the head; must keep the eye closed; pain very severe, coming on at 10 or 11 A.M., and continuing until night; cured by 6th dil. (7). **Chronic headache in nervous subjects; violent pain in the forehead and temples, at times involving the eyes*, attended by vertigo, nausea and vomiting; must hold the head and eye down (7). **15.** Pressing pain in the sinciput with vertigo, immediately (7). *Pain in the sinciput and confusion of the head (7). *Disagreeable headache in the sinciput (7). Sensation of dulness across the forehead just over the eyes, third day (8). *Violent headache, mostly confined to the forehead, with fever, second day (2). **20.** *Burning and throbbing in the head aggravated by motion and stooping, temporarily relieved by pressing the head firmly with the hands, with occasional sweat for some hours (2.) Dull pressive headache in the upper part of the forehead as if it would burst, extending to the temples (11). *Violent pressive pains in the forehead and temples for several days (7). *Dull, heavy headache on rising, continued till 3 o'clock P.M., second day (11). Oppressive headache when in a warm room and reading (2). **25.** Boring pains in the temples, continued for several days at intervals, lasting only a few minutes at a time, commencing the third day, after taking 3 drops of the third att. every morning (11). *Slight aching in the left temple (7). *Violent sharp pain in the left temple (7). Violent aching pains through the temples, and organs of causality, comparison, mirthfulness, and ideality (2). Boring pains in the temples every morning on waking, for three mornings (11). **30.** Dull heavy pain in the right temple on waking in the morning, soon changing to the left, first day (11). Throbbing, painful sensation in the temples (3). °Sharp pricking pains in the temples and across the forehead (3). Dull ache in the occiput (6). Aching in the occiput increased by shaking the head (7). **35.** Slight pressure in the occiput (7). Sharp tensive pain from the neck up back of the left ear, extending forward over the left side of the head, first day (7). Headache with fulness and heaviness in the occiput (7.) Falling out of the hair all through the proving.

EYES. Transient biting itching in the right, and sometimes left eyebrow (7). **40.** **Burning stinging* in the right eye, commencing with a dull heaviness and causing flow of water; twice repeated (7). **Stinging itching in the eye, eyelids and around the eyes*, on the left side, and more at the internal canthus (7). Itching of the right eyelid, continuing all day at intervals. (This symptom repeated in several provings) (7). *Itching and prickling of the lids of the right eye, 1st day (11). Violent stinging in the lower right eyelid, in the morning (7). **45.** Burning stinging and sensation of swelling around the left eye, and in the superciliary ridge (7). *Pain around the orbits of the eye (7). °Pricking sensation as if from a foreign body (3). Aching pressure in the orbit of the left eye, mostly the lower portion, continuing for several hours; twice repeated (7). *Slight agglutination of the eyes at night; had to pick them open in the morning (7, 11, 6). **50.** Sensation as if there was a mass of mucus in the left eye, continuing all day (7). Flow of mucus and lachrymation of the right eye at night in bed (7). °Soreness, redness of the eyes and eyelids, secretion of mucus and agglutination of the lids, attended with nettlerash over the surface (7). °STYES (7 et al). °Soreness of the margin of the lids and canthus (7). **55.** °Erysipelatous inflammation of the eyelids (7). A sensation of whirling around in the sight, with difficulty of seeing at the same time, lasting only for a moment (2). *Dull, heavy feeling, inclination to close the eyes, desire to rub them forcibly, making pressure with the fingers when closed for some time (3). **Weak eyes;* for several days the light is painful (7). The eyes are weak, and an indisposition is felt to use them; they are painful and easily fatigued when employed; only regain their strength and vigor the 10th or 12th day; this was experienced by one who had never had weakness of sight before or since (7). **60.** Tremulous twitching in the left eye, more at night, and continuing for several days (7). °Inflammation of the eyes and lids attended with burning and biting pains and itching; many cases (11). °Œdematous swelling of the eyelids (7). °*Smoky opacity of the cornea*, occasioning almost entire loss of sight; several cases (7). °Opacity of the cornea with congestion of the sclerotica, obscuration of sight of several months' duration (11). **65.** °Inflammation of the cornea (7).

EARS. Burning of the superior portion of the left ear (7).

NOSE. Violent sneezing immediately (7). Frequent sneezing for many days, eleventh day, in two provings (7).

FACE. Sore elevations like the sting of insects, very tender to the touch, at the external corner of the eyebrow (7). **70.** Burning stinging, as of fire, on the chin and malar bones (7). Burning stinging at the left superciliary ridge (7). Swelling of the lips, and sensation of swelling for several days, followed by a fine eruption around the lips, and dryness and peeling off of the lower one (7). Roughness and feeling of tension in the lips, especially the upper one (7). Dark streak along the epithelium of the lips, they are rough, chapped and peel off (7). **75.** Prickling in the lips, and sensation as if they had received a severe contusion, with sensation of swelling; in a few hours (7). °Burning, biting, stinging heat, assuming a purplish hue, in about 24 hours (3). °Erysipelas of the entire face, with light redness, swelling, heat, burning fever, coated tongue and thirst; in a girl of 9 years, cured by the 6th dil., every 4 hours (7). °Erysipelas of one entire side of the face and nose, swelling under the eye, resembling that from a sting, cured by the third att. in water, rapidly and permanently (5).

TEETH. Jumping pain in the superior molars of the left side (6).

MOUTH AND THROAT. **80.** Contraction and erosion in the throat in the morning (7). Extreme sensation of rawness and scalding all around the margin of the tongue, as if it had been scalded, and slight pimples on the edge from taking the tincture, at 4 hours (7). Increased feeling of contraction in the throat, rendering deglutition difficult, at 8 hours (7). *Rawness, burning and blisters along the edge of the tongue, which are very painful, accompanied with stinging, at 8 hours, from the tincture (7). Scalding of the mouth and throat for two days (7). **85.** Stinging itching deep in the throat at the lower part of the neck, accompanied with a sensation of constriction (7). Great accumulation of viscid mucus deep in the throat in the morning, which requires repeated hawking, eleventh day (7). Dryness and heat in the throat, first day (11). Dryness in the mouth and throat, the tongue feels as if burnt, second day (11). Prickling heat on the tongue, 1st day (11). **90.** Sensation of dryness in the mouth and throat, 2d day (11). Copious accumulation of soapy saliva in the mouth and throat, in the morning, second day (11). °Burning stinging sensation in the mouth and throat (3). *Dryness of the tongue, red, fiery appearance of the buccal cavity, with painful tenderness (3). An aching pressure as if from a hard body, back in the upper part of the throat and fauces, continuing for some hours, at half an hour. (Occurred in two provings) (7). **95.** °Very appropriate in various kinds of angina, with redness, swelling, and stinging pains (7). *Glossitis.

APPETITE AND STOMACH. Violent eructations (6). Eructations tasting like the yolk of eggs (6). Nausea, apparently from the throat (6). **100.** Nausea and inclination to vomit at night, and disagreeable rumbling in the abdomen as if a diarrhœa would come on (7). Prickling pain in the stomach, as from needles (6). Sensation of heat and burning in the stomach 1st day (11). °Bilious vomiting, with a single dose in 15 to 30 minutes, 4 cases (3).

ABDOMEN. Aching and pressing pain in the hypogastrium, with bearing down in the uterus, as if the menses would come on, in two persons (7). **105.** Rumbling in the abdomen, as if diarrhœa would ensue (6). Sore feeling in the abdomen in the morning (6). Sickly feeling in the abdomen which disposes a person to continue in a quiet sitting posture (6). Dull pain in the bowels (6). Soreness of the bowels felt when sneezing or pressing upon them (6). **110.** Fulness and evident enlargement of the abdomen, from many and large doses, in a female (7). *Fulness and sensation of bloating in the abdomen as if she were puffed up* (7). °Ascites following enteritis; abdomen distended with serum; countenance sunken, pale, sickly; urine scanty, high colored; pulse quick, wiry; deficient appetite (5). Has proved curative in several cases of ascites (7). °Enlargement of the abdomen, with swelling of the feet and scanty urine, in a lady of fifty (7).

ANUS AND STOOL. **115.** Sensation of stuffing in the anus (6). Throbbing in the rectum (6). Heat in the anus (6). Loose lumpy stool (6). *Loose stool in the morning (7). **120.** Loose, urgent stool in the morning (6, 7). Bowels confined from the 8th to the 12th day (7). Stools soft and pappy, mixed with serum, as though soft fæces had been beaten in water but not dissolved; the color that of an orange (8). Loose stools eight days in succession (11). Several loose stools daily (7). **125.** Several loose yellow stools, with extreme weakness and prostration; stools coming on at every movement of the body as though the anus were continually open; in a lady of 40 affected with chronic ascites, from the 6th dil. (7). Two loose stools daily for five days (11). °Painful diarrhœa (3). Yellow, watery diarrhœa, griping, 12 movements in as many hours (3). *Frequent yellow, watery evacuations, from a single dose (3); several other similar cases. **130.** Hemorrhoidal affection with constipation, small tumors upon the verge of the anus; biting, boring, stinging pain, indescribable, insupportable, with extreme nervousness and irritability; pain relieved in 4 hours, cured in 24 hours (3). °Involuntary dark bloody oozing from the rectum, with swelling of anus (3). °Hemorrhoidal tumors attended with soreness and burning, stinging pains (3, 8, 11, et al). Sensation in the rectum resembling an electric shock, slightly painful, succeeded by urging to stool (6). Stool natural, preceded by emission of flatulence and a small quantity of almost colorless water, containing lumps or fragments of jelly-like mucus, streaked with blood (6).

URINE AND GENITALS. **135.** Repeated urination every few minutes, continuing through the entire day, in a person never subject to such attacks. The medicine, 1 drop, 2d, was taken at night, the symptoms appeared the day following (7). Frequent and excessively profuse discharge of natural urine through the day and night in a dropsical and pregnant subject, from 3 doses of the 30th (7). Frequent and copious discharge of urine (7). Somewhat frequent desire to urinate, attended with uneasiness in the spermatic cord, fifth day (8). More frequent inclination to urinate, attended with some burning before and after emission, second day (11). **140.** Urine high colored with more frequent emission, small in quantity, third day (11). Burning in the urethra before and after urination, third day (11). A pustule sore as a boil, surrounded by a red areola, and maturated in the centre, arises in the hair of the pubes, remaining sore and painful some days (7). °Urine scanty, with burning, smarting pain; several cases (3).

Stitch-like pain in the urethra (6). **145.** Frequent desire to urinate, attended with burning in the urethra with uneasiness in the spermatic cord, sixth day, from large doses (8).

MENSTRUATION. *Bearing down pains and sensation as if the menses would come on, in many cases* (7). Bearing down pains as in the early stages of parturition, in several cases (3). Bearing down pains in the uterus as if the menses would come on, with aching and pressing in the hypogastrium (7, 11). Metrorrhagia at the second month with profuse flow of blood, heaviness of the abdomen, faintness, great uneasiness, restlessness and yawning (7). **150.** Hemorrhage from the uterus, occurring in a lady who was always regular and healthy, occurring one week after the cessation of the usual menstrual period, and three days after taking the medicine (7). *Miscarriage at the second month;* from drop doses of the second dilution (7). *Miscarriage at the third month* (7). Miscarriage *at the fourth month* in a healthy young married female during an attack of mild fever; on giving *Apis* 6, abortion came on, attended with profuse flooding (3). Should only be given to pregnant females with the utmost caution (7). °Amenorrhœa in young girls; many cases (7 et al.). *Suppressed menstruation, many cases (7 et al.). °Great increase of pain and tenderness in the ovarian region in two cases, one of large induration, the other in a supposed incipient stage of development (3). °Has proved curative in several cases of enlarged ovaria and also in ovaritis (7, 11). Ovarian dropsy? (7).

LARYNX AND COUGH. **160.** Hoarseness and rough voice through the day and night, second day (7, 6).

CHEST. Pressure in the chest, soon (7). Sharp pains in the chest at night (7). Stitches through the chest and back at night. *Stitches in the left side of the chest (6). **165.** Several stitch-like pains just below the heart (6). Hurried and difficult respiration with fever and headache, second day (2). Pain near the heart, which almost arrested the breathing at night, continuing at intervals for some days (11). Sensation as though he should not be able to breathe again (11). Short rapid breathing at night (2). **170.** Sensation of warmth or burning in the chest, first day (11.) Pains as of a bruise, and sensation of weight in the chest for several days (7, 3.) Sensation of fulness, tension and pressure in the chest, first day (11). Dull aching pains in the left side of the chest near the middle of the sternum, several times during the day, with sensation of fulness in the chest, with short breath first day (11). Sensation of burning heat in the chest and stomach early in the morning, second day (11). **175.** Sensation of soreness, lame, bruised feeling, as if from recent injury from being jammed, bruised or beaten; confirmed in many provers (3). *Sensation of melting heat in the region of the diaphragm, as if from running violently (3 et al.). Slight oppression of the chest, with frequent desire to draw a deep inspiration (6). Slight pain in the left side of the chest under the short ribs (6). °Has proved curative in hydrothorax, in several cases (7, 11).

BACK AND NECK. **180.** Rheumatic stitches in the muscles of the right side of the neck, worse when moving the head in that direction, came on when rising in the morning, very painful; not so much noticed when moving the head in any other direction, second day (7). Tension in the right side of the neck, beneath and back of the ear, soon (7). Sudden flush of heat over the back, as though sweat would break out, accompanied by a pain at the left ileo-sacral junction (3). Dull pressure under the scapula, with sore feeling on moving the parts (6). Slight sensation of stiffness in the nape of the neck and small of the back (6).

SUPERIOR EXTREMITIES. **185.** Aching in the right shoulder and upper portion of the arm, soon (7). °Erysipelas of the left arm and wrist, with redness, swelling, heat, and tumefaction of the part; cured with 6th dil. (7). Burning as of fire in small circumscribed spots on the hands, continuing for some minutes, second day (7). Fiery burning at the points of the finger (7). Tingling of the fingers of the left hand, soon (7). **190.** Darting pains in the left elbow for an instant, third day (8). Great increase and intensity of the odor from the axillary glands, fourth day (8). Dull pains apparently in the bones of the arms and fingers (6).

INFERIOR EXTREMITIES. Fine burning stinging on the knee (7). Darting, transient pain in the external malleolus of the left ankle for four days (8). **195.** Dull pains as if in the bones of the lower extremities (6). Sore feeling of the flesh of the lower extremities, disappearing on walking, returning again while sitting (6). Burning of the toes and redness like erysipelas and heat of a circumscribed patch on the foot, while the remainder of the feet are cold; continuing half an hour (7.) At night, on removing the boots and socks, the feet were found swelled full, with a sensation of heaviness and rigidity, the upper part of the feet felt bungling and itched, and were of a bright red color. The soles of the feet and balls of the toes had a feeling of painful fulness, and in walking gave the sensation as if cushioned; sixth day, as from many large doses (8). Burning of the feet, first day (11). **200.** *Œdematous swelling of the extremities (7).

SKIN. *Prickling all over the body, most on the back and palms of the hands, the face, forehead, and under the eyes, mostly in circumscribed points, immediately on taking the drug (6, 7 et al.) *Eruption resembling nettle-rash came out all over the body of a man, soon after being stung (7). °Nettle-rash in a lying-in woman (7). °Large hard elevations like mosquito bites, upon the back and legs of a child, accompanied with stinging, itching and burning (7). **205.** *Blotches on the body and back of the hands, attended wilh stinging like nettles, second day (11). Portions of the surface as large as a dollar swell up without discoloration, and become excessively sore and tender to the touch; 1st att. and tinct. (7). Itching pricking in the skin on different parts of the body, more on the lower extremities, and continued through the day, 1st day (11). °Eruptions upon the whole surface of the body somewhat resembling measles, with great heat and purplish circumscribed hue upon the cheeks (3). Eruption like nettle-rash over the whole body, second day after taking the 30th att., attended with burning and itching (11). **210.** °Retrocession of eruption in scarlatina, with violent fever, extreme heat, injected eyes, congestion to the head, and violent delirium continuing for many hours; *acon.*, *bell.*, *bry.* and other remedies did no good; *apis* every three hours brought out the rash, relieved the congestion and delirium, and cured the case (10). °A ringworm on the neck of a girl aged 12, inflamed and excoriated by the clothing, with one dose 30th att. (11). *Sensation of burning heat and stinging in various portions of the surface of the body, at the same time (3). The entire surface becomes exceedingly tender to the touch; every hair is painful on contact, from 6th dil. (7). °Hard, livid purplish tumors, or small elevations upon the forehead, face, and lower limbs (3). **215.** **Furuncles*, and LARGE SWELLINGS *of every description*, or local inflammations attended with them, and accompanied *with stinging pains* (7 et mult. al.). *NETTLE-RASH in numerous instances (7 et mult. al.). *Œdematous swelling of the extremities (7 et al.). °Puffy swelling of the face, hands, forehead, temples, about the eyes, neck and upper arms, with inability to swallow food, nasty taste in mouth, fever, thirst; can drink water constantly; commenced with a violent shaking chill: cured with *apis* 30, then 6, every three or four hours (7). °Post-scarlatinal dropsy, several cases after *ars.*, *bell.*, *dig.* and *acon.* had failed (9). **220.** °*Anasarca* and *ascites* after scarlatina (7 et al.).

SLEEP. *Fidgetty restlessness in the latter part of the night (7). Fidgetty restlessness the entire night with inability to sleep (7). Night sleep is full of dreams (7); *this symptom repeated in every proving.* Night sleep is yet full of dreams, mostly of travelling, eleventh day (7). Disagreeable dreams about fiends (11). **225.** Frequent waking, first night, and dreams with vexatious cares about various kinds of business (11). Sensation as of movement from place to place, mostly travelling by railroad (11).

FEVER. Pulse 95, full and strong (2). Pulse increased 20 in a minute, full and strong, second proving (2). Sweat breaks out occasionally (2). **230.** Sweating and dryness of the skin, alternately (2). Occasional feeling of chilliness (2). Inclination to yawn (2). Slight chill soon passing off, followed by fever at night (2). Pulse accelerated, first day (11). **235.** Heat at night with agitation, first night (11). Pulse increased from 65 to 77, first day (11). General feeling of heat, worse in the chest and stomach, first day (11).

GENERALITIES. General feeling of lassitude, second day (11). General feeling of lassitude with trembling (11). **240.** Sudden prostration of the vital force, severe vomiting, profuse diarrhœa, cold extremities, paleness of face, severe griping pains in the abdomen, pulse feeble, scarcely discernible at the wrist; no redness or pain in the part stung. [From a sting on the eyebrow.] *Apis-mel.*, 3, 5 glb., and not repeated; reaction came on in 10 to 15 minutes; improvement continued; some redness of the part stung appeared on the abatement of the general symptoms (3). *Bruised sensation* all over him, sides, hips, back, everywhere, restlessness the whole night and loose urgent stool; in the morning from some pellets of the 6th dil. taken over night for a stye: this train of symptoms repeated 2 or 3 times from similar doses (7).

4. *Clinical Remarks.*

CASE 1. The following case of involuntary proving of the *Apis* is reported by Dr. BISHOP.

Mrs. R., æt. 40, unmarried. Large Ovarian Tumors. Left tumor pressing upon the rectum, interfering with defecation—should think them four inches in diameter, extremely hard to the touch per vaginam and externally—of three years' standing, having been suddenly developed by a powerful emmenagogue. General health not good; subject to nervous headache. At the time she came under my care, July 13th, 1850, she complained much of sharp, lancinating pains in the ovarian tumors; urine scanty; bowels constipated; but no headache or fever. Failing to relieve the lancinating pains in the tumors as I had done before with *Lachesis*, followed by *Platina*, and not succeeding with any other remedy to my liking, I left 3 drops of *Apis-mel.* 2; also the same quantity of the first dilution, directing her to take the first dilution if she received no relief from the second, but if any aggravation occurred to stop the medicine immediately. The symptoms which I will now detail and which I consider pathogenetic, began to be developed before she had taken of the second. But as she had always been notoriously faithful in taking allopathic remedies, come what would, and as my next visit was deferred nearly two days beyond the time I intended, she had taken all the medicine left her.

Symptoms. HEAD.—General headache, very severe, with great sensation of pressure or rush of blood to the head. Throbbing, painful burning sensation in the temples.

EYES.—Smarting burning sensation, great redness of conjunctiva, very sensitive to the light.

FACE.—The patient seemed at a loss for language to express the peculiar burning and heat in her face experienced during the first 24 hours of its continuance; a somewhat livid and purplish appearance came on upon the abatement of the heat and burning.

CHEST.—Nothing of importance developed in the air passages, but some portion of the respiratory muscles, including the diaphragm and mediastinum, indicated a specific impression from the drug. She felt a severe burning pain under the short ribs on both sides, most severe on the left and of longer duration, continuing in the left side more than two weeks, and so severe as to deprive her of sleep nearly the whole time.

I will endeavor to describe the kind of heat and burning which, according to my own experience and the testimony of others, may be regarded as a specific and pathogenetic symptom of the *Apis-mellifica.* 1. On the surface like the sting of bees, or rather the burning heat which follows the introduction of the virus. 2. Upon the serous membranes and muscular tissues, especially in the region of the diaphragm, the pathogenesis of *Apis-mel.* is best described by the peculiar sensation of heat or melting, if I may be allowed the term; a sensation sometimes experienced after running violently, so that one is obliged to sit down exhausted, and in common parlance, feeling as if his vitals were literally melting. 3. Somewhat resembling the effects of *arsenicum*, so far as the mere sensation of heat is concerned, but with actual heat, in addition, and a livid purplish hue.

STOOL.—Greenish, yellowish, slimy diarrhœa, perfectly painless, coming on in about 24 hours after taking the first dose; she had 12 movements during the day; never subject to looseness of the bowels, and never had anything in her life resembling it. The diarrhœa subsided after one day's continuance.

URINE.—Diminished in quantity one half, although scanty before taking the medicine; the scalding burning sensation was very severe while urinating.

FEVER.—The development of heat and fever, which I regarded as pathogenetic in this case, continued to increase for about 36 hours, and was then followed by a severe shaking chill, occurring about 5 o'clock in the morning; she felt very cold, but was not actually so to the touch of another person.

GENERAL REMARKS.—The pain in the ovarian tumors was much diminished in a day or two, and at the end of two weeks she had not much disturbance from that source. I was wholly unable to control the heat and burning pain in the left side, though I made an effort to do so for about ten days, at which time she took, on her own responsibility, a large dose of epsom salts and soon after was bled, but with no benefit or abatement of the symptoms. After waiting rather patiently against time for improvement, she so far recovered as to visit relations at some distance, which, I must confess, somewhat relieved me, to say the least, from positive proximity to the subject of experiment with *Apis-mellifica.*

The following examples of the clinical use of the *Apis* have been furnished from various sources.

CASE 2. *Ascites;* reported by Dr. BARKER.

A gentleman of 70, feeble constitution, lymphatic temperament, light. skin, blue eyes, was seized, after an attack of influenza, with dropsical swelling of the chest, abdomen, feet and legs. He was unable to lie down without panting, and was always worse towards morning; urine reduced to a half pint per day. *Apis* 3 (dec. dil.); after three days the urine began to flow freely; between 3 and 9 A. M., two quarts would frequently be discharged, and under the use of this remedy, subsequently alternated with *Ars.* 60, the patient entirely recovered.

CASE 3. *Ascites;* reported by Dr. GREENE.

W. C., æt. 3½ years. Abdomen very much distended with serum, countenance sunken, pale, sickly, pulse quick, rather wiry, appetite poor, urine scanty and high colored. He had an attack of enteritis in September last, from which he rapidly recovered. I supposed that to be the cause of the present difficulty. I administered in their turn *ars.*, *dig.*, *dulc.*, *merc.*, *china* and *sulph.*, but with no decided effect. The effusion still continued to increase up to Feb. 10th, at which time there was much difficulty of breathing except in nearly an erect position. At this time I performed the operation of paracentesis, drawing off some 7 or 8 lbs. of a dark, sizy, muddy looking serum. I then gave one drop *apis* three times a day, for five or six days, with two doses *merc. sol.*, intermediately, at which time the urine became more free, although there had been some more sensation of fluid in the abdomen during that time.

Finding the quantity of urine increased and the general symptoms better, I gave 4 or 5 pellets of *apis*, 3, three times a day, and continued that treatment five or six days, his health still improving. I then reduced it to twice a day, which he has continued to the present time; there are now no dropsical symptoms and the boy is lively, appetite good, bowels regular and every way in a promising condition for perfect health. Repeated *med.* only every third night.

CASE 4. *Ascites;* reported by DR. HUMPHREYS.

An elderly lady of light complexion, lymphatic temperament, had long suffered from dropsical swelling of the abdomen and extremities. The ankles and feet were quite œdematous and clumsy, the urine scanty and high colored, and she suffered from general depression and weariness. She had used several remedies to no purpose. *Apis-mel.* 30, rendered prompt and decided service, and has since always relieved her when from extra fatigue or other cause the dropsy has manifested itself.

CASE 5. *Ascites;* reported by DR. MARCY.

The following case occurred in the practice of DR. TAFT of Hartford, Conn.: The patient, a boy of 12, was attacked in July, 1849, with dysentery. After several weeks of medication under an allopathic physician, the acute symptoms subsided and the evacuations gradually assumed their natural state, but there remained an unnatural fulness and tenderness of the abdomen, some difficulty of respiration, especially on assuming the recumbent position, a dry and harsh skin, and a materially diminished secretion of urine. Notwithstanding the persevering employment of the usual allopathic routine of cathartics, mercurials and diuretics, the patient continued to grow worse, his abdomen became very much distended with serum, and very tender to the touch, or from even the pressure of the bed clothes; the respiration became exceedingly laborious and difficult, obliging the sufferer to remain for a good portion of the nights in his chair; impaired appetite, an almost entire suppression of urine, emaciation, debility, small and rapid pulse, anxious expression and other signs accumulated.

In this condition he came under the care of Dr. Taft, who administered *dig.*, *ars.*, *dulc.*, *merc.*, *chin.*, *sulph.*, *hell.*, but without amelioration. In the meantime, the increasing difficulty of respiration, loss of rest, of appetite and pain, had reduced the patient to so serious a condition that I was called in council with Dr. Taft in order to decide respecting the propriety of tapping. In consideration of the urgency of the symptoms and the inefficiency of the remedies which had been used, I evacuated the effused fluid, amounting to sixteen pounds, and advised a second trial of *arsenicum* and *digitalis.* No effect resulted and there began to be signs of thoracic effusion. Recourse was now had to the first trituration of the honey-bee, (5 to 100), and after two or three doses a large quantity of urine was passed, and the symptoms were all ameliorated. After the remedy had been continued for two weeks, all traces of effusion disappeared, the appetite and strength began to improve and the respiration became natural and easy. The patient was restored to perfect health.

Case 6. *Asthma;* reported by Dr. Wells.

Mr. N. P., æt. 70, had shortness of breath, oppression of the chest on taking an inspiration, and sensation of heat in the chest. These symptoms had been gradually increasing several weeks. Took *apis* 3, once a day, and was completely relieved in one week.

Case 7. *Bronchitis;* reported by Dr. Bishop.

Mary C., æt. 2 years. High fever, hot, dry skin, full pulse, laborious respiration resembling croup, painless diarrhœa, yellowish, sometimes greenish and slimy, tongue slightly coated white, disturbed sleep at night with muttering, incoherent talking. Gave *aconite*, *bry.*, *hep.* and other remedies, for three days without any benefit. Respiration very laborious, requiring unusual aid from the abdominal muscles; face flushed with increasing livid appearance. Fourth day; pulse not as frequent, but feeling under the finger like shot or some spherical body, gliding along the artery; cough attended with the ringing sound peculiar to affections of the upper portions of the respiratory tubes. Prognosis unfavorable, deeming it probable the patient would die in spite of all my efforts. Left her three doses of *apis* 3. Next day found her much better, face natural, pulse much improved, fever nearly gone, appetite improved, had slept well and without the usual mutterings, fright, &c. Continued the medicine in diminished doses, and next day found her so much better that I dismissed her as cured.

Case 8. *Cephalalgia;* reported by Dr. Bishop.

S. A. W., æt. 36. Took one drop of *apis* for periodical headache, with direction to repeat *ad libitum.* The first dose promptly suspended a paroxysm in its incipient stage. No homœopathic remedies had ever before had any effect in stopping his headache. The same result was obtained the second and third time. He then requested a supply of the remedy to be used as occasion required, which was furnished him, with directions not to use too much of it. This advice he did not heed. He got an aggravation of his complaint, and at length developed in his chest the true pathogenetic symptoms of the virus, viz.: sensation, as of having been bruised, jammed or beaten.

Dr. Kellogg has given the *apis* with decided benefit in the case of a female who had suffered for years under symptoms of general prostration, particularly in cold weather, attended by asthmatic symptoms, as cough, choking pain in the chest, with coldness and deadness of the extremities, and purplish livid hue. Also, in some cases of chronic sick headache, where there seemed utter prostration of the central ganglionic nerves.

Case 9. *Diarrhœa;* reported by Dr. Bishop.

J. M. B. Sept. 1st., 1850. Yellowish, greenish diarrhœa; some griping pain; pain in the eyeballs and across the forehead, more on the right side for some years past, but formerly in both temples alike, languid, listless, unaccountable feeling. A year ago had partial development of intermittent fever. At the time, said he had "the blues." Could not bring his thoughts to bear upon anything definitely. Hands bluish, inclined to coldness; appetite poor. Was promptly cured of all these symptoms by a single dose of *apis* 3.

REMARKS.—The action of *Apis-mellifica* in the case of Mr. Butler (a single dose) remained about two months, and then the symptoms seemed to require its repetition. A single dose relieved him as before, and he had no occasion for repeating it for four or five months. A single dose has always been sufficient for him, and in no case do I recollect the improvement which set in, to have continued for less time than two months. Mr. B. is 23 years of age, light complexion, spare and thin, muscular power not great, uses a good deal of tobacco.

CASE 10. *Diarrhœa chronic;* reported by Dr. BISHOP.

J. S., æt. 6 years. Chronic diarrhœa and general emaciation. Sequelæ of measles. In this case there had been only a partial development of measles upon the surface, attended with fever and cough for two months, and then general emaciation, with tenderness of the bowels, loss of appetite until he was reduced to a mere skeleton. He then received from me a few drops of *apis*, which immediately improved his appetite, bowels became regular, his flesh returned, and he continued quite well for some months. Dec. 28th, 1850, saw him again; dry white tongue, loss of appetite, feverish heat during the night, and other times pale, emaciation going on. A few doses of the same remedy again set him right.

Saw him again about the 1st of January, 1851, and, at the request of his mother, left him a number of doses of *apis*, in case he should need it at any time in future. He soon after got a dose and grew worse, got another and then another, resulting in the development of a tumultuous action which, for nearly 24 hours, seemed to threaten his life. At this time I was from home attending the meeting of the Central Association, at Utica, and did not see him until the paroxysm of excitement had nearly subsided. From his mother I learned the following particulars of the case: general heat and redness of the surface, like scarlet fever, with some eruption like measles, cough and laborious breathing resembling an alarming stage of croup, muttering, delirium, &c. He got an emetic of Ipecac. from an allopathic physician, which seemed greatly to mitigate the symptoms, and when I saw him the next day he was quite comfortable.

CASE 11. *Diarrhœa;* reported by Dr. BISHOP.

Mrs. C., æt. 40. Gastralgia and bilious diarrhœa. Pain and tenderness at the pit of the stomach, with burning sensation, as in some cases of acidity; fæcal discharges, yellowish, bordering on green, nearly painless. This lady had occasionally been subject to long and severe affections of the stomach, sometimes connected with obstinate constipation, at other times diarrhœa. She attributed it to erysipelas, which at times made its appearance upon the lower limbs and upon various portions of the body. I have seen it occupying the lower limbs in the form of dark purplish and painful tumefactions attended with much constitutional disturbance. I have treated her homœopathically for what she called "Erysipelas in her stomach." From these attacks she would, after a long time, recover, but the results of medical treatment were not at all satisfactory to myself. At this time she had been laboring under the usual precursory symptoms, which had often ushered in a long and protracted disease of the stomach. For about two weeks the symptoms, it is true, did not indicate *per se* anything of peculiar interest or difficulty, except in connection with past experience and observation in her particular case. I left her three doses of *apis* 3, with directions to repeat once in twelve hours if no aggravation of symptoms occurred, but if any occurred to omit the medicine entirely. The first dose increased the burning sensation in the stomach, also the diarrhœa. This aggravation subsided in eight or ten hours, with great improvement in all the symptoms.

She took the second dose, which brought up the burning pain in the stomach, as did the third; the aggravation soon subsided, and I never knew a more perfect and speedy cure than was produced by the three doses of *apis* in this case. Her erysipelatous affection has never made its appearance since.

CASE 12. *Eruptions;* reported by Dr. BISHOP.

Mr. J. M. Eruptions upon the inner portion of the thighs, also below the knees, upon the hands, face, and back of the neck, but more upon the central portions of the body, with the following characteristics: commencing with small pustular formations just under the cuticle, with burning, smarting, stinging sensation; in coming to maturity, deposition of dry, scabby matter, laminated form, scaly, brownish and sometimes light straw colored. Looseness of the bowels in the morning, thin, watery, yellowish; some griping at times, but generally painless. The looseness of the bowels had continued three or four weeks. Treatment for the last ten days, *rhus* and other antipsoric remedies: no abatement of symptoms, either of skin or bowels.

On further examination I found the burning, stinging sensation in the eruption more severe than I had imagined, and was, in consequence, induced to try the *apis*. I had no attenuation of the remedy with me, and accordingly medicated a portion of sugar with the mother tincture, much less than one drop, then rubbed with another portion and dissolved a s n a part of this in a cup full of water. Dose, one tea-spoonful twice in twenty-four hours. Cured immediately and effectually of both diarrhœa and eruption; no return for eighteen months.

CASE 13. *Erysipelas;* reported by Dr. GREENE.

Erysipelas of the whole of one side of the face and nose; swelling under the eye resembling that produced from the sting of the honey-bee. *Apis* 3, ten or twelve drops in a glass of water; dose, a spoonful repeated in one to three hours until better. Swelling subsided entirely, and the next morning the young lady returned to her school and has had nothing of the kind since to my knowledge.

CASE 14. *Metastasis of Eruption;* reported by Dr. BISHOP.

J. C. R., æt. 35. Saw him at the commencement of his illness; symptoms indicated the fever peculiar to the locality where he resided; chills for five or six days, not much febrile re-action; after some days improved so much as to be out and oversee his business in part; did not visit him again in a week, and when called again his wife thought I had been mistaken in the nature of his complaint, and that he was laboring under inflammation of the lungs. On examining the case again I found the following symptoms:

CHEST.—Sensation of soreness, as if from a recent mechanical injury. Sensation as if the chest had been jammed, beaten, or bruised, especially on the left side. Full inspirations did not particularly increase these sensations. Tendency to chilliness and increase of these symptoms every other day; pulse 65, soft and feeble; cough harrassing, especially at night; shortness of breath, respiration much disturbed by exercise; bowels natural; appetite good.

Mercurius relieved his cough, and with the aid of *ars.*, the periodicity was suspended for nearly two weeks. Some remains of the lame, sore, bruised feeling about the chest, also feeling of prostration and shortness of breath, partial return of chills and slight aggravation of the symptoms every other day. In this state he continued about two weeks, doing some light labor without any medical treatment, except a few doses of *merc.*, which he took for his cough.

I was called to see him again in the night of Nov. 10th. Found him with symptoms (apparently) of inflammation of the pleura and diaphragm; but little cough, respiration extremely painful, pulse rather full and somewhat accelerated. He got a single dose of *aconite*, followed by *bry.* 3., in drop doses once in 3 hours: next day much improved. *Bry.* 6, once in 8 hours. Pain and soreness much better for several days, but shortness of breath and feeling of prostration continued. The former symptom soon returned, viz.: the peculiar sensation in the left side of the chest, also under the short ribs and in the mediastinal region, respiration not increasing the pain. I had supposed the present symptoms to be connected in no small degree with chronic rheumatism, but at this time my attention was called to what he denominated salt rheum, which had for many years troubled him more or less. Its retrocession from the surface had always been attended with what he termed rheumatic pains; but when the eruption was upon the surface he was free from them. I then recollected giving him *ars.* some 5 or 6 years before, for the eruption upon the hands, with much benefit, as he assured me it had never made its appearance since on his hands, but sometimes upon his body, especially about the chest. There had been nothing of it upon any portion of the surface for some time previous to his present illness. I made a pretty thorough trial of *ars.* and other remedies, but without any particular benefit; and at length he made up his mind to either go South and spend the winter, or try hydropathic treatment. On a careful re-examination of the chest symptoms, I found they corresponded with the pathogenesis of *Apis-mel.*, according to my own provings of that remedy, more perfectly than I was aware of, and in the following particulars: sensation in the muscles of the chest as of having been bruised, jammed, or beaten, pain in the left side under the short ribs, shortness of breath, especially on exercise, disposition to chilliness and a peculiar prostration of the great central organic nervous power, or that anomalous condition of the vital forces of the nervous centres, which, in its details, is often so perplexing to the practitioner, especially if pressed by the patient to give his disease a *name*. This consideration, as well as the clinical test of the remedy, in some cases of psoric disease induced me to try *apis* 3, in doses of a quarter of a drop. The first dose was attended with the disturbance in the region of the diaphragm and stomach already described, followed by the looseness or painless diarrhœa to which I have already alluded in the proving of *apis*. I saw him the next day after my prescription, and he assured me *this* was emphatically *the* remedy: that he felt every way better than he had done for some weeks; that he began to feel strong and like himself; was not troubled with shortness of breath, or any sore feeling or pain about his chest. He took the remedy once in a day or two for a time, and has remained perfectly sound and healthy ever since.

Case 15. *Gastro-enteritis*; reported by Dr. Bishop.

M. T., æt. 8 years. Gastro-enteritis, ushered in by vomiting, extreme pain and tenderness in the region of the stomach and upper portion of the abdomen, fetid breath, foul tongue, constipation, disturbed sleep at night, muttering, &c., much disturbed from dreams, pulse frequent, wiry. After one week's treatment, during which time there was not much abatement of the vomiting, or even of any of the prominent symptoms, I gave *apis* 3, three doses; next day found him better, rested quite well during the night, tenderness and pain much less; and from this time, the prominent and troublesome symptoms abated, passing off entirely in a week.

CASE 16. *Incipient Hydrocephalus;* reported by Dr. BISHOP.

Miss F., æt. 8 years. Dull, stupid state during the day, much inclined to sleep. At night, during sleep, talking, dreamy state; sleep in the morning profound—cannot be waked without being taken out of bed, shaken and forced about for a time. Great languor and lassitude, pale face, slight constipation, urine small in quantity—has been ill about two weeks. The mother informed me that, eight years before, a daughter of the same age sickened in precisely the same manner, and, at length, died of dropsy of the brain. I prescribed various remedies for ten days without any apparent benefit to the patient. The child inherited from her mother a psoric taint, which, in the parent, generally manifested itself in the form of urticaria, and sometimes on the lower extremities in detached and isolated elevations, painful and tender to the touch, and always assuming in their progress a purplish or livid hue. A few such spots were faintly visible upon the neck and forehead of the child, not having attained any elevation above the surface, or hardness.

I left her three doses of *apis* 2. She got one dose at 11 A.M., one at 3, and the other at 7 P.M. Her sleep, for the first time since her illness commenced, was comparatively quiet that night; awoke early the next morning, was lively and somewhat disposed to play and amuse herself about the house—had much more color in her face than at any time for two weeks. She began to improve visibly soon after taking the second dose. Next day left three more powders of the third—had more disturbance that night in her sleep than in the preceding one, but awoke early in the morning, and was out to play in the afternoon. Hard purplish spots upon the face, forehead and neck, and lower limbs, made their appearance in the second and third days after taking the medicine. These remained hard and painful some ten or twelve days, and disappeared. She was some time in regaining her strength and bodily activity, but at length became entirely well.

CASE 17. *Hydrothorax;* reported by Dr. WELLS.

Mrs. J. H. C., æt. 58, has been troubled with anasarca several years, and more recently, has had decided symptoms of hydrothorax, as sensation of fulness in the chest, shortness of breath, pains, sometimes dull and sometimes sharp, in the chest, inability to lie in the horizontal posture. Dec. 10th, 1850, commenced taking *apis* 3, every two days for two or three weeks, and then at longer intervals, with complete relief to all of the symptoms. Saw her in June, 1851, quite well.

CASE 18. *Inflammation of the labia;* reported by Dr. HUMPHREYS.

A lady of 38, mother of several children, had an extremely large and painful swelling of the labia, attended with violent heat and stinging pains. She received *apis* 30, a spoonful every three hours in the afternoon, and before the next morning the swelling and pain had disappeared and she was rapidly restored.

CASE 19. *Ophthalmia;* reported by Dr. HUMPHREYS.

A young lady, æt. 18, fair complexion, rather lymphatic temperament, was attacked in Oct., 1850, with a violent inflammation of the right eye. It came on suddenly without apparent cause, and she went into the hands of a skilful allopathic practitioner, who treated her five months, when my advice was sought. During his treatment three ulcers had formed on the cornea, one in December and two others in February. She had taken considerable medicine internally, frequent blisters behind the ears and had used various washes, &c. When I was called in, the ulcers, which had been nearly healed, were worse, the vessels of the eye injected, dreadful pain darting through the eyes, intolerance of light in both eyes, keeping them constantly closed; the entire cornea was scattered over with dark, smoky clouds, and thickened and covered with a film.

She could only discern the light of a window when turned towards it, and the pupil could not be discovered through the smoky and discolored cornea. The albuginea was dark red, the redness running insensibly into the cornea, tears of scalding water ran from the eye; cold feet, hot head, delaying menses. I commenced treatment in February. She received *merc.-cor.* and *bell.*, *merc.*, and *hep.* 3, until March 20th, at which time the temperature of the surface had become normal, the intolerance of light less, yet the general appearance of the eye and sight indicated no very marked improvement.

March 20th. She took *apis* 30 in water, a spoonful morning and evening. The effect was immediate. The following morning the eye looked clearer and she remarked that she could even see the eyes of her sister. From thence the improvement was rapid and permanent, and on the first of May she was discharged. There remained only a slight opacity of the cornea, which has since entirely disappeared. I have never witnessed so rapid, perfect and brilliant a cure in my experience. She took no other medicine, with the *apis* 30, except an occasional dose of *acon.*, when the pain in the extremities and heat became too violent.

CASE 20. *Ophthalmia;* reported by Dr. HUMPHREYS.

A woman of 50, dark complexion, bilious temperament, had suffered from ophthalmia for three years, and had been, with little benefit, under the care of several oculists. Her eyelids were swelled, dark red, everted, denuded of the lashes, granulations along the edges, the conjunctiva reddened and full of dark vessels, the cornea darkened and smoky, vision very indistinct, eyes intolerant of light, running and agglutinated. *Apis* 30, every three or four days, changed the entire aspect of the case. The eyelids were relieved entirely, the conjunctiva lost its dark vessels, the cornea became clear, vision improved, and she left almost entirely well.

CASE 21. *Tonsillitis;* reported by Dr. HUMPHREYS.

A lady, æt. 26, subject to frequent attacks of quinsy, which, despite the application of the usual remedies, *bell.*, *lach.* and *merc.*, generally ended in suppuration, was taken with one of the old attacks, viz., chilliness, then heat, violent pain in the temples, redness and swelling of the tonsils, uvula and fauces, painful difficulty of swallowing, stinging pains in attempting to do so. She received first *aconite*, then *apis* 30, which soon afforded relief, and under its use in 24 hours every vestige of the complaint disappeared. She declares that she has never received such marked and substantial relief from any other medicine as from it.

CASE 22. *Tonsillitis ;* reported by Dr. HUMPHREYS.

An unmarried lady, æt. 28, frequently subject to sore throat, was attacked with one of her usual ill turns, viz., violent pain in the forehead, lachrymal disposition, discouraged, desponding mood, very greatly enlarged tonsils with redness and swelling of the uvula and entire fauces, also great difficulty of deglutition, and smarting pain in the throat; no appetite, tongue coated. *Acon.* and *bell.* were given for twenty-four hours with no particular relief, when I resorted to *apis* at intervals of four hours either alone or in alternation with *merc.* An immediate and decided effect was produced, and in twenty-four hours she was dismissed with only a few doses of *apis* in case of relapse.

CASE 23. Reported by Dr. WELLS.

Mr. N. B. has had pains in the left hypochondriac region, extending upward into the chest. This case of several years' duration, had not been benefitted by the usual remedies, *arnica, sulph.*, &c. Took a few doses of *apis* 3, which entirely removed the disease.

The following cases by Mad. De Bonneville were communicated to Dr. Humphreys by Dr. Hering. The guide in the choice of the remedy was the symptom of SWELLING.

CASE 24.—An old woman, some 80 years of age, sanguine nervous bilious temperament, had a white puffy swelling of a paralyzed arm and hand. Three doses of the *apis*, one given daily, produced an entire removal of this symptom. About three months afterwards the same person from excessive grief became paralyzed upon her entire right side. Some ten days after her second stroke, the same symptom, swelling, occurred over the entire side, entirely closing her right eye. A few doses of the *apis* entirely removed this symptom.

CASE 25.—A woman about 37 years of age, sanguine nervous temperament, had both her eyes closed with a purplish, white swelling, preceded by intense pain in the right eye. One dose of the *apis* removed the swelling and when it returned a fortnight or so afterwards it was again removed by one dose, and has not returned again in eleven months.

CASE 26.—A girl of 13 years. Gave the *apis* for a dark, puffy swelling under the eyes; a dose every three days for about a fortnight, with success.

CASE 27.—A child of nervous temperament, fifteen months old, had a whitish, red swelling of the lower portion of the anus, attended with intolerable itching. Two doses of the *apis* at an interval of six days, entirely removed the affection.

CASE 28.—A man of 28 years; sanguine nervous bilious temperament.—Sudden paralysis of the entire right side, with violent delirium, at times amounting to phrensy. Gave the *apis* the first medicine, as I learned from his wife that he had, before his attack, sudden whitish swellings that itched violently upon his head, and sometimes upon his neck. In less than an hour after giving the *apis* he was broken out in countless places upon his head, and much quieted in his mind. The swellings subsided before morning, and his phrensy was such as to require three men to hold him from throwing himself headlong from the bed.—Gave *hep.-sul.* one dose and the *apis* fifteen minutes afterwards; and he become rational for the most part of the day, and much broken out upon the calves of his legs. Used the *apis* several times afterwards in this case, always with marked success.

CASE 29.—Used it for a lad fifteen years of age, lymphatic sanguine temperament, who had been poisoned in the woods, upon the face and hands without benefit. Used *rhus-rad.* with complete success.

Case 30.—A woman of about 30 years. Sanguine nervous temperament. Swelling of the tongue, with a dry, glossy, yellowish appearance, accompanied with excessively painful vomitings of bile, &c. Gave *nux* and *bryonia* until the vomiting was subdued, the swelling of the tongue continuing, gave *apis* twice, once in three hours, with a decidedly good effect. A few months afterwards for the same symptoms gave the same medicine with good results.

Case 31.—A young man about 20 years old, of sanguine bilious lymphatic temperament, had been thrown from a horse and his left knee badly sprained. Gave the *apis* for the swelling, one dose. Some two weeks afterwards from standing upon it too much, the knee again swelled, and the use of the *apis*, one dose, immediately removed the swelling.

Case 32.—A woman of about 30 years had swelled eyes every morning for a long time. Cured by three doses alternated with *sulphur*. I never saw her.

Case 33.—A man of about 45 years, nervous sanguine temperament.—Painful, puffy swellings of the knees. Five doses alternated with *iodium*, a dose once in three days, cured the affection.

7.—ARISTOLOCHIA MILHOMENS.

ARIST.-MIL. A. Grandiflora (Gom.). A. Cymbifera (Mart.). Snakeroot.

1. *Description and Preparation.*

Very many species of *Aristolochia* have been used in medicine in different countries. Among these the *A. serpentaria*, a very common plant in the United States, has become so popular that the root (the part employed medicinally) is sold by the bale, and forms an extensive article of traffic. The species used by Mure in the following provings is an inhabitant of Brazil, and is thus described by him (*Pathogénésie Brésilienne*, 315):

"A climbing plant; stem glabrous; leaves alternate, uniformly cordate, ribbed, presenting between the ribs reticulated veins; petioles long, furnished with a large, entire, uniform, sheathing stipule; flowers solitary upon a sulcate peduncle, eight or ten centimetres long; perianth single, very large, of a yellowish brown, tuberculated, curved, divided into two lips; the upper acute and lanceolate, bent a little outwards; the lower twice as long as the other, dilated at the base, and expanding into a large oval disk with waved edges. The whole flower is covered with prominent nerves. Stamens six, epigynous; ovary glabrous, surmounted by a stigma with six very short and rounded lobes."

The part employed in the following provings was the flower.

2. *Prior Knowledge of its Effects.*

We are not aware of any experiments with the particular species employed by Mure. The *A. pistolochia, longa, clematitis* and *serpentaria* have been long employed in medicine both in Europe and in this country. They are considered, in the undistinguishing jargon of the old school, to be "stimulant tonics, acting *also* as diaphoretics or diuretics, according to the mode of application. The *A. Serpentaria* too largely taken occasions nausea, griping pains in the bowels, sometimes vomiting and dysenteric tenesmus * * . It has been highly recommended in intermittent fevers, and though itself generally inadequate to cure the complaint (!), often proves serviceable as an adjunct to Peruvian Bark or the Sulphate of Quina. It is sometimes given in dyspepsia, and is employed as a gargle in malignant sore throat." (*Wood and Bache* Dispensatory, 660.)

It is not worth while to accumulate matter of this sort, especially as both the species and part of the plant used in the provings were different.

3. *Provings.*

There was but one prover; his name is not given, nor is he described, nor are the doses taken particularly stated. The experiments of the Brazilian School were generally made with the fourth or fifth dilution.

1st day. Disturbed rest. He dreams that he can neither eat, nor drink, nor walk. Throbbing in the right frontal eminence for a minute. Mouth pasty through the whole morning. Thirst. Pain in the right groin. Swelling of the left leg. Swelling of the lower part of the calf. Borborygmi in the stomach and intestines. Lancinations through the whole extent of the left inferior extremity. The left leg is red and inflamed. Head heavy. Great thirst, with bitterness of the mouth. Anorexia. Stinging in the hypothenar eminence of the left hand; half-past 3 P. M. Sensation of torpor at the vertex. Pricking in the right testicle. Pricking in the right thigh. Prick as from a pin in the lower part of the left leg. Itching on the internal surface of the left thigh. Prickings in different parts of the body. Pain in the hypothenar eminence of the right hand at 7 P. M. Sensation of torpor in the cerebellum. Prick under the heel. Itching on the external malleolus of the left foot; 8 P.M. Itching on the skin of the prepuce. Cramp-like pain in the right internal malleolus. Bruised pain over the left pectoral muscle, which is sensitive to the touch at night.

2d day. Unquiet sleep. He dreams of a sheep and a dog covered with red scarves; the first, elevated above the ground, shook his head, and was seized by the dog in the middle of his back; the dog himself was suspended by the back by a man accompanied by many other individuals. Afterwards a very amorous dream, with pollution. Painful spot under the scapula, as if from having received a blow. Disagreeable sensation behind the left internal malleolus. Uneasiness, then pricking in the thighs at 2 P. M. Bruised pain in the left knee. Lancinations in the anterior part of the left external malleolus, at 7 P. M. Fulness of the stomach. Acute pain in the right thigh. The leg is swollen and violet-colored in the morning; it becomes inflamed by fatigue, and turns a blackish red towards evening. Want of appetite. The whole leg is covered by large irregular patches, formed by extravasated blood. He makes water more frequently than usual. The head is burning hot. Continual thirst and bitter mouth. Excoriations of the lips and gums. Complete anorexia. The left leg is painful, as if excoriated; the pain passes to the right internal malleolus, and becomes more acute.

3d day. Lancinating pain at the apex of the heart, which takes away his breath at night. His temples are very sensitive to touch during the whole day. Stiffness of the leg, with impossibility of standing up for a few minutes. Sharp pain between the shoulders. Dull pain at the lower part of the lumbar region, and in the hypogastrium. Burning pains at the anus. Excoriations of the lips and gums as yesterday. Itching above the bend of the right arm. Cramp-like pain in the left tendo Achillis. Partial swelling around the malleoli. Bruised pain under the left patella at 3 P. M. Lancinations in the lower part of the right leg and internal malleolus at 3½ P. M. The upper and lower parts of the left arm are painful to the touch at 4½ P. M. Painful lancinations in the internal part of the left knee. Pricking in the joint of the first phalanx of the little finger at 8 P. M.

4th day. Pain in the dorsal portion of the left index. Colic, followed by a stool first soft, then diarrhœic twice in succession, in the morning. Malaise, as if something were collected in the internal part of the right leg above the knee, during the evening and part of the night.

5th day. Uneasiness in the lumbar region. Feeling as if the lower part of the right leg had a tendency to fall down upon the malleoli, as a stocking might do; he often carries his hand there, as if to raise it up. Itching on the anterior part of the right leg. Pricking on the internal surface of the right leg. Uneasiness in the lower part of the tendo Achillis. Easy stool.

6th day. Itching on the internal malleolus of the left foot. Itching on the right thigh. Pain above the right internal malleolus. Disgusting dreams.

7th day. Malaise after waking in the morning; he cannot go to sleep again; he feels as if something incommoded him about the malleoli for several hours. This pain increases, becoming a bruised pain towards 3 P.M. The malleoli appear swollen. Acute pain in the sacro-lumbar region. Pain in the right side.

8th day. Pain at the scrobiculus. The pains in the legs continue. Persistent pain above the left internal malleolus. Smarting on the interior, superior part of the right thigh in the evening. Acute lancination in the head in the evening.

9th day. Acute lancination in the left side of the head in the evening.

10th day. Severe lancination behind the head. The upper part of the left leg is painful to the touch. Shootings in the cerebellum.

4. *Digest of the Symptoms.*

AUTHORITY. *Pathogénésie Brésilienne*, 315.

The figures refer to the day on which the symptom was observed.

HEAD. Head heavy (1). The head is burning hot (2). Throbbing in the right frontal eminence for a minute (1). Sensation of torpor at the vertex (1). **5.** His temples are very sensitive to touch during the whole day (3). Acute lancination in the head (evening, 8). Acute lancination in the left side of the head (evening, 9). Severe lancination behind the head (10). Shootings in the cerebellum (10). **10.** Sensation of torpor in the cerebellum (1).

MOUTH. Mouth pasty through the whole morning (1). Excoriations of the lips and gums (2). Excoriations of the lips and gums as on the second day (3).

APPETITE. Anorexia (1). **15.** Want of appetite (2). Complete anorexia (2). Thirst (1). Great thirst with bitterness of the mouth (1). Continual thirst and bitter mouth (2).

STOMACH. **20.** Borborygmus in the stomach and intestines (1). Fulness of the stomach (2). Pain at the scrobiculus (8).

STOOL AND ANUS. Colic, followed by a stool, at first soft, then diarrhœic, twice in succession (morning, 4). Easy stool (5). **25.** Burning pains at the anus (3).

URINARY AND GENITAL. He makes water more frequently than usual (2). Itching on the skin of the prepuce (1). Pricking in the right testicle (1).

CHEST. Lancinating pain at the apex of the heart which takes away his breath at night (3). **30.** Bruised pain over the left pectoral muscle, which is sensitive to the touch at night (1).

BACK. Painful spot under the scapula, as if from having received a blow (2). Sharp pain between the shoulders (3). Pain in the right side (7). Uneasiness in the lumbar region (5). **35.** Dull pain at the lower part of the lumbar region and in the hypogastrium (2). Acute pain in the sacro-lumbar region (7).

SUPERIOR EXTREMITIES. The upper and lower parts of the left arm are painful to the touch (4½ P.M. 3). Itching above the bend of the right arm (3). Stinging in the hypothenar eminence of the left hand (3½ P.M. 1). **40.** Pain in the hypothenar eminence of the right hand (7 P.M. 1). Pain in the dorsal portion of the left index (4). Pricking in the joint of the first phalanx of the little finger (8 P.M. 3).

INFERIOR EXTREMITIES. Pain in the right groin (1). Lancinations through the whole extent of the left inferior extremity (1). **45.** The left leg is red and inflamed (1). Swelling of the left leg (1). The leg is swollen and violet-colored in the morning; it becomes inflamed by fatigue and turns blackish red towards evening (2). The whole leg is covered by large irregular patches formed by extravasated blood (2). Malaise as if something were collected in the internal part of the right leg above the knee (evening and part of night, 4). **50.** The pains in the legs continue (8). Uneasiness, then pricking in the thighs (2 P.M. 2). Stiffness of the leg, with impossibility of standing up for a few minutes (3). Pricking on the internal surface of the right leg (5). Smarting on the internal superior part of the right thigh (evening 8). **55.** Pricking in the right thigh (1). Acute pain in the right thigh (2). Itching on the right thigh (6). Itching on the internal surface of the left thigh (1). The upper part of the left leg is painful to the touch (10). **60.** Itching on the anterior part of the right leg (5). Bruised pain in the left knee. Bruised pain under the left patella (3 P.M. 3). Painful lancinations in the internal part of the left knee (3). Prick as from a pin in the lower part of the left leg (1). **65.** Swelling of the lower part of the calf (1). Cramplike pains in the left tendo Achillis (3). Uneasiness in the lower part of the tendo Achillis (5). Prick under the heel (1). Malaise after waking in the morning; he cannot go to sleep again; he feels as if something incommoded him about the malleoli for several hours (7). This pain increases, becoming a bruised pain (towards 3 P.M. 7). **70.** Partial swellings around the malleoli (3). The malleoli appear swollen (7). Feeling as if the lower part of the right leg had a tendency to fall down upon the malleoli as a stocking might do; he often carries his hand there as if to raise it up (5). Cramplike pain in the right internal malleolus (1). Pain above the right internal malleolus (6). **75.** Lancinations in the lower part of the right leg and internal malleolus (3½ P.M. 3). The left leg is painful as if excoriated; the pain passes to the right internal malleolus and becomes more acute (2). Lancinations in the anterior part of the left external malleolus (7 P.M. 2). Itching on the left external malleolus (8 P.M. 1). Itching on the left internal malleolus (6). **80.** Persistent pain above the left internal malleolus (8). Disagreeable sensation behind the left internal malleolus (2).

SLEEP. Disturbed rest (1). Unquiet sleep (2). **Dreams.** Disgusting dreams (6). **85.** He dreams that he can neither act nor drink nor walk (1). He dreams of a sheep and a dog, covered with red scarves; the former, elevated above the ground, shook his head and was seized by the dog in the middle of his back; the dog himself was suspended by the back by a man accompanied by many other individuals (2). Afterwards, a very amorous dream with pollution (2).

GENERAL. Prickings in different parts of the body (1).

8.—ARSENICUM-METALLICUM.

ARS-MET. Metallic arsenic.

1. *History, Description and Preparation.*

The various preparations of arsenic have long been known. Aristotle, Dioscorides and Theophrastus are said to have been acquainted with the compound which it forms with sulphur, called *auri-pigmentum* or *orpiment.* It is most frequently found in composition, but sometimes in the metallic state. It was first carefully examined by Brandt in 1733, and has since been very thoroughly investigated by succeeding chemists.

Arsenic is a brittle metal of a bright steel-gray color, and a density of about 5·7. Its attraction for oxygen is considerable, as when exposed to the air it soon tarnishes; it is said to be perfectly preserved under water. At 356° Fahr. it volatilizes without fusing, and may be obtained by condensing the vapor, which has a strong smell of garlic, in crystalline scales. It is isomorphous with phosphorus, tellurium and antimony, and seems to have relations of a similar kind with nitrogen.

The metal may be obtained in a state of purity by heating in a glass retort a mixture of one part of white arsenic and three parts of black flux; it condenses, in the neck of the retort, into a metallic crust.

2. *Prior Knowledge of its Effects.*

This may be summed up in the words of Christison: "*In conformity with what appears to be a general law in toxicology,* THE METAL ITSELF IS INERT."

3. *Provings of Metallic Arsenic.**

FIRST PROVING.

Dec. 24, 1850. For three successive evenings one grain of the third trituration was taken.

*The metal used in the following provings was prepared in perfect purity at the laboratory of Professor Lehmann, in Leipzig, in 1845, by Dr. Buchheim, now professor of Materia Medica, in Dorpat. It had not altered, and had its full metallic lustre when in 1847 triturations were made in dry weather by Rademacher,

Dec. 25. First day. Slept unusually well last night, cannot keep awake in the evening. Ulcer on the right inner side of the underlip sore, when the tongue touches it. Gums swollen and painful to the touch.

Dec. 26. Second day. On awaking in the morning, sensation as if the head was swollen. The normal pulse being 55, is accelerated to 68 in the morning, with pulsations all over the body. Sensation of lameness in the *right* hip-joint, as if he could not use the right limb, but can walk well enough after using it. Pulsation all over, especially in the right hip-joint, *worse* in the morning, better in the evening.

Dec. 27. Third-day. Has slept better and longer than usual, is very reluctant to rise in the morning. The same ulcer on the inside of the lip as on the first day, only on the left side.

SECOND PROVING.

Jan. 3, 1851. *Same prover.* Every evening for three days one grain of the first trituration.

Jan. 4. First day. At nine o'clock A. M., pulsation all over the body, especially under the sternum, pulse (the normal pulse being 55) is 68, heavy and dull feeling in the forehead, eyelids slightly inflamed and swollen. Dry heat in the palms of the hands. Dry mouth; tongue coated with whitish mucus. Bloated feeling and burning in the feet. Lumbago.

Jan. 5. Second day. Pulse 68 in the morning, 53 in the evening. In the afternoon tension and sensation of swelling in the abdomen, with feeling of heaviness of head, like vertigo.

Jan. 6. Third day. Last night, sensation of swelling of hands, fingers and feet, feels as if he could not close the hands, cracking of all the finger-joints. Slept little, with great inclination to sleep. Sensation of swelling of the head, face feels as if bloated. Pain in the left side of the head, extending to the left eye and left ear, with nausea. Pulse in the morning 68. Hot eructations as of bile. Headache, worse when laughing. Soreness of the scalp when pulling even but one hair; bloated abdomen. Debility and general sensation of prostration.

Jan. 7. Fourth day. Restless sleep, with sensation of fulness of the head, felt while sleeping, and worse when awaking. At night burning of hands and feet; eyes so painful that he cannot read much. In the morning pulse 68, in the evening 43. Dreams of danger, principally danger of water.

Jan. 8. Fifth day. Pulse 72 in the morning, 64 in the evening. Feels pulsations all over. Slept better last night, but still restless.

with his usual exactness. A new mortar was used and kept for further triturations in the same manner as I have done with all other chemicals.

All the following provings were made under the direction of Dr. Lippe; and most of the symptoms were taken from a thesis of Doctor Stevenson, a graduate of the Pennsylvania Homœopathic College, in 1851, with his permission.

C. HERING.

Feels all the time while sleeping as if he would have headache in the morning on awaking.

Jan. 15. Twelfth day. Varices on the *right* side of the anus; painful after stool, but not bleeding.

THIRD PROVING.

Jan. 16, 1851. *Same prover.* For five successive evenings every evening six pellets of the 30th potence of *Ars.-met.*

Jan. 17. First day. At 6 this morning pulse 49, at 9 A.M., pulse 64, full and strong with throbbing sensation all over the whole body. Piles still external, but better. At 10 P.M., pulse 48. Burning sensation in the feet.

Jan. 18. Second day. Feet burning hot last night without any moisture; he was compelled to hold the feet out of bed all night. At 6 A.M., pulse 48. At 9 A.M., pulse 68, with throbbing sensation all over; feeling of drowsiness also; he slept well last night; feeling of despondency and lowness of spirits, which is found difficult to shake off; gums swollen, feel as if scalded, with accumulation of water in the mouth; slight pains in the left side of the chest near the heart; piles still external on the right slde of the anus.

Jan. 19. Third day. Slept well last night; feet did not burn so much; in the morning tongue is coated white; the imprints of the teeth are seen on the edges of the tongue. Pulse, 9 A.M., 68, full and hard. Piles have nearly disappeared; gums not so much swollen and feel not as scalded as yesterday; red sandy deposit in the urine; *throbbing sensation like that of yesterday.*

June 20. Fourth day. Pulse in the morning 64; itching and burning in the lower part of the face; piles bleed a little.

June 21. Fifth day. Pain in the muscles of the left chest; great lassitude; throbbing all over. Coryza; scalding water runs from the nose, excoriating the nostrils; great lassitude and prostration of strength; a burning itching in the lower part of the face as if an eruption would come out.

June 22—27. Sixth till eleventh day. Itching, burning, stinging in the face, with swelling; worse at night. Relieved by washing the face in cold water. On the right forehead and in the right groin it is worst. Forehead feels much swollen; the skin is stiff drawn over the forehead, immovable. The itching is relieved by pressing (and pinching), not by scratching. For many nights past very unpleasant dreams, full of danger by water, he is in imminent danger of being drowned, &c.

Later. Desquamations of skin in very small scales. A scab which he had had for twenty years on the first joint of the third finger of the left hand healed entirely; when formerly the scab had been torn off, a liver-colored spot remained, on which a new scab formed.

Feb. 8. No more medicine had been taken, but the same coryza as before returned again, accompanied with hoarseness, and on the 9th with very intense inflammation of the throat for which one dose of *belladonna*, 400, was successfully administered.

FOURTH PROVING.

Dec. 11, 1850. *Another prover.* For six successive nights one dose of one grain of the third trituration was taken.

Dec. 12. First day. Feels as if the fumes of whiskey had gone to his head; great drowsiness in the afternoon, and irresistible sleepiness early in the evening.

Dec. 13. Second day. From 11 A. M., till evening, irresistible sleepiness; feels as if he should fall asleep while walking in the street in the afternoon. The following five days great lassitude, weakness, and depression of spirits.

FIFTH PROVING.

Jan. 16, 1851. *Same prover.* Took for six days, every evening, six pellets of the 30th potence of *ars.-met.*

Jan. 17. Pulsations in the umbilicus and right anterior tibial artery at the superior extremity of its inferior third. Deep-seated numbness in the region of the right hip-joint, extending to the pubes.

Jan. 18—26. The feet, usually icy cold, have become warm and sweat more. Numbness in the right lumbar region and inside of the right thigh down to the knee, extending from the vertebræ down to the crest of the ilium.

Jan. 27. Œdematous swelling of the forehead and face, with itching which can only be allayed by pinching the skin. Itching in the right groin down to the knee.

SIXTH PROVING.

Feb. 7. *Same prover.* One dose of six pellets of *ars.-met.*, 30.

Feb. 9. Awakes in the morning at six o'clock with a distressing, lancinating, griping pain in the bowels; afterwards one sharp, burning, watery stool, relieving the abdominal pains, but leaving great weakness; he falls asleep after sitting down; pulse 60, full.

Later. Sensation of dryness in the right knee-joint. In the right groin a painful, swelling pain goes up to the hip and is worse when the leg is extended; worse when sitting, the leg then goes to sleep; better when walking. This pain continued for a long time in the same place. Where this painful swelling is felt a bubo suppurated 24 years ago.

4. *Digest of the Symptoms.*

The figures indicate the attenuation by which the symptoms were produced.

MENTAL. **1.** Depression of spirits. Despondency. Indifference. HEAD. A sensation as of vertigo (2d d.) (1). **5.** Sensation as if the fumes of whiskey had gone to the head (1st d.) (3). Heavy and dull feeling in the forehead (1st d.) (1). Pain in the left side of the head extending to the left ear and left eye, with nausea (3d d.) (1). Head feels as if swollen in the morning when awaking (2d d.) (3). Sensation of fulness in the head while sleeping, and worse when awaking in the night (4th d.) (1). **10.** Headache worse when laughing. Itching of forehead which cannot be allayed but by pinching up the skin (12th d.) (30). Soreness of the scalp when even pulling but one hair (3d d.) (1).

EYES. Sensations of heaviness in the eyes. Eyelids slightly inflamed and swollen (1st d.) (1). **15.** Eyes so painful that he cannot read much.

NOSE. Fluent coryza. *Vide* 52. Scalding water runs from the nose, excoriating the nostrils (5th d.) (30). The coryza returns in fifteen days with heat in the face and hoarseness, lasting three days, when it became accompanied with angina faucium, for which *bell.* 400, one dose, was successfully administered.

FACE. Itching and burning in the lower part of the face, as if an eruption would break out (4th d.) (30). **20.** Face feels as if bloated (3d d.) (1). Bloated face (3d d.) (1). Itching all over the face, which can only be relieved by pinching the skin (for some days). Burning, itching, stinging in the face, with swelling; skin feels as if stiff, relieved by bathing the face with cold water; later, desquamations in small scales. The itching is relieved by pressing, but not by scratching.

MOUTH. **25.** Ulcer on the right side of inner under lip (1st d.) (3). Ulcer sore when touched with the tongue (1–2d d.) (3). Ulcer on the left inner side of the under lip (1st d.) (3). Dry mouth. Tongue coated white, covered with mucus (12th d.) (1). Tongue coated white, showing the imprint of the teeth on the edges (3d d.) (30). **30.** Gums swollen and painful to the touch (1st d.) (1). Gums swollen and feeling as if scalded, with accumulation of water in the mouth; aversion to wines and liquors.

STOMACH. Nausea (3d d.) (1). Hot eructations as of bile (3d d.) (1).

ABDOMEN. **35.** Bloated abdomen (1–3d d.) (1). Tension and sensation of swelling in the abdomen (3d d.) (1). Pulsation in the umbilicus. Numbness and sensation of paralysis in the right lumbar region, extending from the vertebræ to the crest of the ilium (1st d.) (30). Lumbago. **40.** Varices on the right side of the anus, painful after stool (not bleeding) (12th d.) (1). Varices bleed a little (4th d.) (30.) Varices feel only sore, but neither pain after stool nor bleed (16th d.) (30.) After awaking in the morning at 6 o'clock, distressing, lancinating, griping pain in the bowels; afterwards, one sharp, burning, watery stool, relieving the abdominal pain, but leaving much debility; he falls asleep sitting on a chair, and has no appetite; pulse 60, much fuller than in health (2d d.) (1). **45.** Constipated (16th d.) (30).

GROINS, URINE. Itching in the right groin extending down to the knee (12th d.) (30). In the right groin a painful swelling, worse when extending the leg, pain goes up to the hip and continues for a long time. In the same place where this painful swelling appears, a bubo suppurated 24 years ago. Red sandy sediment in the urine (3d d.) (30). Offensive sweat on the genitals (for some weeks).

CHEST. Pulsation under the sternum (1st d.) (30). **50.** Slight pains in the left side of the chest in the region of the heart (2d d.) (30). Pain in the muscles of the left chest (2d d.) (30.) Hoarseness with coryza (21st d.) (30). *Vide* 17.

UPPER EXTREMITIES. Sensation of swelling of hands and fingers (3d d.) (1). Hands and fingers feel stiff; they feel as if they could not be closed (3–9th d.) (1). Cracking of all the finger-joints (2d–14th d.) (1). **55.** Dry heat in the palms of the hands. *A scab which had been on the first joint of the third finger of the left hand for 20 years, healed entirely; when formerly the scab had been torn off, it left a spot of liver color, and a new scab soon formed.

LOWER EXTREMITIES. Sensation of lameness in the right hip-joint (2d d.) (3). Sensation as if he could not use the limb, but he can walk well enough after he has been on his feet a short time (2d d.) (3). Pulsation in the right hip joint, worse in the morning, better in the evening (2d d.) (3). **60.** Deep-seated numbness in the right hip-joint (1st d.) (30). Sensation of paralysis in the right hip-joint, extending to the pubic symphysis down inside of the thigh to the knee. Pulsation in the right anterior tibial artery at the superior extremity of its inferior third (1st d., **1** and 1st d.) (30). Sensation of dryness in the right knee-joint (4th d.) (3). Feet burning hot, feel as if bloated (1st d.) (1). **65.** Feet burning hot, without the least moisture (2d d.) (30). *Feet usually icy cold, have become warm and sweat much. Feet burning more at night; he has to hold them out of bed, cannot have the least cover on them (1–14th d.) (1 and 3).

GENERAL. **70.** Emaciation. Pulsation all over the body. The symptoms appear first on the right and then on the left side. Morning exacerbations. The symptoms recur again after two weeks. Aggravation after drinking a small quantity of brandy, for which he had not the slightest desire.

SLEEP. **75.** Unusually sound sleep at night (1st d.) (3). Irresistible inclination to sleep in the day-time and early in the evening (2d d.) (3). Great drowsiness in the morning after rising, having had a sound sleep (2d d.) (30). Very reluctant to rise in the morning after a good night's sleep (3d d.) (3). Feels as if he should fall asleep while walking in the street in the afternoon (2d d.) (3). **80.** Stupor in the morning notwithstanding a good sleep all night (3d d.) (30). Very sleepy but cannot fall asleep (2d d.) (30). During sleep a sensation as if he would have a headache when awaking in the morning. During sleep dreams of danger, especially of danger on the water (5th d.) (1). On awaking in the morning sensation as if the head were swollen (1st d.) (1).

FEVER. Normal pulse being 55, is accelerated to 68 in the morning (1st d.) (1). Normal pulse being 55, is accelerated to 68 in the morning (2d d.) (1). **85.** Normal pulse being 55, is accelerated to 68 in the morning (1st d.) (30). Normal pulse being 55, is accelerated to 68 in the morning and falls down to 53 in the evening (2d d.) (3). Normal pulse being 55, is accelerated to 68 in the morning and lowered to 43 in the evening (4th d.) (1). Normal pulse being 55, is now 72 in the morning, 64 in the evening (5th d.) (1). Normal pulse being 55, is now, in the morning, 64, in the evening 48 (1st d) (30). **90.** Pulse after midnight 48, in the morning after rising 68 (3d d.) (30). Pulse 64 in the morning (4th d.) (30). The pulse continues to rise in the morning and to fall in the evening for 30 days longer, without taking more medicine.

5. *Remarks on the Foregoing Provings, by* C. Hering, M.D.

The proving of metallic arsenic is of the greatest consequence to the scientific development of our Materia Medica. It will furnish answers to questions of fundamental importance.

Christison says in his Index: "Arsenic acts in all its chemical forms *except in its metallic state.*" (American reprint, page 230). "In conformity with what appears to be a general law in toxicology, *the metal itself is inert.*"

The foregoing provings are sufficient to satisfy even the most sceptical that the metal is not inert, and it would be absurd to re-assert the inertness of metallic arsenic and deny or reject our experiments without at least repeating them.

As regards the "general law in toxicology," we have only to say that it is a fair example of what have been styled general laws, and even of most of those which have been called "special laws." So-called experiments, rude and rough, in which a few rabbits, cats or dogs have been tormented, either to death or not to death, in the coarsest possible way, such is the *ultima ratio* of "toxicology." Christison furnishes proof of this by quoting: "Bayen and Deyeux, however, found that a drachm, carefully prepared, might be given in fragments (!) to dogs without injuring them; and they once gave a cat half an ounce (in fragments ?) without any other consequences than temporary loss of flesh."

I should think loss of flesh was something like an effect, as it very likely appeared rapidly or it would not have been regarded at all; because the "general law" in Orifila's "model" experiments and in nearly all the rest seems to be, that what does not follow within a few minutes does not follow at all. The giving metals in the form of fragments, *i. e.*, little pieces, in order to test "a law," is, to say the least, a childish experiment.

We know that all metals, *i. e.*, every one thus far proved, in the metallic form and in the state of the finest powder, not only produce decided effects, but symptoms of longer duration and characteristic peculiarity.

Aurum, Argentum, Stannum, Zincum have been proved by Hahnemann and others; and *Platinum* by Stapf, to which have been lately added *Cadmium, Palladium, Osmium, Tellurium,* &c.

Notwithstanding the repetitions of these experiments by others, for instance the proving of metallic silver by Huber, with the same results, the old school takes no notice of it. With a stubborness which borders on stupidity they stick to their "general laws," no matter how much they are shaken by all the new discoveries in the natural sciences, nay even by their own experience. While I was attending Schönlein's clinical lectures in the hospital at Wirzeburg, I induced a fellow-student to make an experiment with triturated gold, which, he said, was absolutely inert. A few days after, he was obliged to keep his room, having an awfully swollen red nose, exactly confirming Hahnemann's observation. He is now a professor and a man of importance in pathology, but he keeps his mouth shut; he has not the courage to come out and acknowledge the truth; he is afraid to come forth as a witness, afraid to touch the superstitions of the age. He will not read this reproach, but even if he should, his face will not turn as red as his nose was; he is hardened like the rest.

Christison, in the same paragraph, says; "Of the different preparations of arsenic it may be said, in general terms, that those are most active which are most soluble." And further: "It is difficult to put this—the inertness of the metal—fairly to the test, because it is not easy to pulverise the metal without a sufficient quantity being oxidated to cause poisonous effects.

Both assertions are worthy of consideration, as they have had much influence even in our homœopathic pharmacy. I will only remark that Christison seems to have forgotten that the sub-oxide of arsenic is as insoluble in water as metallic arsenic, and thus ought to be considered as inert. And he does not know that arsenious oxide (AsO^3), the arsenic of the shops, which is less soluble than arsenic acid (AsO^5), acts with decidedly more violence than the latter. It seems to be the same with sulphur, in its corresponding oxidations, and with phosphorus. If a healthy person takes, at proper intervals, the different grades of oxidation, the highest will always be found to act the mildest. But we will not declare this to be a general law, until further experiments have been made.

We will now consider the two very important rules of the old school;

1. *Solubility as a condition of effect.*

2. *Oxidation of the metals as a condition of increased effect.*

The fluid state is favorable if violent symptoms are to be produced in a short time. It is an old chemical law: *corpora non agunt nisi fluida.* The immediate production of violent effects is the result of chemical action; some essential and constituent parts of the body are to be destroyed by chemical action; and it may be that such effects are dependent on the fluid state of the agency. But effects, in general, must be ascertained by experiment, separate from the experiments which test the solubility of the agent. It would require a long series of experiments to enable us to reach a sound conclusion, that the effects observed were dependent on the solubility. The one has thus nothing to do with the other. Suppose we were even to allow the conclusion, we have still no right to conclude, negatively, that what is insoluble is inert.

The most striking fact against the inertness of insoluble substances is afforded by osmic acid. Any one can soon ascertain that it has an effect, by inhaling it through the nose or trying it in the stomach. But as soon as it comes in contact with organic matter it is decomposed, and metallic osmium or its sub-oxide blackens the mucous membrane. As both the smell and the effect are peculiar, the latter cannot depend altogether upon the mechanical influence.

The only conclusion, then, which can be drawn from the experiments of the toxicologists is, that that which is soluble produces an effect; to conclude the converse, that that which is insoluble can produce no effect at all, is, like all hasty *negative* conclusions, not only unwarranted, but extremely foolish and injurious.

Every chemist knows that the experiments hitherto made in regard to solubility are very imperfect, meagre, and insufficient; and until the vital importance of an accurate knowledge of the different degrees of solubility is seen by the chemists, it will be in vain to expect them to undertake the long and tedious labor of searching for the laws of solubility.

It is known that solubility has relations to the *temperature*, the *motion* or shaking and the *quantity* of the solvent. Small proportions have not been sufficiently regarded.

Sobrero, when he saw that his oil—which I have called Glonoin—precipitated in water, inferred that it was insoluble in it. Dr. Zumbrock, taking such water and feeling the powerful influence, analysed and measured it accurately, and found that 0.128 parts of Glonoin are soluble in water at a medium temperature.

The solubility of mercury in water is still denied, but the decided mercurial effect of water boiled with mercury allows no doubt on the subject. But the chemists, accurate as they are, have generally been too hasty in denying such facts as may fall within the *errors* of observation. Liebig himself came to the most absurd conclusion, that as the homœopathic doses fell within the unavoidable errors of the scales, they were nonsensical things; as if the errors of chemical observation had anything to do with the observation of effects on the living! At the same time he is perfectly aware that plants contain substances taken up in such small quantities that no chemist of our days can discover a trace of them; fluoride of calcium exists in the teeth in sufficient quantity to be detected, and must be derived from plants, in which no chemist could detect it. It would be unscientific to suppose that fluorine forms a part of a plant, without any other function or use than that cattle may use it to give hardness to their teeth. As plants contain it, they must require it for their own existence, and to say that it is merely accidental, would only be a higher degree of absurdity. Whatever has a function must be capable of producing an effect, and as it has a function in quantities falling within the admitted errors of chemical analysis, similar quantities must be powerful enough to produce effects.

It is a well known fact that a solvent saturated with one substance is still capable of dissolving a certain proportion of another and even of several others in succession. For instance, if we take 8 ounces of water and saturate it completely with sulphate of iron ($FeOSO^3$c. aqu.), which will require 9½ ounces, we can afterwards dissolve in the same solution 1½ ounce of the sulphate of magnesia, and the liquid will still take up three ounces of sugar, and perhaps other substances after this. While every one is familiar with this, there is another fact not so well known, which is one of the most important in chemistry, and will explain innumerable phenomena in organic chemistry, physiology and especially in the science of effects or Materia Medica.

Sometimes the presence of one substance in a solution will increase its power of dissolving another, or if one is already dissolved, another may not only be added, but in increased quantities. Lithia is the least soluble in water of all its relatives, ammonia, potassa and soda; but its solutions will dissolve urates, which are insoluble in pure water. Uric acid, the morbid product, which causes, besides innumerable other troublesome symptoms, gravel in the kidneys, stones in the bladder, and the deposits on the joints of the fingers in gout, and which is formed and kept in solution in the blood and urine under conditions of which we are ignorant, requires 10,000 parts of water for its solution. In a solution of carbonate of potassa the solubility of some urates and uric acid increases about a hundredfold; in a solution of carbonate of soda it doubles, and in a solution of carbonate of lithia it doubles again. Lithia being the least soluble among its relatives (only 1 to 1,000), increases the solubility of uric acid in water four hundredfold. The same quantity of water which would have dissolved $\frac{1}{100}$ part of a grain of uric acid will, after one grain of carbonate of lithia has been dissolved in it, receive 4 grains of uric acid.

This opens a field for the most important researches, and until it has been sufficiently cultivated, we have no right to say of any substance that it is insoluble, in the fluids of the organism; and it is evidently perfectly absurd to contend, that because it is insoluble in water it is therefore inert when introdnced into the vital economy.

Cinnabaris is rejected by the so-called rational schools, 1st, because we do not know of any agent capable of dissolving it in the animal body, and has been declared by the toxicologists not to be "possessed of any deleterious action of the animal body," founded on the disgustingly absurd experiments of Orfila. These philosophers are themselves, however, so much the subjects of deleterious action that they can reason backwards; thus, in the experiments of Smith, who found that the Cinnabar acted, an impure article was used. It is possible, and even probable, that the high estimation in which Cinnabar was held by the ancients in a great many diseases, may have resulted from its containing arsenic; but even a mixed sulphuret and arseniuret of mercury is not capable, so far as we know, of being dissolved by any agent present in the body.

Ten years ago I took a trituration of chemically pure Cinnabar, and observed a most decided and unmistakable action. I repeated the experiment several times; the 3d trituration always acted the same day. Others repeated those experiments with nearly the same results, particularly Dr. Lippe, who observed the same peculiar congestions of the head which we have ever since permanently cured in a number of cases.

Finally, Dr. Neidhard undertook to prove the *Cinnabaris*, fully, with the assistance of the students of the Homœopathic College in this city, and with such a brilliant result that it is now one of our most important and best proved medicines.

Still we do not know any agent in the animal body capable of dissolving Cinnabar, but we know with a certainty equal to any other in natural sciences that it acts upon the organism, and we know the mode of its action so that we can make use of it as an agent to cure the sick.

Shall we reject it and wait until chemists please to detect "an agency capable of dissolving it in the animal body?"

Having shown that solubility, or what is known about it, has no conditional connexion with effect, as the latter must be ascertained separately by independent experiments, we have now to consider the remaining point, oxidation as a condition of increased effect.

It is said that arsenic is not easy to pulverize without a sufficient quantity being oxidated to cause poisonous effects. We have already remarked that if solubility is required, the sub-oxide of arsenic being also insoluble, the oxidation explains nothing. But, it is also too hasty a conclusion to say, that oxidation necessarily follows pulverization. It is true, most metallic arsenic in damp air changes into a black powder which is supposed to be AsO; but better prepared metallic arsenic does not, especially not in dry air.

I expect to decide the question very soon, if time will allow me to examine the trituration of metallic arsenic which was used in Lippe's experiments by the microscope, as the metallic particles will be seen either with the strong splendor and tin-whiteness which this metal possesses, or with the dull black color of what is called the sub-oxide. It may be both are mixed.

But let us suppose that it is in the condition of sub-oxide; does that explain its efficiency? We know that a great many metals do not combine with oxygen if pulverized or triturated according to our way of preparing; with some metals it is even a difficult thing to produce a combination with oxygen; some combine with rapidity even when simply exposed to the air. We know the first mentioned class to act powerfully, and we know the latter would poison or destroy parts of our organism, if brought in contact with it in the metallic state. Between these two extremes lie all the rest, some oxidizing rapidly, some slowly. We know of some that they have a decided effect, notwithstanding they are reduced to the metallic state in the body; thus while the opposite process takes place. Furthermore, we know that those which act in the metallic state—like mercury—will act in the state of oxides —red precipitate—but it would be preposterous to assume that they acted more violently in the latter state. We refer to the case reported by Burnett in the Philosophical Transactions, 1823, page 402, where the whole of 200 persons on board of two ships and all the animals on board were poisoned by mercury; there being in the hold of the vessels leather bags filled with quicksilver, of which some had burst. As we know that mercury is soluble in air in the metallic state, and even that a small quantity of quicksilver in a bottle will amalgamate a gold leaf hanging from the stopper (Faraday), it requires the stubbornness of an old school doctor to suppose oxidation necessary in order to produce or explain these effects.

Not a single series of experiments has ever been made, to prove that oxides act more readily than their metals.

We would not have spoken of such absurdities of the old school had we not before us propositions to introduce into Homœopathy the oxides instead of the metals. We refer to *Oesterreichische Zeitschrift*, Vol. 1, No. 1, p. 174, where several reasons are given, not one of which will stand real criticism.

We come now to a proposition of some consequence.

We all know that every drug taken by a prover or a patient, may undergo chemical changes sooner or later after it comes in contact with the body. We know, beyond a doubt, of some substances, that as soon as they come in contact with animal tissues or fluids, they combine with them or are decomposed. We know of some, that they are not, and of others that they are, expelled unaltered, from the body; of a great number we do not *know*, but have a full right by a sound analogy to conclude, that they also will. We know there are no exceptions to a mathematical rule; the same is the case with natural laws, so-called exceptions being only apparent, and if properly studied either confirming the law or proving that it is no law. Every substance will follow the laws of chemical affinity, in contact with unorganized bodies as well as with organized. As fast as careful researches are made, apparent exceptions always disappear. It has been supposed, for instance, that the organism could produce chemical elements. Careful experiments have shown clearly that it cannot. It has been supposed that chemical laws were overruled by the dynamic influence or life, as by something higher, and were obliged to submit, but there is not a single fact known to confirm this.

It is the manifold influences present in organisms, the great combination of influxes, which makes it rather a difficult problem, in some instances, to decide. Still, in every case in which the scrutiny of natural philosophers has been directed to such a question, the answer, without exception, has confirmed the higher power of the chemical laws.

Thus, every substance taken by a prover or given to a patient, as soon as it comes in contact with the tissues or fluids, will follow its chemical laws.

Single elementary substances will combine with others if they meet them and have an affinity for them. Nitrate of silver is immediately decomposed, and the metal forms an albuminate of silver; the nitric acid, a nitrate of albumen; both, we are allowed to suppose, are dissolved; the first, certainly, enters the blood and is deposited in the skin, the second, if dissolved, is decomposed and nitrates of the alkalies formed. What we call the symptoms of nitrate of silver is thus the combined effect of these two or more combinations. Single elementary substances may combine with oxygen, hydrogen or carbonic acid, or with other free acids or alkalies; or they may decompose some of the parts of the animal fluids or tissues.

If a certain substance combine with oxygen and is oxidized, either by taking the oxygen from air or water, or other contents not essential to life, the effect of such a substance taken in a chemically pure state, must be identical with the effect of the oxide, and it would be indifferent whether we give the patient the one or the other.

If a certain substance combine with hydrogen in the system, the effect will be the same as if this combination had been taken. As there is an essential difference between the combinations of an element with hydrogen, and of the same with oxygen, it is a question of great importance to know which will take place, or, if both are possible, what are the conditions for the one or the other. According as the one or the other happens, the opposite cycles in the time of the day, and the opposite direction with regard to the sides of the body in electro-positive or negative bodies, would be manifested in such combinations. The gaseous hydrogen combinations would act like alkalies, the oxygen combinations like acids; this I suppose to be a fundamental law in *Materia Medica.*

The difference between the effects of carburetted hydrogen and carbonic acid, is as great as a difference possibly can be. There is, in fact, no similarity whatever. It is like the difference between ammonium and nitric acid.

Sulphuretted hydrogen acts also very differently from sulphurous or sulphuric acid, and we should not suppose it could be the same substance in both, if we did not know it.

Arseniuretted hydrogen acts very differently from arsenious acid, according to the cases of poisoning and to my own provings, but the difference is not as wide as in the case of carbon and sulphur.

We may conclude that the other corresponding combinations have also more differences than similarities; thus, phosphuretted, seleniuretted, and telluretted hydrogen have very different effects from phosphoric, selenic, and telluric acids.

Thus if the same substance can combine in the body with oxygen or hydrogen, there must be a considerable difference in the effects.

Sulphur applied to the skin, for instance, as a powder put in the stockings under the soles of the feet, combines with hydrogen, and is expelled as sulphuretted hydrogen from the skin and the lungs. It is this experiment which induced me to propose it as an antidote or preventive to Asiatic cholera (1833).

The books will tell us that sulphur could not exist in the blood as sulphuretted hydrogen; that the sulphur would be changed into sulphuric acid and form sulphates. All this is not sufficiently proved, but the combination with hydrogen is a certain fact, and can be ascertained by experiment. It may be that under certain conditions the one, and under other conditions, the other affinity would come in play, and if so we ought to know what these conditions are.

While proving the *tellurium* in the metallic state, I had reason to suppose it had combined with hydrogen in the body. The same may have been the case with *selenium*. *It may be the same with metallic arsenic*, or it may be not; the similarity between the effects of arseniuretted hydrogen and metallic arsenic may have another cause. According to a French chemist, arseniuretted hydrogen is decomposed by contact with the animal tissues, and metallic arsenic is precipitated. Experiments would *soon decide the point*, and whether the combination take place or not, the metal would probably be our best agent. At all events it is theoretically and practically a question of importance to make the following series of provings and comparisons:

HYDROGEN.		ELEMENTS.	OXYGEN.
Sulphuretted Hydrogen.		*Sulphur.*	*Sulphuric Acid.*
Seleniuretted	"	*Selenium.*	Selenic Acid.
Telluretted	"	*Tellurium.*	Telluric Acid.
Phosphoretted	"	*Phosphorus.*	*Phosphoric Acid.*
Arseniuretted	"	*Arsenic.*	*Arsenic Acid.*
Antimoniuretted	"	Antimonium.	Antimonic Acid.
Carburetted	"	Carbon.	Carbonic Acid.

Those in *italics* have been already more or less proved.

The practitioner already finds a remarkable difference of effect between sulphur and sulphuric acid, between phosphorus (which changes mostly into phosphorous acid while preparing it, or after its contact with the mucous membranes) and phosphoric acid. We have reason to suppose this will be the case with the other acids.

The combination of the same substance with hydrogen must give us very important medicines, not only on account of their quickness and intensity of action, by far superior to the effects of the uncombined elements or the acids, but especially on account of their very marked and characteristic differences. Their general characteristics must be not only different, but opposite, and what we know thus far of the sulphuretted and arseniuretted hydrogen confirms this. The diseases in which the acids are of use, are of an opposite character to such as are helped by the hydrogen combinations.

The Red Sulphur Springs of Virginia are famous for "reducing the pulse;" it is the slow development of small doses of sulphuretted hydrogen in the stomach on which this effect depends, as experiments with sulphuretted water have proved.

The difficulty, and in some instances the impossibility, of using the other hydrogen combinations, have hitherto prevented their introduction into our Materia Medica. If we should prescribe such mixtures as would produce the gas in the stomach, we should have a mixed effect. The very ingenious apparatus of Drysdale (*British Journal*, 7, 559; 8, 152;) has overcome the apparently insurmountable difficulties, but it is only for such desperate cases or diseases as cholera and the like. My experiments with the arseniuretted hydrogen have shown in 1846–7, that the millionth of this gas, taken by inhalation, caused a dangerous illness, lasting several weeks. But experiments could be made with still smaller doses, and this difficulty overcome, and we intend to do it as soon as possible.

Still, on either supposition, that metallic arsenic forms arseniuretted hydrogen in the body, or that arseniuretted hydrogen is decomposed in contact with the tissues, depositing metallic arsenic, it would be better to use Metallic Arsenic, at least in chronic diseases.

The proving of *Metallic Arsenic* has been one of the most important steps towards the solution of this question, and as soon as my time will allow, I will publish the known effects of the *arseniuretted hydrogen*, and a comparison on the one hand with *arsenious acid*, and on the other with *Metallic Arsenic.*

It would be of great service in these investigations, if we could find provers to repeat and augment the experiments; the 3d trituration acts very strongly, and I would recommend that preparation, as the effects are of long duration. I will, with great pleasure, supply any one with the drug who wishes to assist in repeating the provings.

9.—ARTEMISIA-VULGARIS.

ARTEM. Mugwort.

1. *Description and Preparation.*

This common and very bitter plant belongs to the large natural family of *Compositæ.* The American *A.-vulgaris* is thought by Nuttall not to be identical with the European species; they are, however, very similar.

The whole plant should be gathered at the season of flowering, and the juice expressed.

2. *Knowledge of its Effects.*

We have as yet no provings of the *Artemisia*, though it is much to be desired that some were undertaken. It is a popular remedy in Germany against Epilepsy, and has been used in many cases with success; in Catalepsy and Somnambulism; in Chorea and in one case of Strangury.

NOACK and TRINKS give the following summary of what is known about it. *Arzneimit.* 1, 141.

Aggravation of the epileptic paroxysms.—Excitement of the nervous system.—Profuse, specifically fœtid, putrid, garlic-smelling sweat.—Violent contractions of the uterus; labor-pains.—Prolapsus, rupture of the uterus.—Abortion.—Profuse menstruation; metrorrhagia.—Increased flow of the lochia.

10.—ASTERIAS-RUBENS.

AST. Star-fish, Sea-star, Finger-fish. *Fr.* Etoile de Mer.

1. *Description and Preparation.*

This well-known animal belongs to the general division *Radiata*, class *Echinodermata*. It is very commonly found on the sea-coasts of France and England. It has five fingers or rays symmetrically disposed about a common centre, the under surface of which contains the mouth of the animal. Their anatomy has been most patiently and minutely investigated by Tiedemann. The calcareous coat, with the numerous spines and processes, was found by Mr. Hatchett to consist of carbonate of lime with a little phosphate of lime.

Dr. Pétroz, who has given us the proving of this remedy, has unaccountably omitted to state how his preparation was obtained. The entire animal was probably brayed alive in a mortar until it was reduced to a magma, which was then digested with alcohol to produce a tincture. A better mode would be to triturate the magma with sugar of milk.

2. *Digest of the Symptoms.*

AUTHORITIES. DR. PÉTROZ (*Journal de la Société Gallicane*, vol. 1, p. 225) states the following provers. **1.** M. P. **2.** M. P. J. **3.** M. T. **4.** M. M. **5.** Mad. B. **6.** Mad. T. **7.** Mademoiselle M.

MIND. **1.** Sadness alternating with almost insupportable cerebral excitement; she is desirous of undertaking some intellectual or corporeal labor, walking or taking violent exercise; this state has no resemblance to that produced by spirituous liquors, it is rather a moral intoxication; (2d and 3d days) (7). Slight disturbance of the intellect with general weakness; (6th day) (2). Feeling of extreme anxiety from noon to three o'clock; it seems as though some misfortune were impending, as though some bad news were about to arrive; then tears are felt to be a relief; (6th day) (4). Irritability, anger, necessity of quarrelling with somebody; from noon to 2 P.M.; (6th day) (4). **5.** Depression, ennui, he thinks he is about to meet with misfortune; he perceives that if it should arrive, he would sooner weep than fret or get angry; (6th day) (4). The symptoms disappear by degrees, leaving behind them a moral sensitiveness that impels him to weep under the influence of the least emotion; (11th day) (1). Extraordinary gaiety in the evening; (1st day) (6). Tears, with despair, succeeded almost immediately by a calm; (3d day) (7). He does not like to work in the afternoon; (6th day) (1).

HEAD. **Vertigo.** **10.** Transitory vertigo (3). Vertigo when walking; (1st day) (3). Vertigo; (10th day) (5). **Fulness and Heat.** Sensation of fulness as though from congestion, and sometimes even as if from a rush of blood to the head; (2d day) (7). Determination of blood to the head, sensation of fulness, heat; it feels as if it would split; (2d day) (7). **15.** Heat in the head; it seems as if the air about her head were hot; (1st day) (7). Heaviness of the head; after one hour; (1). Heaviness of the head, heat, throbbings, redness of the face; (1st day) (1). Fulness of the head, which seems to distend the sides of it; (1st and 2d days) (7). The blood determines more strongly to the head; (4th day) (7). **Forehead.** **20.** Acute, transitory lancinations in the forehead and temples, especially in the occiput; (1st day) (3). Pressive pain in the forehead, sensation of fulness, contraction of the muscles and pressive constriction above the eyes; (1). Violent pressive pain in the sinciput, in the morning; it is with difficulty dissipated in the course of the day by a walk in the open air; (7). Very violent pressive pain in the forehead, above the eyes; (4th day). Violent pressive pain in the forehead which seems to crush the eyes by an enormous weight; (4th day) (7). **25.** Boring pain above the left eye, coming and going suddenly, and producing contraction of the eye-brows; while this pain lasts she seems to look through a mist; (2d day) (7). **Head generally.** Feeling of distress in the brain; (1st day) (1). Transitory pain in the right half of the head; (3d day). Sudden pain on the right side of the head; (3d day) (7). Slight lancinations in the brain; (7). **30.** Lancinating pain in the right temple; (2d day) (5). Lancinations in the brain, when blowing his nose, during the first half of the night; (4th day) (3). The headache disappears suddenly towards noon and the ideas are clearer; (7). Pressive pain on the right side of the occiput, making it difficult to walk; (5th day) (7). Pressure in the temples; (1st day) (3). **35.**

Throbbing in the head; (2d day) (7). Throbbing in the head when ascending or walking; (2d day) (1). Pain, during the continuance of which her head seems as though it were being crushed; (3d day) (7). Pain in the vertex as if the skull would break; (3d day) (7). He wakes in the night in great distress; it seems to him as if his brain were shaken by electric shocks, his head seems empty, almost deprived of consciousness; thinks he is attacked with apoplexy (night between the 6th and 7th day); this lasts several minutes; when he recovers his consciousness his pulse is hard and much accelerated; the right carotid beats violently; this febrile state continued to the end of the next day; (2). **40.** During the severe pains the whole cranium is sore; (5). The headaches increase towards afternoon and oblige her to go to bed; they are more violent behind than before, the head is painful all night; (9th day). Agitation, spasms, sense of uneasiness in the upper part of the brain, especially on making a mental effort; the feeling is similar to the feeling of lassitude in a limb the muscles of which have been severely exercised; (10th day) (5). Difficulty in enduring labor in the afternoon; (6th day) (1).

EYES. Heat in the eyes; (1st day) (7). **45.** Bloodshot eyes; (4th day) (1). Light fatigues the eyes; (1st day). Difficulty in bearing the light; (4th day) (7). The eyes are drawn backwards; (3d day) (7). Fatigued look. **50.** Twitching of the lids, the edges are red; (7th day) (7). Pain in the eyes from within outwards; (7th day) (7).

NOSE. Epistaxis; (9th day) (1). Epistaxis renewed three times in five days; (2). Sneezing and coryza on waking in the morning; (9th day).

EARS. **55.** Lancinating pain in the meatus, perceived for some seconds, is concentrated in the occiput, and ceases; these pains returned in the course of the day, but less violently; (3d day) (3). Sudden, very violent noise in both ears lasting less than a second; (3d day) (3). Dulness of hearing, more marked on the right side; (2d day) (5). Dulness of hearing, noise of rushing of water in the ears; (7th day) (1).

FACE. Face red; (4th day) (5). **60.** Face red and swollen; (3d day) (5). Stupid look, a stupid expression in the attitude and look; (7th day) (5).

MOUTH. Swelling of the tongue; (3d day) (5). Drawing pain in the tongue (5). Embarrassment of the tongue, dislike to speak; (5th day) (5). **65.** Saliva more abundant, disposition to bite; (5th day) (5). Irritation of the throat, short-lasting sensation of heat; this feeling returns several times during the day; (1st day) (2). Irritation of the throat, at first very slight, becoming more perceptible on the 5th day (5). Dryness of the throat; (6th day) (5). Sore throat (constriction) on waking in the morning; (8th day).

APPETITE. **70.** Want of appetite, no taste; (4th day) (7). Disgust for meat; (7th day) (1). Capricious appetite, she desires highly seasoned dishes, strong cheese, liqueurs, coffee, tea; (8th, 9th, 10th days) (7).

STOMACH. Dull pain extending the whole length of the œsophagus; (1st day) (3). Frequent forcible eructations in the morning; (1st day) (1). **75.** Nausea; (2d day) (1). Weariness and great heat in the stomach in the morning, with many violent eructations; (7th day) (1). Dull pain in the muscles of the præcordial region; (2d day) (3). Constriction in the præcordial region (4).

ABDOMEN. Dull pain in paroxysms in the right side of the abdomen near the navel; (7th day) (1). **80.** Flatulence after every meal, which is very troublesome, as it cannot be expelled either upward or downward; (3d day) (7). Violent colic, with shivering, alternating with flushes of heat in the face; (5th day) (7). Alternation of swelling and diminution of the abdomen during the twenty-four hours; (3d day) (7). Drawing in the abdominal walls; (3d day) (7).

RECTUM; ANUS; STOOL. Heat in the rectum. **85.** Slight hæmorrhoidal swelling; (3d day) (7). Hæmorrhoidal flow, lasting two days; (5th and 6th days) (7). **Stool.** Constipation, fruitless desire to go to stool, a symptom she never before experienced; (1st day) (7). Difficult, consistent stool; (3d day) (7). Colic followed by diarrhœa; (3d day) (5). **90.** Brown, liquid stool discharged in a violent jet; (4th day) (5). Several soft stools during the day (4).

URINE. Frequent, limpid urine; (2d day) (7). Frequent desire to urinate, urine more abundant; (7th day) (1). Thick, viscid urine; heat in the urethra on urinating; (8th day) (1).

GENITAL ORGANS. **Male.** **95.** Frequent erections during sleep (4). Erection in the morning; (3d day) (3). **Female.** Sensation of pressure upon the lower abdominal organs, impeding locomotion; (3d day) (7). General feeling of distress in the womb as though something were pushing out; (2d day) (7). General feeling as if the menses were about to appear; (2d day) (7). **100.** Twitching in the uterus; (2d day) (7). Unusual degree of moisture in the vagina, which is soothing; (3d day) (7). Menses retarded eight days, during all which time the colics and other sufferings which usually accompanied them continued, but ceased on their coming on; they were more abundant than ordinary. Excitement of the venereal appetite every morning in bed; (3d day) (7). Besieged by desires, fearful of inability to sustain these painful sensations; nervous commotion (3d day).

CHEST. **105.** Lancinating pain in the anterior inferior portion of the chest to the right and left of the sternum; this transitory pain was diminished by carrying the upper part of the body and the shoulders backwards; (4th day) (5). Drawing pain towards the internal part of the chest from before backward, extending, under the left nipple, into the whole internal part of the arm to the extremity of the little finger; (5th day) (1). The whole left side of the chest is painful; motion aggravates the pain; (1st day) (3). Substernal pain (6). Feeling of fulness in the chest causing fear of syncope; (7th day) (1). **Palpitations.** **110.** Anxiety caused by undulating throbbings in the chest, in the night (6th day). Frequent violent palpitations. Dull palpitations, scarcely perceptible, distant; it seems as if his heart had ceased to beat

(4). Twitching palpitations; (3d day) (1). When the palpitations are most violent, they extend to the epigastrium with a sensation of constriction; (3d day) (1). **115.** Anxiety in the heart during the night and morning; (7th day) (1). **External.** Feeling as if the left breast were drawn inwards (4). Drawing pain in the breast; (2d day) (7). Swelling and distension of the breasts as if before the menses; (3d day) (7). Very slight eruption between the breasts (6). **120.** Slight redness with floury efflorescence on the chest; (4th day) (7). A spot as large as the palm of a child's hand upon the chest, causing violent itching; the redness disappeared at the end of five or six days (7).

BACK. Drawing pain in the sacrum (1st and 2d days). Drawing pain in the back.

UPPER EXTREMITIES. Restlessness in the limbs, especially in the bends of the arms; it is scarcely endurable to have the arms covered; (4th day) (7). **125.** Pain extending from the thumb-joint into the shoulder (which?) (7th and 8th day) (2). Pain in the right shoulder; (2d day) (3). Coldness in the left arm, it seems as if a cold wind were blowing on it; (3d day) (7). Pain in the left elbow joint; (7th day) (3). A red circular spot of the size of a franc on the left olecranon, causing neither itching nor smarting, becoming covered with a dry, furfuraceous, friable coat, which falls off in two days, without leaving any mark; a similar but smaller eruption on the anterior portion of the same arm; (11th day) (7). **Hands and Fingers.** **130.** Numbness of the hands and fingers; (6th, 7th and 8th days) (2). Numbness of the left hand, extending into the arm; (2d day) (7). Numbness of the hypothenar eminence and little finger; (5th day) (4). Pain in the flexor tendons of the left hand; (2d day) (3). Severe itching around the left thumb-nail; (7th day) (3).

LOWER EXTREMITIES. **135.** Lassitude in the lower limbs; (4th day) (1). Weakness in the legs when standing so that she needs assistance in walking; (3d day) (5). Painful lassitude of the lower limbs (6). Pain in the right hip and whole left side up to the scapula, lasting to the sixth day and giving rise to fever (2). Dull pain in the left coxo-femoral joint in the morning; (2d day) (1). **140.** Burning lancinations in the great trochanter and left coxo-femoral joint, extending like lightning into the external side of the ham; (3d day) (1). Same symptom; (9th day) (5). Sensation of drawing in the right hip as if the leg were too long and drawn downwards; (5th day) (7). Formication in the lower limbs; (11th day) (1). Great uneasiness in the lower limbs when in a closed apartment. **145.** Desire for fresh air; (3d day) (7). **Thighs and Legs.** Deep lancinations in the anterior part of the thigh; (6th day) (1). Dull lancinations in the anterior part of the thigh; (1st day) (5). Drawing pain on the external side of the left thigh; (7th and 8th days) (2). Very lively itching in the thighs and legs, exceedingly uncomfortable, renewed towards 6 P.M. in the open air; (7th day) (3). **150.** A little excoriation on the leg caused by scratching becomes the seat of a pretty severe lancinating pain; (8th day) (3). Diminution of sensibility of the limbs, especially of the thighs and legs; (4th day) (3). Pain in the left knee; (2d day) (3). **Feet.** Painful drawing in the soles of the feet and toes (8th day). Pain in the joints of the left foot; (2d day) (3). **155.** Lancinating pain in the toes, especially in the great left toe, with very great heat and extreme sensibility, which cannot endure the ordinary covering; increased after sunset and in a closed room; redness of the skin; it is increased by heat; the cold air or cold water assuages the pain at once, but the heat of the bed renews it, although it ceases during the first part of the night (3d day). This pain continued to appear in a troublesome manner for several afternoons, and finally disappeared like the other symptoms (7). Pain in the left foot, concentrated at the metatarsal articulation of the great toe, lasting all day (6th day). It is aggravated by motion, renders walking impossible, and has a gouty character (3). Acute pain in the joint of the left foot, increased by walking; (7th day) (3). Insupportable pain in the left foot and in the muscles of the leg; (8th day) (3). Violent cutting pain in the left great toe, sensibility of the left sole, toes very painful; (3d day) (7). **160.** Pain in the joint of the right foot (6). Burning heat in the feet; (11th day) (1). The pains in the joints, particularly those of the left great toe, return three days after having ceased to take the drug (3).

FEVER. **Temperature.** Aversion to everything which increases the heat of the body, great desire to wash with cold water; (3d day) (7). Desire for the open air, anxiety, impatience of being shut up; (5th day) (7). **165.** The general heat is increased during the whole period of action. **Fever.** After the evening meal, general malaise, heat of skin and fulness of pulse; (1st day) (1). Violent heat in the head, then over the whole body, desire for cold drinks and for cold both internally and externally; (3d day) (5). Shivering with somnolence, hot skin, restless night; (3d day) (1). Heat of skin, fever toward the close of the day, shivering, heat followed by coldness; (10th day) (5).

SLEEP. **170.** She slept from 2 A.M. to the middle of the day; (3d day) (7). Agitated sleep; (11th day) (1). Need of rest and disposition to sleep after reading a moment; (10th day) (1). Many dreams about persons and events; the images are extraordinarily vivid and lifelike; she thinks she sees, touches and hears the persons of whom she is dreaming as though she were awake, but without any painful impressions; (2d and 3d days) (7).

GENERAL. General malaise, lassitude; feels better after eating. **175.** The symptoms are aggravated in the after-part of the day, especially in the evening. Great lassitude from heat, especially the heat of the bed. It is difficult to remain doing nothing.

3. *Clinical Remarks.*

Some clinical remarks on the *Asterias*, with illustrative cases by Dr. PÉTROZ, may be found; *N. A. Hom. Journ.*, vol. 2.

11.—CINNABARIS.

BY C. NEIDHARD, M.D.

CINNAB. Cinnabar, Vermilion, Sulphuret of Mercury, Hydrargyri sulphuretum rubrum.

1. *Preliminary Remarks.*

Our annual conventions are friendly and pleasant gatherings of the friends of our cause from various sections of the country. Eloquent addresses have at least informed the people, that Homœopathy is not yet defunct, as it has been predicted it would be, for the last twenty years. But have they been really able to effect anything for the general advancement of homœopathic science, as was their principal duty to do? Where are the provings which would confirm the symptoms of our *Materia Medica?* Where are the provings of new remedies, as still many diseases occur for which no homœopathic *simile* has been discovered? Where are the monographs of individual diseases enriching its archives? Has there ever been a well-concerted plan for the advancement of our cause submitted to the convention, that has been thoroughly acted out? To all these questions a negative answer must be given. Under these circumstances each one must work in his own individual sphere as far as he is able, and admonish all those with whom he may have any influence to do likewise.

By doing everything we can for the scientific improvement of Homœopathy, we can best and most permanently establish our own success. But when had the morally benighted ever intellectual insight enough to understand this simple truth?

It has been for some time my desire to make a series of provings with substances which are found in a naturally compound state, as being probably better calculated to eradicate the many complicated chronic diseases, than the simple substances. A number of students, perceiving the importance of the step, were at once willing and ready to engage in these experiments. It is my plan to prove every year one or two of these compound remedies of either entirely new substances or such as have only been imperfectly experimented with before. Occasionally, also, an American plant will be proved.

I have commenced with *Cinnabaris*, because the experiments of Hahnemann with this remedy were but few in number, and he had expressed a wish to have them perfected.

The symptoms contained in the following provings were principally obtained from the 30th and 6th dilutions and from the 3rd trituration, centesimal as well as decimal.

My main object was to enjoin upon the provers, to record the symptoms in the order in which they experienced them, so as to obtain a complete history of the pathogenesis of the remedy. Another important point with me was, that no new dose should be taken by the prover so long as symptoms were felt from the first dose.

The difficulties to be encountered in establishing, on paper, an efficient arrangement, are not a few. It would have been no doubt easier to separate the different symptoms belonging to each organ. But as this could only have been effected at the risk of omitting many important groups, by which alone the action of the remedy in different organs is to be perceived, I preferred the laborious task of tracing the connection of the symptoms in all the organs, as far as possible. Whatever symptoms, then, the different provers experienced at the same hour or hours, or which returned after a certain interval of time, at the same time, have been grouped together in the order in which they appeared, however remote from each other might be the organs affected.

I would suggest, that an analysis of the symptoms of a remedy may be made in the following manner:—Place the heads of the different organs on single sheets of paper, as *head*, *eyes*, *mouth*, etc., etc., and put down at once every group, that has some reference to each organ. The same may be done with regard to the conditions. By these means we may save a great deal of writing and re-writing.

My conviction is, that the progress of the Homœopathic Materia Medica can better be promoted by still more accurate provings, and faithful provers, than by any other method.

2. *Description and Preparation.*

The *Cinnabaris* I employed in the following provings was carefully prepared by Mr. John, apothecary. I should have preferred, as I do in every instance, to have proved the native Cinnabar also, but I was unable to obtain any. According to "*Schrœder's Arzneischatz*:" Cinnabaris consists of mercury one part, sulphur two parts, well triturated together and heated.

The native Cinnabar is of the same nature as that prepared by art, and is only distinguished from it by its stony part varying according to the mines in which it grows. The best is said to be found in the Hungarian gold mines. That which is found near the city of Grems (Kremnitz?) is preferred to others. The natural is often suspected, because it contains particles of arsenic. According to modern writers "the best-defined crystals are found in the coal formation of Moschel, Landsberg and Wolfstein in the Palatinate* * * * Well-crystallised specimens are mentioned also from Japan, Mexico, and Brazil. The principal repositories of this ore, however, are Almaden in Spain and Idria in Carniola, where it occurs almost exclusively massive, and whence it is obtained in large quantities, as an ore of mercury."—*Alger's Phillip's Mineralogy.*

3. *Provings.*

Precaution was taken that none of the provers should be acquainted with the remedy he was experimenting with, until all the provings were finished.

First Proving.

Dr. Smith Armor.—1851. January 25th.—Six hours after taking $\frac{1}{1000}$ part of a grain of Cinnabaris had a rumbling through his abdomen below the transverse colon, which lasted about one hour and a half.

Jan. 26th. *2d dose.*—Taken in the morning, and in three or four hours after, his abdomen, below the transverse colon, felt hot, his tongue is covered with a white fur, and there is a beating burning in both temples, which he felt all day.

Second Proving; Sixth Attenuation.

A. J. Brewster, aged 26, enjoys good health.

1851. Jan. 11th. Took at bed-time twenty pellets of the sixth dilution of *Cinnabaris.*

Jan. 12th. In the morning a sense of general prostration, great weakness of all the limbs. Feeling of depression and weakness of the whole system as after a severe illness. Indisposition for mental labor. The head feels weary as from long mental application—a dull heavy ache in the front of the head; from the front to the back of the head, mostly over the right eye and temple, heat in the head. Occasional darting pains through the head from without inwardly.

Eyes watery and dull, with a sharp sticking pain in the inner canthus of the left eye, as of a sharp stick being stuck in the lower lid.

Loss of sleep during the fore-part of the night. Restless and tossing about during the whole night, with anxious dreams, which he is wholly unable to recall after awaking. Nausea with occasional throbbing in the left hypochondrium. Abdomen distended, stools hard and too large.

Dull aching in the bones of the forearms and legs. Numbness in the left arm from the elbow to the end of the little finger, passing off on using the arm, and returning again while at *rest.*

In the morning appetite greatly impaired. But little appetite for breakfast after taking the remedy the previous night. Feels better in the open air and after dinner. Pulse 60, skin moist and cool.

THIRD PROVING ; THIRD TRITURATION.

A. J. BREWSTER. 1851. Jan. 22nd. Took, a quarter before 11 o'clock A. M., 5 grains of 3rd. trit. of *Cinnab.* (Hahn.)

At 3¼ P. M., felt a sharp steady pain in the forehead, mostly in the right orbital region, soon after felt a sharp throbbing in the left hypochondrium in the region of the spleen. At 10 o'clock P. M., felt a dull aching pain in the bones of the forearm and legs.

Jan. 25th. Took at 11 o'clock A. M. a dose of the third trituration (decimal scale); in half an hour felt a sharp aching pain in the right supra-orbitary region, shooting backwards and downwards to the ear and side of the neck. Front of the head very hot. The pain is worse in the warm room and on moving the eyes and scalp.

Chilliness in the warm room. An uneasy indescribable feeling in the abdomen. Numbness of the left arm from the elbow down to the end of the little finger. 10 o'clock P. M. Pain in the head increased to a heavy, stupefying ache, aggravated by thinking, reading, and pressure. Tenderness of the epigastric region.

Jan. 26th. A. M. Symptoms all better. 8 P. M. The pains in the head return, with a numbness and heavy aching in the arms and knees and lower legs.

Jan. 27th. 11 o'clock A. M. Pains in the head return again, with a disposition to fall asleep while listening to the lecture, several times, notwithstanding his making a great effort to keep awake. Constrictive feeling in the umbilical region. Urine tinged yellow.

Pains all aggravated in the evening. Better in the open air and after eating and sleeping.

FOURTH PROVING ; THIRD DEC. TRITURATION.

DR. J. P. DAKE, subject to indigestion, costiveness, and a dull heavy feeling in the fore-part of the head. Dark hair, dark complexion.

Jan. 28th. Took a powder, five grains of the third trituration (decimal) of *Cinnabaris* at 11 o'clock P. M., about half an hour before retiring. In ten minutes after, he felt a warm glow through his legs, which was soon succeeded by a dull pain in the left arm just above the elbow, and by occasional darting pains in the lower extremities. There was also a dull pain in the lower dorsal portion of the spine, continuing only for a short time. A space about the size of a quarter of a dollar, just above and between the supra-orbital regions (root of nose?), felt as though pressed upon by a cold metallic body; while within the cranium, underneath, there seemed to be more warmth than usual. A dull pain, felt before, in the temple and side of the forehead, disappeared. Urgent desire to urinate.

Although intending to sit up and study longer, yet feeling wearied in body and confused in mind, he soon retired. Upon lying down there were rumblings in the abdomen and pains passing from the epigastric to the pubic region. There was also some nausea and uneasiness in the stomach. Every little noise about the house troubled him, as though it were something serious. Although accustomed to dream much, yet he had more troublesome dreams than usual. He awoke and started up several times without purpose; once with a heavy pain, in the fore-part of the head. Upon arising at 7 o'clock in the morning he felt a little giddiness and pain in the forehead, with a sensation of soreness in the eyeballs. These passed away soon after breakfast. Before noon acidity of the stomach, general headache and heaviness of the eyes came on, somewhat as usual, only much aggravated.

The prover took 3rd centes. trit. previously, and felt nearly the same symptoms as those recorded above, but did not ascribe the effect to the medicine. In one of his dreams, he saw a spider as large as an ox.

Fifth Proving; Sixth Attenuation.

Dr. John H. Henry, aged 22. Light hair, healthy.

From the 6th dilution. (The prover has taken the medicine repeatedly, and alleges that he always has experienced the same symptoms. We have noted them down *bona fide* as they were given to us, although some have expressed a doubt about them, because they were so many and so distinct. This prover is, however, unusually sensitive to the action of all medicines, and we could not do more than express to all our provers the awful responsibility they underwent in diverging even in the slightest degree from the most accurate and truthful statements).

Pain in the region of casuality. A sensation of sticking over the secretive region, which increases and becomes a numb-pain, extending to the right temple (time and locality), with a feeling of warmth on the right side. Disposition to sleep during the day. The pain extends from one temple to the other across the *os frontis* from right to left (time and locality), is mild in the forehead but violent in the organs of locality and time both night and day and on rising in the morning. Before going to bed there is a drawing pain in the head, extending from the crown to the occiput, inclining to the right. Pain deep as if in the centre of the head.

Pain from the right lachrymal duct around the eye to the temple. Drawing sensation from the right inner canthus across the malar bone to the ear. A sensation as if there were something in the eyes, lasting three days. Feeling as if the eyelids were enlarged or puffed, as if the muscles were too short, when looking up to the wall. Pain from the inner canthus of the left eye across the eyebrows (organs of size, color, order, calculation). Itching of the lids of both eyes.

Itching of the nose with bleeding, after blowing it. The blood is very dark. The itching is caused by pimples at the right nostril.

Taste as of tobacco, coffee in the mouth. Pricking sensation in the mouth and fauces. Small spot on the left side of the tongue, which itches. Small sore on the roof of the mouth. Itching on the left side of the face.

On turning the head, pain on the right side of the neck, below the sterno-cleido-mastoideus muscle. Pain in the back part of the neck, when the head is thrown back, extending to the occiput. The muscles of the back part of neck seem as if contracted. General pain all over the back down to the loins, worse after every dose of medicine, aggravated on drawing a long breath.

Pain in the upper part of the left and right lung, an inward soreness over the heart, extending along the left arm on taking a long breath. Mucus which is thrown up, tastes like old tallow, mixed with coffee. Pain under the lower point of the sternum extending to the left side under the short ribs. Pain along the left arm, particularly in the little finger, third finger, and thumb. On supinating the forearm, the pain is worse at the elbow. It feels as if the " crazy bone " were struck. The least twitch causes the elbow-joint and shoulder to crack. Itching in the palm of the right hand. Pain in the little finger of the right hand. Itching in the joint of right hand.

Pain in the kneejoint worse at noon, while walking. Drawing in all the muscles of the lower extremities on the under surface. Sore feeling of the ankle, attended with heat and itching over the whole leg.

Sore feeling extending from the small of the back around both sides over the ossa ilii, worse on pressure.

Pain in the lower part of abdomen, attended with diarrhœa and also flatulence after taking the first dose. (Colic from eating boiled cabbage.)

Sensation as if there were a raw spot in the centre of the urethra, which woke him up two nights in succession. (Pain in the molar teeth of right side. Increase of urinary discharge. Dreams with much talking during sleep, which is very restless. Lassitude, weariness. Feeling as if an attack of typhoid fever were to come on. Irascibility. Livid circles around both eyes.)

Jan. 19th to 27th. *One hour after taking twenty pellets of the 6th dilution.* Rush of blood to the back part of the head, attended with violent itching and heat extending to each ear, and behind the left ear there came three hard lumps, one the size of a small shot, the other that of a buckshot, and the last a size larger. On the same night he felt a sharp pain in the region of the kidneys, as if some one had driven a nail on each side of the vertebræ. More profuse discharge of clear water. Flow of mucus from the right nostril, lasting for three days.

Pain on the seventh rib of each side in a spot as large as a quarter of a dollar, more on the left side. Violent constipation lasting all the time he took the medicine, and for a long time after. Bleeding piles for two days. Violent itching in the anus, worse at night in bed. A whitish furred tongue in the morning.

Jan. 28th. Violent itching of the corona glandis, with a profuse secretion of pus; the itching was so violent as to cause him to rub it, which only eased it for a short time, to return with tenfold violence. Two small red spots made their appearance on each side of the glans, secreting a large quantity of lardaceous matter. It had the appearance, according to his opinion, of herpes preputialis.

Profuse sweating between the thighs. Violent erections in the evening. After finishing the medicine all desire for an embrace is lost, which was not the case before he took the medicine.

All the above symptoms except the perspiration were most violent at night in bed; the perspiration about 12 o'clock in the day. He had also a constant pain in the left arm joint, when turning and straitening the arm and when writing. (Every evening hoarseness, with croup-like cough. Right middle finger and palm of hand scurvy tetter exedens.)

Sixth Proving; Sixth and Third Attenuations.

Dr. Albert Lindsay, dark hair, aged 28, uses no coffee, tea, spices, nor any other stimulants.

Jan. 11th, 1851. Twenty pellets of *Cinnabaris* 6th on going to bed.

Great restlessness at night, continual dreaming and waking. He would be scarcely lost in a drowse, before he would be dreaming. Vivid dreams of studies and business, etc. Drawing, aching pains in the thighs from the hipjoints nearly down to the condyles, aggravated by moving and accompanied with great lameness experienced on getting up and attempting to walk, getting better after walking a short distance.

Jan. 12th and 13th. Symptoms of a cold in the head (?), with lameness of the thighs, much mucus in lumps of a dirty yellow color from the posterior nares, during the whole week.

Jan. 13th. *Took twenty globules* at bed-time. Had many dreams and waked up often. (Increased dryness of throat and mouth, being obliged to moisten and rinse the mouth every time he wakes up.)

Jan. 14th. *Took twenty globules of Cinnab.* 6, at 7 o'clock A.M. Shooting, aching pain on posterior side of right thigh from the hip-joint to the middle of the os femoris, about 9 A.M., on straining at stool. In the evening of the same day, took again thirty globules. Continual restlessness, and dreams that a lump is in his throat and right ear.

Jan. 16th. At night *twenty to thirty globules.* In addition to the restlessness and dreaming, woke up with a throbbing pain in the organ of conscientiousness, extending to forehead, over the eye.

During the day and night of the 17th of January he was troubled with aching pains in the thighs; soreness in the umbilical region, obliging him to turn during the night as well as during the day of the 18th. A weak sensation in the left eye during the 18th.

Vivid dreams of the lectures, particularly the anatomical, during the night of the 18th. He could not believe that he was not actually there.

Almost every morning after waking, a kind of dull pain (some mornings more intense and sharper) in the forehead and top of the head, worse when lying on the left side and back, going off when turning to the right side and pressing the forehead into the pillow. As soon as he turns to the left side or the back the pains return. On turning to right side or getting up and washing, the pains disappear.

(The prover had formerly some dulness of the head and sometimes some pain on waking, especially after drinking milk the night before, also some dryness and foul taste in mouth, but these symptoms were far less decided than since he has been taking the medicine.) Violent itching and pricking on the inner side of the knee-joint ever since he has commenced to take the medicine, worse in the night and the morning before getting up.

Jan. 21st. Violent itching on the inside of the thighs, knees and legs, worse at the knees, especially at night.

Jan. 22nd. At bed-time took 5 *gr. of 3d trit.* Had several dreams and awoke several times through the night.

On waking up in the morning had an aching pain in the whole of the forehead and top of the head, aggravated by lying on the left side and back, relieved by lying on the right side and pressing the forehead with the pillow. A dull, heavy, and at times a sleepy feeling during the day.

Jan. 24th. Restless sleep with many dreams, feels very tired in the morning, aching across small of the back and in the limbs. A kind of throbbing pain in the forehead on waking, going off on pressing the head on the pillow.

Jan. 25th and 26th. Same pain in a diminished degree.

Jan. 27th. Symptoms of cold in the head—fulness of the head—discharge of much mucus from the nostrils. Aching pain in the small of the back and legs. Uncommon tiredness and weakness. Sensation of emptiness in the stomach and very hungry two hours after eating a hearty breakfast. Sore on the inside of the under lip towards the left.

Jan. 28th. Severe aching and drawing pains in the back from the region of the kidneys to the sacrum, and in the thighs and legs all last night and to-day. Drawing up of the legs affords relief. He did not wake up with headache in the morning, but about 9 o'clock A.M. a kind of a sore pain commenced at the crown of the head and extended as far front as the organ of veneration (at times there is a slight sensation of throbbing); it is very sensitive to touch, he cannot even touch the hair without causing a sore pain. This pain continued all day. Weakness and sleepiness in the eyes about noon; could scarcely keep them open.

Jan. 29th. No pain this morning but the scalp is sensitive to touch. Slight pains in back and legs, but much better than yesterday.

(The prover here remarks that when he was from thirteen to seventeen years of age he took large quantities of calomel, and was in consequence for years afflicted with terrible drawing aching pains in the legs, especially twelve or twenty hours before a storm. He was a regular barometer. The pains he experienced from the effects of the medicine were exactly like those he suffered years ago from calomel. He was of course entirely ignorant, like all the others, of the nature of the medicine he had undertaken to prove.)

SEVENTH PROVING; SIXTH ATTENUATION.

DR. C. L. MERRIMAN, aged 31, light hair, nervous sanguine temperament.

1851, Jan. 28th. Twenty pellets of the 6th dilution of *Cinnab.* 10 o'clock A.M.

In two hours felt a fulness and general pressure in the whole head as after taking cold, with dull, aching pain in the region of benevolence —better in the open air.

Great drowsiness and lassitude in the warm room. Occasional shooting and prickling pain in the two middle fingers of left hand, better by firm pressure upon the thumb. The above symptoms continued about eight hours.

Jan. 30th. *Twenty pellets of* 6*th.* Symptoms similar in kind, but somewhat less in degree, and passed entirely away in about eight hours.

EIGHTH PROVING; THIRD AND FIRST DEC. TRITURATIONS.

DR. J. L. MULFORD, of good constitution, not predisposed to any acute or chronic disease.

1851, Jan. 25th. Took 5 *gr. of* 3*rd trit.* ($\frac{1}{10}$) of Cinnab. on going to bed, but without producing the slightest effect.

Feb. 2nd. Took 5 *gr. of* 3*rd* ($\frac{1}{10}$) without any effect.

Feb. 3rd. Took 10 *gr. of* 1*st* ($\frac{1}{10}$) *trit.* Shooting pains in the forehead with great heaviness. Shooting pains in the inner canthus of the right eye with a burning and itching.

Hoarseness of the voice in the morning, going off in two or three hours.

Shooting pains in the bowels at intervals during the day. Flashes of heat, confined to the abdomen, with great flatulence.

All the above symptoms more in the forenoon and less in the afternoon and evening.

Feb. 4th. Pain in the bowels before each evacuation, all the other symptoms as detailed above in a less degree.

NINTH PROVING; THIRD DEC. TRITURATION.

DR. D. S. PRATT, aged 24, dark hair. (Has been subject to irritation in the throat, posterior nares, tonsils and fauces for three years, considerable inflammation after taking the slightest cold, worse at night, secretion of tenacious mucus during the day and dryness at night, much soreness in the morning. Inclination to empty deglutition, fits of violent sneezing; has also derangement of the stomach, much flatus, with disturbed sleep, &c., &c.)

The prover took 5 *gr. of the* 3*rd trit.* of Cinnab. ($\frac{1}{10}$) at three different times, followed by much improvement in the throat.

The only symptom of an unusual character that he observed, was a pressing pain in the right temple.

Tenth Proving.

Dr. J. M. Randell, dark hair, dark complexion, aged 20.

1851, Jan. 13th. *Twenty globules* of the 6th dilution. Seems to lower the pulse in the forenoon and make it irregular. Twenty min. of 12 o'clock pain in the left side of the head, temple and supra-orbital ridge. Sensation as if the abdomen were too large, and wishes to have everything loose about the bowels.

Numb pressing pain in the eyes. Numb feeling in the elbows, as if the ulnar nerve was compressed, also numbness in the knee-joints. Hands cold. Pain in the forehead. Sticking in the chest just beneath the sternum. Griping pain in the bowels. The pulse, which was at 12 o'clock M. from forty-four to fifty-two, rose at 4 o'clock to eighty. Pain in the organ of tune. Sensation as if there were something in the ear. In the afternoon his friends remarked that he was very cross and sullen. Sleep restless with vivid dreams, but he cannot remember them in the morning; urine turbid. Pain in the tendo-achillis and os calcis after walking. Pain in the left side of the face and teeth.

The above symptoms were produced by a single dose. Several other doses had a similar effect.

Eleventh Proving; Thirteenth Attenuation.

J. C. Raymond, aged 27.

1851, Feb. 3d, Monday evening. *Twenty globules* of the 30th dil. of *Cinnab.*

In about an hour had sharp darting pains like electric flashes passing from the first phalanx of the ring finger of the right hand to the middle of the fore-arm and from the lower extremity of the radius of the left arm up to the elbow.

Restlessness and sleeplessness during the night from a constant flow of ideas, changing from one subject to another.

On Tuesday an increased flow of saliva. From four to five o'clock P.M. a severe pain extending from the cartilage of the seventh rib at its juncture with the sternum, to the right hypochondriac region under the inferior border of the tenth rib.

On Tuesday night he took 40 *globules*; on Wednesday night took 60 *globules*; on Thursday night took 5 *gr. of* 1-10, and on Friday night 10 *gr. of* 1-10, with no perceptible effect until Saturday, when there was increased sexual desire, with erections, which continued at night, terminating by an emission of semen.

Feb. 9th. On Sunday night, took 20 *pellets* of the 30th attenuation. An increased flow of saliva during the day on Monday, so much so, that when he attempted to speak, he found some difficulty from his mouth being constantly filled with saliva. He had some pain of a dull character in the forehead, over the eyes in the afternoon, which became severer in the evening, and was aggravated by motion. Had occasional pains in the left side of the chest between the cartilages of the 5th and 6th ribs.

Tuesday. The increased flow of saliva still continues.

In the afternoon pain of a dull aching character, in the right frontal region, aggravated in the evening. Also a return in the evening of the pains in the left side of the chest, in the region of the heart, of a sharp cutting character, producing difficulty in getting breath, while they continued.

Wednesday night he was awakened several times from sleep by a severe pain in the right arm. It continued in the morning and during the day of Thursday, at times very severe, commencing about the centre of the os humeri and extending to the elbow, and along the radius to its inferior extremity; the pain was of a heavy aching character, deep-seated, and caused lameness and difficulty in moving the arm. In the forenoon he had also a return of the sharp cutting pains in the region of the heart, followed by wandering pains throughout the whole chest.

Twelfth Proving.

Dr. Hamilton Ring. Aged 29, light hair.

1851. Jan. 14th. 20 *pellets* of 30th dilution of *Cinnab.* at 4 P. M., and on the 15th also, 20 pellets of the same dilution at 9 A. M.

In the course of the day (15th), he experienced on the bridge of the nose, a sensation similar to that produced by touching it with a metallic substance. Sticking pain about the punctum lachrymale of left upper eyelid.

Next day, Jan. 16th, he noticed a small pimple (like a transparent vesicle), sore to touch, on the inner edge of the eyelid, near the spot where the pain was, which latter had disappeared.

Jan. 17th. 10½ A. M. Took 30 pellets of 6th dilution.

Soon after, *aching and somewhat sharp pain in the left hypochondrium, in front, over a space as large as may be covered by the hand;* worse on moving about and in the open air. *Pain soon extending around the lower border of ribs behind, and to region of left kidney, where it seems dull and somewhat oppressive.* (All felt and disappeared in four hours).

Soon after this appearing in *right hypochondrium, in front, and extending around to back, and region of right kidney, where the pain is of the same character as in the left kidney.*

The dull pressive pain is felt in one and then in the other region of the kidney alternately.

The pains intermit in severity, and those in the hypochondria are relieved by bending forward.

Occasional flashes of pain in right temple from in front backwards (organ of mirthfulness).

Soreness in roof of the mouth.

Heaviness in head, desire to sleep during the day, restlessness at night, indisposition to mental exertion.

The above symptoms appeared nearly, if not exactly, in the order in which they are written; those in *italic* were felt most severely

Jan. 18th. (In the evening, occasional shootings in upper part of left temple, along temporal ridge, dulness in the whole head, especially in the forehead just over the eyes, lame sensation in right shoulder joint.

Jan. 19th. At 10½ A. M., took one powder of 1½ trituration (centesimal), after which the following symptoms were experienced.

An hour after, an uneasy, creeping and pressive sensation about the ossa nasi, lasting about an hour, and is the sensation experienced by most persons on putting on a pair of heavy spectacles, if not accustomed to wear them. Also for a short time a pain and sensation of fulness in the meatus of the left ear.

In the evening a sensation of approaching looseness of the bowels.

Itching in various parts of the body, while walking in the open air.

Jan. 20th. In the forenoon head full, nervousness and irritability about noon, for a short time; also, for a short time, sticking pain in the back part of left knee joint; in the afternoon a slight pain in right knee joint (similar to the pain in the left one), with a creeping sensation above and below it, seemingly about the bone, lasting about an hour; (during the day itching over the body).

Jan. 21st. Frequently itching over the body, and itching and sticking in the internal and external canthi; head full, heavy, with strong pulsations of temporal arteries, great inclination to sleep during the day.

Jan. 22d. Itching on body and in the canthi, as before; a spot on right side, on one of the ribs (7th and 8th), as large as a wafer, very sore to touch, with occasionally a sore pain in and around it, head less heavy than the day before, a sore spot on the tip of the tongue.

Jan. 23d. About 4 A. M. was awaked by a dull sticking pain in region of left kidney, which lasted but a short time. Afterwards tossing about and sleeplessness for an hour; after rising from bed, a fulness and pressure in the occiput and back of the neck, continuing with much severity until about noon; after which the symptom somewhat abated; heaviness and sleepiness during the day; pains of short duration in the right hypochondrium, in middle of left breast, in front in the left kidney, occiput; itching over the body at times.

In the evening, sticking pain in the region of left side of 5th and 6th dorsal vertebræ; the sore spot on the right side has continued with the characteristic symptoms before mentioned; during the day there were pains at a corresponding spot in the left side of the same character as pains connected with the other, but without a *sore* spot.

Jan. 24th. Occasionally a sticking pain on the right side of the same dorsal vertebræ (5th or 6th); pain sometimes in the left side of occiput (organ of amativeness); itching of eyelids, and of various parts of the body; sore spot on the right side continues.

The *pains in the knee-joint*, mentioned as having been experienced on the 20th inst. have been occasionally felt in a slight degree every day since.

The sore part on the right side continued 3 or 4 days.

The itching in various parts of the body and in the canthi of the eyes were felt for 5 or 6 days.

The dulness of the head and unfitness for mental exercise have not, after the lapse of a week, entirely disappeared.

The severest *pains* experienced were those in the hypochondria and kidneys.

The pains mentioned as felt on the 23d and 24th, on the side of the 5th or 6th dorsal vertebræ, were occasionally felt until the 27th.

Has been disposed to costiveness during the whole time of taking the medicine.

On the 27th after dinner had a feeling of weight in the lower part of the rectum and a sensation like aching.

Thirteenth Proving; Fifth Attenuation.

Dr. C. E. Toothacher, of lymphatic nervous temperament, brown hair, general health good. In childhood affected with rachitis. In youth with burning sensation in chest, with colic in umbilicus and stomach; subsequently he had pains in the face, itching, burning in throat and roof of the mouth. At present ringing, humming or roaring in the ears, with frequent itching sensations over the whole body, slight dull pain in the back of the head and neck, sense of dull pain in one or both ears. Some remains of a former severe chronic bronchitis, causing frequent hawking and spitting, with thick pus-like mucus in the morning. Disposition to flatulence in the bowels; passes water frequently. Frequent sleepiness when sitting. Languor.

1851, Jan. 18th. 9 o'clock A. M. took 30 *pellets* of the 5th dilution of *Cinnabaris.* 6 o'clock P. M. Sensation of soreness on the left side of the root of the tongue on swallowing, accompanied by roughness and stiffness, continuing through the night.

Jan. 19th. At 9 o'clock A. M. took 30 *pellets* more; at 10 o'clock, slight pain in the sinciput. Sense of elevation on walking in the open air; never felt better in his life; like the effects of a cordial. At 8 o'clock P. M., after tea, a peculiar metallic taste in the mouth, not much unlike sulphate of zinc, or the taste left after a metal or salt, continuing more or less one hour.

Jan. 20th. 5 o'clock next morning, a peculiar agreeable sensation of *exhilaration*, and with fulness extending from all sides of the chest, particularly the thorax, towards the stomach and heart, accompanied or followed by a similar sensation in all the joints, continuing with intermissions till 8 o'clock; occasional pain in the sinciput. A peculiar drawing in the mouth after rising, until breakfast. A small sore on the right side of the tip of the tongue, also one on each lip, continuing several days.

At 2 o'clock P. M. sensation in the mouth and continued since 8 o'clock, modified by a continual tendency to hawk and spit, with unusually copious flow of saliva and mucus, also a sensation of warmth under the sternum, and sense as if secretions were flowing from the stomach and all the mucous surfaces, as well as from the salivary glands.

A peculiar nervous thrill pervading the whole frame, even to the fingers and toes, affecting especially the joints. Sense of languor and depression, as after excessive exhilaration or intoxication. The above sensation continued with intermission for 3 days.

In the eyes for two days excessive itching in the inner canthi from 6 o'clock the first evening.

From 9 to 12 o'clock, itching in the outer canthi, severe and frequent, with a sense of stiffness in the upper eyelids.

In the afternoon, when sitting in the house, a sensation as if a breeze of cold air was blowing upon the eyes, very marked. Eyes very sensitive to cold air in walking out.

Frequent pain in the lower side of the left knee near the inner side of the tibia; lameness and frequent stitches on walking, particularly inner side of knee-joint.

FOURTEENTH PROVING; SIXTH ATTENUATION.

DR. DANIEL WILDER, æt. 39.

1851. Jan. 13th. 20 *globules* of *Cinnabaris*, 6th dil., on going to bed. Restless, uneasy sleep.

Jan. 14th. 20 globules of 6th dil. on going to bed. Increased restlessness, with constant dreaming; seemed to dream before getting asleep.

Jan. 15th. Pain in all the joints, with lameness during the day. Dull pain in the forehead, which is cold and is relieved by the warm hand—aching soreness of the eyes, worse in the evening. Pulse at noon 60, in the evening 80. Aching soreness in the teeth. Regurgitation of wind from the stomach; sores in the mouth on the underlip—severe pain in the forehead, which lasts all night; great restlessness and nervousness. A good deal of mucus at the posterior nares, which comes away in lumps.

An eruption on the inner and lower part of the thigh, with itching. Unusual irritability during the whole time since he took the medicine.

FIFTEENTH PROVING.

MR. JOHN R——T, aged 27, nervous, sanguine temperament.

1851. Jan. 14. Tuesday. Took 20 *globules* of the 30th dil. before going to bed. Slept very well, but had very vivid dreams, which he could not remember.

Next day, general nervous uneasy sensation—feels desirous of improving spiritually, but is rather disconsolate.

Jan. 15th. Wednesday, 10 P. M. Took 20 *globules* of 30th dil. Felt a drowsy sensation as though he could readily sleep—went to bed at 12 o'clock. He still had the drowsy sensation and very strong desire to sleep, but he could not sleep on account of a disagreeable, nervous sensation, which caused him to toss about in bed for an hour and a half. He sleeps not so well as the night before, and his dreams are vivid and rather pleasing, but he cannot bring them to his recollection. (He dreams more or less every night, but thinks his dreams were rather unusually vivid.)

Jan. 16th. Thursday. His mind is in a morbid state, he is disposed to fret at trifles, and is not at all satisfied with himself. At night the same day he took 40 *globules* of 30th dilution. He is again restless and has vivid dreams.

Jan. 17th. Friday. A still more aggravated morbid state of the mind, fretfulness. Also sexual excitement on the least provocation. At 10 P. M. took 5 *gr.* of 3*d trit.* (centesimal). He felt no desire for sleep, but sat up and read until half past one on Saturday morning. He did not sleep for half an hour after going to bed. He dreamed continually, but not so vividly as before.

On waking at 8 o'clock his throat is dry, he is thirsty, sensation as if he had not had a refreshing sleep.

He has no particular sensations on Saturday. His moral and mental state is rather improved.

At 2¼ P. M., sexual excitement as if he were to have an emission, but is able to combat the feeling.

From the first time he took the medicine, he felt as if pimples were to come out over his body, with a general uneasy sensation and itching. (The prover has had this feeling for some time, but now in an aggravated form.)

Symptoms of flatulency of the stomach, irregularity of the passages, pressing in the forehead, with a sensation of congestion, to which the prover had been subject for some time, have now nearly disappeared.

Since taking the medicine it is quite difficult for him to fix his mind long on any subject. He cannot pay attention to the lectures as well as before. This sensation is relieved by the open air. He cannot think long, deeply or clearly on any subject, and his mind seems to be altogether disturbed.

Jan. 19th. Sunday, 12 M., took 5 *gr. of* 3*d decim. trit.* 5 P. M., strange congestive sensation about the head, principally in the forehead.

8½ to 10¼ P. M., fulness and pressure in the forehead.

10¼ P. M. sensation of water in the left ear, which soon passes off. Pain and tired feeling in the right hip and afterwards in the left. Tired feeling in all the joints of the lower extremities, better from rising and walking; sensation of having taken cold, and general feeling as not being fit for any mental labor; depressed, melancholy, cynical state of mind, nervous system excited.

Jan. 21. Tuesday, 8 A. M., took 40 *globules of* 6*th dilution.* No symptoms observed until 7 P. M. Left cheek flushed, and in left eye watery sensation; soon passed off; congested sensation over the whole head, particularly in the forehead; great difficulty of collecting ideas and studying usefully, and even aversion to close study; after retiring did not sleep for over an hour, but tossed about, very nervous and mentally vexed.

Jan. 22d. Wednesday. Symptoms of mind and head much the same as Tuesday evening. Eruption on posterior cervical region and soreness from right ear into the middle of the posterior cervical region, as if the glands were affected.

Jan. 23d. Thursday. Increase of the soreness, very severe in the evening. The left eye still continues to water several times, passing off each time in a few minutes.

The soreness in the posterior cervical glands continues until Jan. 27th, but it gradually decreased in severity. Has also occasionally fever and fulness in the forehead. Itching at night, especially on the inside of the thighs.

Sixteenth Proving.

T. took 20 globules of 30th dil. *Cinnab.* at night. Had an increase of the flow of saliva, and a pain running near the ensiform cartilage from the 7th rib on the right side diagonally through to the chest.

No farther effect was produced from 40 to 60 glob. of same dil., nor from 5 gr. and 10 gr. of the 1st decimal trit.

Seventeenth Proving.

Mrs. H. took the 6th dil. and experienced a great increase of the flow of urine and saliva, lasting one hour; with shooting pain in the left side of the head from the occiput to forehead—flow of tears.

Eighteenth Proving.

Miss F. took one dose of *Cinnab.* 6th, and had a dizziness and lightness of the head—soreness in the stomach, with tightness in the temples.

Nineteenth Proving.

Mrs. F. took at 8 A. M. 20 *drops* of the 5th dil. of *Cinnab.* At half past 8 A. M. sensation of fulness and weight across the temples, with sometimes throbbing over right temple, worse on motion. These symptoms disappeared before noon. Aching in small of the back, as if bruised.

* There are days in the evenings of which, she feels unusually well and strong.

Feb. 5th. Took at 8 A. M. 10 *drops* of 5th dil. Aching in both ears, lasting about fifteen minutes. At 11 o'clock unusual drowsiness and heaviness over the eyes. (In the evening nervous trembling of the heart with anxiety, to which she had formerly been subject, again returns.)

From 1 gr. of 5th decimal trit., unusual drowsiness in the morning. In the afternoon, two passages of the bowels, the last one with straining.

* Mind clearer and more cheerful.

Unusually vivid dreams of a sensual nature.

Twentieth Proving.

A patient of light complexion who received *Cinnabaris*, 1st trituration, for a phimosis, soon complained of the following most obstinate symptoms, which he never felt before, and which may be clearly ascribed to the effect of the medicine.

He took it for two weeks with constant improvement to phimosis. After discontinuing it for ten days he still had the severe pain in the head, which was mitigated by *Sulph.* and *Bellad.*, but only finally relieved by *Iodine. Nitric Acid* aggravated it.

Intense headache, relieved by external pressure. This pain was so severe that he could hardly endure it. Noises in the ears after eating.

Head excessively sore on the outside to every touch. Pain darting through from the sides of the head and the temples. The pain is near the outer edge of the orbit of the right eye, and more frequent on the right side of the head than the left. Constant pain in the right side of the head. From the temples the pain goes to the occiput. Excessive lachrymation.

Dryness in the mouth, with desire for cold water. Bad taste in the mouth, with phlegm and ptyalism; loss of appetite; eats very little; constipation, only one passage in a week; soreness under the right breast near the last true rib, particularly on drawing breath. Feeling of coldness and sensation of inertia; drowsiness; nightly sleeplessness; hears the clock strike every hour; redness of the skin, like a chronic eruption. He wakes up suddenly as from a dream. The headache is much worse after sleeping.

4. *Digest of the Symptoms.*

The following are the abbreviations used :—

1. S. A.—Dr. S. Armor.
2. B.—Some women and girls proving under the direction of a friend of Dr. Hering's (3d trituration).
3. A. J. B.—A. J. Brewster.
4. J. P. D.—Dr. J. P. Dake.
5. H.—Hahnemann.
6. C. Hg.—Dr. C. Hering.
7. J. H. H.—Dr. J. H. Henry.
8. Ktz.—from Koschwitz's translation of "*Schroeder's Arzneischatz.*"
9. L.—Dr. A. Lippe.
10. A. L.—Dr. Albert Lindsay.
11. C. L. M.—Dr. C. L. Merriman.
12. J. L. M.—Dr. J. L. Mulford.
13. Nd.—Dr. C. Neidhard, including symptoms from three ladies, and from a patient of Dr. N.'s.
14. D. S. P.—Dr. D. S. Pratt.
15. J. M. R.—Dr. J. M. Randell.
16. J. C. R.—Dr. J. C. Raymond.
17. H. R.—Dr. Hamilton Ring.
18. Rt.—a prover who does not permit the use of his name.
19. C. E. T.—Dr. C. E. Toothacher.
20. D. W.—Dr. Daniel Wilder.

The asterisk (*) is prefixed to curative symptoms.

Antidotes.—*Sulph. and Bellad.* mitigated the severe pain in head, but *Iodine* finally cured it. *Nitric-acid* aggravated it. (Nd. 1st.)

Moral Symptoms and Head.

(1.) Indisposition for mental labor. The head feels heavy as from long mental application; a dull heavy ache in the front of the head to the occiput, mostly over the right eye and temple, with heat; occasional darting pains through the head from without inwardly. (A. J. B., 6th dil.)

Although intending to sit up and study longer, yet he felt so wearied in body, and confused in mind, that he soon retired. Upon lying down there were rumblings in the abdomen, and pains from the epigastric to the pubic region. There was also some nausea and uneasiness in the stomach. Every little noise about the house troubled him, as though it were something serious. Although accustomed to dream much, yet he had more troublesome dreams than usual. He awoke and started up several times without purpose: once with a heavy pain in the forepart of the head. Upon rising at 7 o'clock in the morning he felt a little giddiness and pain in the forehead, with a sensation of soreness in the eye-balls. These passed away soon after breakfast. Before noon acidity of the stomach, general headache, and heaviness of the eyes came on, somewhat as usual, but only much aggravated (J. P. D., 5 gr., 3d trit.)†

Heaviness in the head, desire to sleep during the day, restlessness at night, indisposition to mental exertion (H. R., 6th dil.)

The dulness of the head and unfitness for mental exercise have not, after the lapse of a week, entirely disappeared (H. R., 6th).

Since taking the medicine it is quite difficult for him to fix his mind long on any subject. He cannot pay attention to the lectures so well as before. This sensation is relieved by the open air. He cannot think long, deeply and clearly on any subject, and his mind seems to be altogether disturbed (Rt., from 5 gr. of 3d cent. trit.)

Left cheek flushed, and left eye watery, sensation which soon passed off. Congested sensation over the whole head, particularly in the forehead; great difficulty of collecting his ideas and studying usefully, and even aversion to close study. After retiring did not sleep for over an hour, but tossed about very nervous, and mentally vexed (Rt., 40 glob., 6th dil.)

The above symptoms of mind and head continued the same the next day (Rt.)

Sensation of having taken cold, and a general feeling as not being fit for any mental labor; depressed, melancholy, cynical state of mind; nervous system excited (Rt., 3d.)

Restlessness and sleeplessness during the night from a constant flow of ideas changing from one subject to another (1st day. J. C. R. 30th.)

†(These and similar groups I have thought best not to separate, as they disclose the consecutive action of the remedy in different parts of the body, forming true medicinal diseases. I did this at the risk of many repetitions at subsequent divisions.)

Forgetfulness of things which he has to do, and which, under other circumstances, he would not easily forget—as, neglecting to extinguish the light.

Forgets to notice the symptoms (C. Hg., 1st day, 3d trit.)

Inattention to the symptoms (C. Hg.)

Fretful and inclined to weep; he reproaches others (B.)

* Mind clearer and more cheerful (5th, Nd.)

His mind is in a morbid state; he is disposed to fret at trifles, and is not at all satisfied with himself (1st day, 30th, Rt.)

Next day a still more aggravated morbid state of mind; fretfulness; also sexual excitement on the least provocation (Rt. 30th.)

Great depression of spirits after meals (B.)

Pain in the organ of tune; sensation as if there was something in the ear. In the afternoon his friends remarked to him that he was very cross and sullen (1st day. J. W. R., 6th dil.)

Irascibility (J. H. H., 6th).

Involuntary thoughts and imaginations without occasion; fear of his or others falling, etc. (C. Hg.)

* Mistakes of the imagination (Ktz.)

Yawning; not inclined to speak, and an intolerable feeling when spoken to (3d trit. L.)

Desire to be alone (3d, L.)

Giddiness, particularly on stooping (B.)

Vertigo and lassitude, particularly in the morning after rising (B.)

Giddiness, with nausea; pressing pain in the forehead disappearing after lying down and during sleep (B.)

Upon rising at 7 o'clock in the morning, he felt a little giddiness and pain in the forehead, with a sensation of soreness in the eyeballs. These passed away soon after breakfast (J. P. D. 3d, 1st day).

Dizziness in the head in the morning after rising (2d day, B.)

Dizziness and lightness in the head; soreness in the stomach, with tightness in the temples (Nd., 6th dil.)

Roaring in the head, half an hour after dinner, and in the evening before retiring, causing dizziness (H.)

Fulness and determination of blood to the head.

Fulness of the head very frequently (1st, 3d day, C. Hg.).

Fulness of the head and eyes, eyes reddened (C. Hg., 3d trit.).

Fulness in the head and about the eyes, which are red (3d L.).

In the evening occasional shootings in the upper part of left temple, along the temporal ridge; dulness in the whole head, especially the forehead, just over the eyes; lame sensation in right shoulder joint (2d day, H. R., 30th).

Unusual drowsiness and heaviness over the eyes (Nd. 5th, 1st day).

In the forenoon, head full; nervousness and irritability about noon for a short time; also, for a short time, sticking pain in the back part of left knee joint; in the afternoon, sticking pain in the right knee joint, with a creeping sensation above and below it, seemingly about the bone, lasting about an hour (H. R. 1½ trit., 2d day).

Frequently itching over the body and itching and sticking in the internal and external canthi; head full, heavy, with strong pulsations of the temporal arteries; great inclination to sleep during the day (H. R., 1½ trit., 3d day).

Head less heavy the fourth day (H. R., 1½ trit.)

Symptoms of cold in the head; fulness of the head, discharge of much mucus from the nostrils; aching pain in the small of the back and in the legs. Uncommon tiredness and weakness. Sensation of emptiness in the stomach, and very hungry within two hours after eating a hearty breakfast; sore on the inside of the under lip towards the left (6th day, A. L.).

Symptoms of cold in the head, with lameness of the thighs; much mucus in lumps of a dirty yellow color from the posterior nares during the whole week (A. L., 6th).

Fulness and pressure in the forehead in the evening (Rt., 30th).

Occasionally, fever and fulness in the forehead (Rt., 6th).

* Symptoms of flatulency of the stomach, irregularity of the passages, pressing in the forehead, with a sensation of congestion to which the prover had been subject for some time, have now disappeared (Rt., 30th dil., and 3d trit.)

Determination of blood to the head the whole day (12th day, C. Hg.)

Flatulence after congestion to the head in the forenoon, during the first day (C. Hg.)

Left cheek flushed and left eye watery sensation, which soon passed off. Congested sensation over the whole head, particularly in the forehead; great difficulty of collecting his ideas and studying usefully, and even aversion to close study. After retiring, did not sleep for over an hour, but tossed about, very nervous and mentally vexed (Rt., 6th.)

At 5 P. M., strange congestive sensation about the head, principally in the forehead, after taking 5 gr. of 3d trit., at 12 M. (Rt.)

The determination of blood to the head, particularly to the vertex, is aggravated when eating, so as to interrupt his meal (C. Hg.)

At 10 o'clock in the forenoon, when rising from the stooping posture, so violent determination of blood to the head and neck, accompanied by dizziness, as nearly to deprive him of his senses (1st day, C. Hg.)

Rush of blood to the back part of the head, attended with violent itching and heat, extending to each ear, and behind the left ear there came three hard lumps, one of the size of a small shot, the other that of a buck-shot, and the last a size larger; on the same night he felt a sharp pain in the region of the kidneys, as if some one had driven a nail on each side of the vertebra. A more profuse discharge of clear urine. Flow of mucus from the nostril, lasting for three days (one hour after taking 20 pellets 6th dil. J. H. H.)

*A great number of persons have been relieved by Cinnabaris, of congestion of blood to the head (Nd.)

In two hours after taking the medicine, he felt a fulness and general pressure in the whole head, as after taking cold, with dull aching pain in the region of benevolence; better in the open air (C. L. M., 6th).

Intense headache, relieved by external pressure. This pain was so severe that he could hardly endure it. The pain in the head is so severe that he can scarcely raise his head from the pillow. It lasts from ½ past 12 to 6 P. M. (1st Nd.)

The headache is much worse after sleeping (1st Nd.)

Dull feeling in the head and pressing headache; ameliorated in the open air; disappearance of the pain after bleeding of the nose; after bleeding ceases, general uncomfortable feeling (in 8 days, B.)

(He had formerly some dulness of the head, and sometimes a pain on waking, especially after drinking milk the night before; also some dryness and foul taste in the mouth, but these symptoms were far less decided since he has been taking the medicine.) (A. L., 6th.)

Pressing headache, occasionally a digging and gnawing in small spots, for the most part in the upper and left side of the head (300, C. Hg.)

Forehead, pains over the eyes, and concomitant symptoms.

Occasional pains in the sinciput (C. E. F., 5th, 2d day.)

A sharp steady pain in the forehead, mostly in the right orbital region; soon after, felt a sharp throbbing in the left hypochondrium in the region of the spleen, after four hours. A dull aching pain in the bones of the forearms and legs, in 11 hours (A. J. B., 3d.)

In half an hour, a sharp aching pain in the right supraorbital region, shooting backwards and downwards to the ear and side of the neck. Front of the head very hot. The pain in the head is worse in the warm room, and on moving the eyes and scalp.

In eleven hours, at 10 P. M., the same pain is increased to a heavy stupefying ache, aggravated by thinking, reading and pressure. Tenderness in the epigastric region.

In the morning better, but in the evening the pains in the head return again, with a numbness and heavy aching in the arms and knees, and lower legs, without another dose.

The same pains in the head return also in the morning at 11 o'clock, with a disposition to fall asleep while trying to listen to the lecture, notwithstanding his making a great effort to keep awake; constrictive feeling in the umbilical region, urine tinged yellow. Pains all aggravated in the evening. Better in the open air, and after eating and sleeping (A. J. B., 3d).

In the morning a sense of general prostration, great weakness of all the limbs. Feeling of depression and weakness of the whole system, as after a severe illness. Indisposition for mental labor. The head feels weary as from long mental application.

A dull heavy ache in the front of the head, from before backwards, mostly over the right eye and temple, with heat in the head. Occasional darting pains through the head from without inwardly (A. J. B., 6th, 1st day).

Pain in all the joints with lameness during the day. Dull pain in the forehead, which is cold, and is relieved by the warm hand. Aching soreness of the eyes, worse in the evening (D. W., 6th, 2d day).

During the first day, he experienced on the bridge of the nose a sensation similar to that produced by touching it with a metallic substance. Sticking pains about the punctum lachrymale of the left upper eyelid (H. R., 30th).

A space about the size of a quarter dollar just above and between the supra-orbital ridges (root of nose ?) felt as if pressed upon by a cold metallic body, while within the cranium underneath, there seemed to be more warmth than usual (J. P. D.).

*A dull pain, felt before in the left temple and side of the forehead, disappeared (J. P. D., 3d).

An hour after taking the medicine, an uneasy, creeping, and pressive sensation about the ossa nasi, lasting about an hour, and is the sensation experienced by most persons on putting on a pair of heavy spectacles, if not accustomed to wear them. Also for a short time a pain and sensation of fulness in the meatus of the ear. In the evening, a sensation of approaching looseness in the bowels (H. R., $1\frac{1}{2}$ trit.).

Pain in the forehead (region of causality). A sensation of sticking over secretive region, which increases and becomes a numb pain, extending to the right temple (time and locality), with a feeling of warmth on the right side. Disposition to sleep during the day. The pain extends from one temple to the other across the os frontis from right to left, is mild in the forehead, but violent in the organs of locality and time, both night and day, and on rising in the morning. Before going to bed there is a drawing pain in the head, extending from the crown to the occiput, inclining to the right. Pain deep-seated, as if in the centre of the head (I. H. H., 6th).

Almost every morning after waking, a kind of dull pain (some mornings more intense and sharper) in the forehead and top of the head, worse when lying on the left side and back, going off when turning to the right side and pressing the forehead with the pillows. As soon as he turns to the left side or back, the pains return. On turning to the right side, or getting up, or washing, the pains disappear (A. L., 6th).

On waking up in the morning had an aching pain in the whole of the forehead and top of the head; aggravated by lying on the left side and back; relieved by lying on the right side and pressing the forehead with the pillows. A dull, heavy, and at times a sleepy feeling during the day (W. L., 3d., 1st day).

Although accustomed to dream much, yet he had more troublesome dreams than usual. He awoke and started up several times without purpose: once with a heavy pain in the forehead. Upon arising in the morning he felt a little giddiness and pain in the forehead, with a sensation of soreness in the eye-balls. These passed away soon after breakfast. Before noon, acidity of the stomach, general headache, and heaviness in the eyes, came on, somewhat as usual, only much aggravated. (J. P. D., 3d).

Pain in the forehead; sticking in the chest just beneath the sternum; griping pain in the bowels (J. M. R., 6th).

After taking the medicine the night before, he had an increased flow of saliva the next day, so much so, that when he attempted to speak he found some difficulty, from his mouth being filled with saliva. He had some pains of a dull character in the forehead over the eyes in the afternoon, which became more severe in the evening, and was aggravated by motion. Had occasional pains in the left side of the chest, between the cartilages of the 5th and 6th ribs.

The second day the flow of saliva still continued; in the afternoon he had again a dull aching pain in the right forehead, aggravated in the evening; also a return of the pains in the left side of the chest in the region of the heart of a sharp, cutting character, producing a difficulty of breathing (J. C. R., 30th).

Dull pain in the forehead, which is cold, and relieved by the warm hand; aching soreness of the eyes, worse in the evening; pulse rises from 60 to 80 in the evening; aching soreness in the teeth. Eructations of wind from the stomach; sores on the mouth on the under lip. Severe pain in the forehead, which lasts all night; great restlessness and nervousness; a good deal of mucus at the posterior nares, which comes away in lumps (D. W., 6th).

Dull pain in the forehead the entire day (B., 9th day).

Pressing pain in the forehead, which spreads upwards, seems to be between the external skin and the muscle; it is aggravated by lying and pressing upon the pillow (B.)

Pain in the right side of the forehead, then in the left, where it is more violent, and draws downwards to the chest; it again recurs somewhat later, diminished by exercise and perspiration (B.)

Pressing in the forehead at five o'clock in the morning, before rising, with dizziness and nausea; disappears after rising and eructations of wind (B.)

Throbbing in the forehead at noon (3d day, B.)

Pricking pain in the forehead during the whole night (B.)

Shooting pains in the forehead, with great heaviness.

Shooting pains in the inner canthus of the right eye, with a burning and itching.

Hoarseness of the voice in the morning, passing off in two or three hours.

Shooting pains in the bowels at intervals during the day. Flushes of heat confined to the abdomen, with great flatulence: all the above symptoms more in the forenoon, and less in the afternoon and evening (J. L. M., 1st).

Temples and sides of head.

Pain from the right lachrymal duct around the eye to the temple. Drawing from the right inner canthus across the malar bone to the ear (J. H. H., 6th).

Dulness in the head, mostly on the right side and towards the posterior part, and about the right ear, in the forenoon after some hours (C. Hg.)

Sensation of fulness and weight across the temples, with sometimes throbbing over right temple, worse on motion (for half an hour, Nd., 5th).

Occasional flashes of pain in right temple, from in front backwards (organ of mirthfulness), soreness in roof of mouth. Heaviness in head, desire to sleep during the day, restlessness at night, indisposition to mental exertion (H. R., 6th, 1st day).

Pain darting through from the sides of the head and the temples. The pain is near the edge of the outer orbit of the right eye, and more frequent on the right side of the head than the left. Constant pain in the right side of the head. From the temples the pain goes to the occiput (Nd. 1st).

A sensation of sticking over secretive region, which increases and becomes a numb pain, extending to the right temple, with a feeling of warmth on the right side (J. H. H., 6th).

Pressing pain in the right temple (D. S. P., 3d).

Pain in the left side of the head, temple and supra-orbital ridge. Sensation as if the abdomen was too large, and wishes to have everything loose about the bowels. Numb pressing pains in the eyes. Numb feeling in the elbows, as if the ulnar nerve was compressed; also numbness in the knee joints. Hands cold (J. M. R., 6th).

In the evening occasional shootings in upper part of left temple, along temporal ridge; dulness in the whole head, especially in the forehead just over the eyes; lame sensation in the right shoulder joint (H. R., 6th, 2d day).

Dizziness and lightness of the head; soreness of the stomach, with tightness of the temples (Nd., 6th).

Frequently itching over the body and itching and sticking in the internal and external canthi, head full, heavy, with strong pulsations of temporal arteries, great inclination to sleep during the day (H. R., 1½, 3d day).

Three or four hours after taking the 3d decimal trit. of Cinnab. in the morning, his abdomen, below the transverse colon, felt hot, his tongue is covered with a white fur and there is a beating and burning in both temples, which he felt all day (S. A.)

Occiput and crown of head.

An hour after taking the medicine in the morning, he has a violent pressing pain in the occiput, also in the left side of the head for two hours. In the afternoon she was obliged to lie down and sleep, after which the pain disappeared (B.)

A great increase of the flow of urine and saliva, lasting one hour, with shooting pain on the left side of the head from the occiput to the forehead; flow of tears (Nd., 6th).

On turning the head, pain on the right side of the neck, below the sterno-cleido-mastoideus muscle. Pain in the back part of the neck, when the head is thrown back, extending to the occiput. The muscles in back part of the neck seem as if contracted. General pain all over the back down to the loins, worse after every dose of the medicine, aggravated on drawing a long breath (J. H. H., 6th).

Before going to bed, there is a drawing pain in the head, extending from the crown to the occiput, inclining to the right. Pain deep as in the centre of the head (J. H. H., 6th).

In addition to the restlessness and dreaming, he woke up with a throbbing pain in the organ of conscientiousness, extending to the forehead over the eye (the night after taking 6th, A. L.)

About 4 A. M., was awaked by a dull sticking pain in the region of the left kidney, which lasted but a short time; afterwards tossing about and sleeplessness for an hour; after rising from bed, a fulness and pressure in the occiput and back of the neck, continuing with much severity till about noon, after which the symptoms somewhat abated; heaviness and sleepiness during the day; pains of short duration in the right hypochondrium, in middle of the left breast, in front in the left kidney and in the occiput; itching over the body at times. In the evening, sticking pain in the region of the left side of the fifth and sixth dorsal vertebræ; a sore spot on the right side seventh and eighth ribs, which he had felt before, continues. It is very sore to touch, with occasionally a sore spot in and around it; during the day there were pains at a corresponding spot on the left side of the same character as the pains connected with the other, but without a sore spot (H. R., 1½, 5th day).

The next day, occasionally a sticking pain in the right side of the same dorsal vertebræ (5th and 6th); pain sometimes in the left side of occiput (organ of amativeness); itching of the eyelids and of various parts of the body; sore spot in the right side continues for three or four days (H. R., 1½, 6th day).

Eruption on the posterior cervical region and soreness from right ear into the middle of the posterior cervical region as if the glands were affected, which continues for seven days, but it gradually decreases in severity (Rt., 6th).

Scalp.

About 9 o'clock in the morning a sore pain, commencing at the crown of the head and extending as far as the organ of veneration (at times a slight sensation of throbbing), it is very sensitive to the touch—he cannot even touch the hair, without causing a sore pain (the sixth and seventh day). Weakness and sleepiness in the eyes about noon, could scarcely keep them open (6th day, 3d, A. L.)

Sensitiveness of the head to the touch; even the hairs are sore (H.).

Pricking about the exterior part of the head, only during the day (H.).

Head excessively sore on the outside to every touch (1st, Nd.).

* Has cured thousands as "*specificum cephalicum*" (Ktz.).

Eyes.

Shooting pains in the inner canthus of the right eye, with a burning and itching (J. L. M., 1st).

Head excessively sore on the scalp to every touch; pain darting through from the sides of the head and temples. The pain is near the outer edge of the orbit of the right eye, and more frequent on the right side of the head than the left. Constant pain in right side of head. From the temples the pain goes to the occiput; excessive lachrymation (Nd. 1st trit.).

(Inflammation of the right eye; itching, pressing, and pricking at the inner angle and the lower lid; constant lachrymation on looking steadily, with profuse discharge of mucus from the nose.) (H.)

Pain from the right lachrymal duct around the eye to the temple. Drawing sensation from the right inner canthus across the malar bone to the ear. A sensation as if there were something in the eyes, lasting three days; feeling as if the eyelids were enlarged or puffed, as if the muscles were too short, when looking up the wall. Pain from the inner canthus of the left eye across the eye-brows (organs of size, color, order, calculation). Itching of the lids of both eyes (J. H. H., 6th).

Redness of the corners of the eyes, mostly at the inner angles; right eye more affected than the left; cornea appears encircled by a red ring. All these symptoms are aggravated in the evening during the first day (B.)

Eyes watery and dull, with a sharp sticking pain in the inner canthus of the left eye, as of a sharp stick being stuck in the lower lid (A. J. B., 6th; 2d day).

Pain in the inner canthus of the left eye, with redness and swelling, mostly towards the lower lid (C. Hg.).

Left eye watery sensation occasionally, for three days, passing off each time in a few minutes (Rt., 6th).

Flow of tears (Nd., 6th).

Sticking pain about the punctum lachrymale of the upper eyelid.

A small pimple (like a transparent vesicle) sore to touch, on the inner edge of the eyelid near the spot where the pain was, which latter had disappeared (H. R., 2d day).

Itching of eyelids and various parts of body (H. R., 1st).

Frequently itching over the body, and itching and sticking in the internal and external canthi; felt for eight days (H. R., 1st).

In the eyes for two days excessive itching in the inner canthi, from six o'clock the first evening.

From nine to twelve o'clock; frequent and severe itching in the outer canthi, with a sense of stiffness in the upper eyelids. In the afternoon when sitting in the house, a sensation as if a breeze of cold air was blowing upon the eyes; very marked. Eyes very sensitive to cold air in walking out (C. E. F., 5th).

Redness of the inner angle of the eyes during the 5th day (B.)

Redness of the whole eye, with swelling of the face (3, L.).

Livid circles around both eyes (J. H. H., 6th).

Weakness of the eyes, with redness of the corners; burning pain (3d day, B.)

A weak sensation in the left eye during the 18th (A. L., 6th, 2d day).

About nine o'clock in the morning a kind of sore pain, commencing at the crown of the head, and extending as far front as the organ of veneration; it is very sensitive to touch; he cannot even touch the hair, without causing a sore pain. This pain continued all day; weakness and sleepiness in the eyes about noon; could scarcely keep them open (A. L., 6th day; 3d).

Eyes weak and over-clouded (5th day, B.).

Aching soreness of the eyes, worse in the evening (D. W., 2d day; 5th).

Upon rising in the morning he felt a little giddiness and pain in the forehead, with a sensation of soreness in the eye-balls. Before noon acidity of stomach; general headache and heaviness of the eyes (J. P. D., 3d).

Numb pressing pain in the eyes (J. M. R., 6th).

Fulness of the head and eyes; eyes reddened (C. Hg., 3d).

Ears.

Pressing, forcing pain deep in the right ear, inwardly towards the neck after sitting down; disappears while sitting, with dizziness after two hours in the forenoon (C. Hg.).

Continued restlessness, and dreams a lump is in his throat and right ear (A. L., 6th).

In half an hour felt a sharp aching pain in the right supra-orbital region, shooting backwards and downwards to the ear and side of the neck; front of head very hot; the pain is worse in a warm room, and on moving the eyes and scalp (A. J. B., 3d).

Drawing sensation from the right inner canthus across the malar bone to the ear (J. H. H., 6th).

Much itching in the right ear, and after using the ear-pick a pain deep in the ear the 9th day (C. Hg.).

The right external ear becomes numb whilst sitting in the carriage the 4th day (C. Hg.).

Rush of blood to the back part of the head, attended with violent itching and heat extending to each ear, and behind the left ear there came three hard lumps, one the size of a small shot, the other that of a buckshot, and the last a size larger (J. H. H., 6th).

For a short time a pain and sensation of fulness in the meatus of the left ear (H. R.; 1st day, 1½ trit.).

At 10 P.M., sensation of water in the left ear, which soon passes off (Rt., 3d; 1st day).

Much itching in the left ear from the 1st to the 4th day; scurfy eruption in the right external ear, between the helix and anti-helix, the 4th day (C. Hg.).

Aching in both ears, lasting about fifteen minutes (Nd., 5th).

Noises in the ears after eating (Nd., 1st).

Roaring in the ears, with swelling of the face (3d, L.).

Face and Nose.

Great heat in the face (while triturating the medicine from 11 to 12 o'clock A. M.), which is much swollen, mostly about the eyes (3d, L.).

Heat and swelling of the face; afterwards pain in the back part of the head (3d, L.).

In the evening left cheek flushed; left eye, watery sensation, which soon passed off (Rt., 1st day, 6th).

Itching on the left side of the face (J. H. H., 6th).

Pain in the left side of the face and teeth (J. M. R., 6th).

Tickling in the nose, obliging her to pick it with the fingers, after the 8th day (B.).

(Violent pricking, jerking in the nose, particularly when eating during the 1st day.) (C. Hg.).

(Sore in the nose in both nostrils at the point until fall, and also in the spring, 1848) (C. Hg.).

Itching of the nose, with bleeding, after blowing it. The blood is very dark. The itching is caused by pimples at the right nostril (J. H. H., 6th).

Symptoms of a cold in the head, with lameness of the thighs; much mucus, in lumps of a dirty yellow color, in the posterior nares during the whole week (A. L., 6th).

Symptoms of cold in the head; fulness of the head; discharge of much mucus from the nostrils; aching pain in the small of the back and legs (A. L., 3d, 5th day).

A good deal of mucus at the posterior nares, which comes away in lumps (D. W., 6th, 2d day).

Flow of mucus from the right nostril, lasting for three days (J. H. H., 6th).

* Irritation in the throat, posterior nares, tonsils, and fauces (D. S. P., 3d).

An hour after taking 1st trit. an uneasy, creeping, and pressing sensation about the ossa nasi, lasting about an hour, and is the sensation experienced by most persons on putting on a pair of heavy spectacles, if not accustomed to wear them (H. R.).

During the 1st day he experienced on the bridge of the nose a sensation similar to that produced by touching it with a metallic substance. Sticking pains about the punctum lachrymale of the left upper eyelid (H. R., 30th).

A space about the size of a quarter dollar just above and between the supra-orbital ridges (root of nose), felt as if pressed upon by a cold metallic body, while within the cranium underneath there seemed to be more warmth than usual (J. P. D., 3d).

Teeth and Mouth.

Pain in the molar teeth of right side (J. H. H., 6th).

Aching soreness in the teeth (D. W., 6th; 2d day).

The 11th day much bleeding from the incisor tooth of upper jaw in right side.

*Both corners of the mouth are chapped (C. Hg.)

Sensation of emptiness in the stomach, and very hungry within two hours after eating a hearty breakfast; sore on the inside of the under lip, towards the left (A. L., 3d, 6th day).

A whitish furred tongue in the morning (J. H. H., 6th).

Three or four hours after taking the medicine in the morning, his abdomen felt hot below the transverse colon; his tongue is covered with a white fur, and there is beating burning in both temples, which he felt all day (S. A., 2d).

A small sore on the right side of the tip of the tongue, also on each lip, continuing several days (C. E. T., 5th).

Regurgitation of wind from the stomach; sores in the mouth on the under lip (D. W., 6th, 2d day).

Small sore on the roof of the mouth (J. H. H., 6th).

A sore spot on the tip of the tongue (H. R., 1½ trit., 4th day).

At six o'clock in the evening, after taking the medicine in the morning, sensation of soreness on the left side of the root of the tongue, on swallowing, accompanied with roughness and stiffness, continuing through the night (C. E. T., 5th).

Taste as of tobacco and coffee in the mouth; pricking sensation in the mouth and fauces; small spot on the left side of the tongue, which itches; small sore on the roof of the mouth; itching on the left side of the face (J. H. H., 6th).

Soreness in the roof of the mouth (H. R., 6th, 1st day).

Sensation of contraction, and burning in the roof of the mouth (H.).

Dryness in the mouth, burning of the throat and the whole breast, with general weakness (14th dil., C. Hg.).

Much dryness of the mouth and throat at night; obliged to drink often; some pricking under the back part of the tongue (H.).

Dryness in the mouth, with desire for cold water; bad taste in the mouth, with phlegm and ptyalism (Nd., 1st).

(Increased dryness of the throat and mouth, being obliged to moisten and rinse the mouth every time he wakes up) (A. L., 6th).

*Inflammation, with great dryness in mouth and throat; worse at night. In several cases $\frac{1}{200}$ helped very quickly (Pehrson).

* Dryness and irritation of the throat (posterior nares, tonsils, fauces) at night, with soreness in the morning; secretion of tenacious mucus during the day; inclination to empty deglutition (D. S. P., 3d).

On waking at eight o'clock, after taking the third trituration the previous night, his throat is dry; he is thirsty; sensation as if he had not a refreshing sleep (Rt.).

Pressing contracting pain in the throat during empty deglutition (H.).

Fulness in the throat, creating a desire for constant swallowing; 1st day (C. Hg.).

The cravat presses him uncomfortably, as if the throat was pressed together from below on both sides, and contracted within, so as to impede swallowing; forenoon of 1st day (C. Hg.).

*Dryness and foul taste in the mouth (A. L., 6th).

Bitter taste in the mouth before, during, and after meals (B.).

Bitter eructations (B.).

Bitter taste in the mouth in the morning; remains after eating (B.)

Taste of tobacco and coffee in the mouth (J. H. H., 6th).

At eight o'clock P.M., after tea, a peculiar metallic taste in the mouth, not much unlike sulphate of zinc, or the taste left after a metal or salt, continuing more or less one hour (1st day).

At five o'clock next morning a peculiar agreeable sensation of exhilaration, with a fulness extending from all sides of the chest towards the stomach and heart, accompanied or followed by a similar sensation in all the joints, continuing with intermissions till eight o'clock. A peculiar drawing in the mouth after rising, until breakfast; a small spot on the right side of the tip of the tongue; also on each lip, continuing several days. At two o'clock P.M., sensation in the mouth continued; since eight o'clock modified by a continued tendency to hawk and spit, with unusually large flow of saliva and mucus; also a sensation of warmth under the sternum, as if secretions were flowing from the stomach, and all the mucous surfaces, as well as from the salivary glands (C. E. T., 5th).

An increase of the flow of saliva, and a pain running near the ensiform cartilage, from the 7th rib on the right side diagonally through the chest (Nd., 30th).

A great increase of the flow of urine and saliva, lasting one hour, with shooting pains on the left side of the head, from the occiput to the forehead; flow of tears (Nd., 6th).

Salivation (Noack and Trinks).

Scanty, tenacious, frothy saliva in the mouth, as after long thirst, still without thirst; after drinking, it passes away; during the first day (C. Hg.).

Running of water from the mouth every morning before rising; pressure in the throat as from eating tart pears; vanishes after getting up (B.).

Slight accumulation of very tenacious and yellow saliva at rising in the morning (2d day, C. Hg.).

Less mucus in the throat during third day (C. Hg.).

An increased flow of saliva (J. C. R., 2d day, 30th).

The same day from four to five o'clock P.M., a severe pain, extending from the cartilage of the 7th rib at its junction with the sternum to the right hypochondriac region under the inferior border of the tenth rib.

The two following days he took every night 40 to 60 globules of 30th; then again for two nights 5 gr. of $\frac{1}{10}$, without any perceptible effect until the next day, when there was increased sexual desire with erections, which continued at night, terminating with an emission of semen. The following night again Cinnab. 30th, 20 globules. The next day an increased flow of saliva, so much so, that when he attempted to speak, he found some difficulty, from his mouth being constantly filled with saliva. He had some pain of a dull character in the forehead over the eyes in the afternoon, which became severer in the evening, and was aggravated by motion. Had occasional pains in the left side of the chest, between the cartilages of the 5th and 6th ribs.

The following day the increased flow of saliva still continues; in the afternoon also dull aching pain in the right forehead; worse in the evening, when also the pains in the left side return in the region of the heart, of a sharp cutting character, producing a difficulty of breathing (J. C. K.).

(I have perceived in other cases that the effect of the remedy often only shows itself after repeated doses; the salivation mentioned above is not merely to be considered as the effect of the last dose, but also of those previously taken, and for this reason have kept intact the whole group) (Nd.).

Stomach.

Great appetite and desire for an embrace (H.).

Great appetite, with thirst and strong sexual desires (H.).

Increases the appetite during the first day (C. Hg.).

Good appetite in the morning, somewhat rare with him, the second day (C. Hg.).

Increased appetite in the morning, the 3d day (C. Hg.).

Strong appetite, but very soon satisfied. He feels better than usual after meals, the 1st day (C. Hg.).

Decidedly better appetite, but less eating the 1st to 3d day (C. Hg.).

(Roast veal has a spicy taste, and like mushrooms (C. Hg.).

No appetite; aversion to all kinds of food (H.).

No appetite in the evening the 2d day (B.).

Loss of appetite; eats very little (Nd., 1st).

Aversion to coffee (B.).

In the morning appetite greatly impaired; but little appetite for breakfast after taking the remedy the preceding night; feels better in the open air and after dinner; pulse 60; skin moist and cool (A. J. B., 2d day, 6th).

Symptoms of cold in the head; fulness of head, discharge of much mucus from the nostrils; aching pain in the small of the back and legs. Uncommon tiredness and weakness. Sensation of emptiness in the stomach, and very hungry within two hours after eating a hearty breakfast. Sore on the inside of the under lip towards the left (A. L., 3d, 6th day).

Aching soreness in the teeth. Regurgitation of wind from the stomach; sores in the mouth on the underlip; severe pain in the forehead, which lasts all night; great restlessness and nervousness, a good deal of mucus at the posterior nares, which comes away in lumps (D. W., 6th, 2d day).

After eating, a very uncomfortable feeling as if the body was swollen and distended. Distressed feeling about the breast and stomach (H.).

Although intending to sit up and study longer, yet feeling wearied in body and confused in mind, he soon retired. Upon lying down there were rumblings in the abdomen, and pains passing from the epigastric to the pubic region. There was also some nausea and uneasiness in the stomach. Every little noise about the house troubled him, as though it were something serious. Although accustomed to dream much, yet he had more troublesome dreams than usual. He awoke and started up several times without purpose; once with a heavy pain in the forepart of the head. Upon rising at 7 o'clock in the morning, he felt a little giddiness and pain in the forehead, with a sensation of soreness in the eyeballs. The acidity in the stomach, general headache and heaviness of the eyes, to which he is subject, is much aggravated before noon (J. P. D., 3d).

At 5 o'clock next morning, a peculiar agreeable sensation of exhilaration, with a fulness extending from all sides of the chest towards the stomach and heart, accompanied or followed by a similar sensation in all the joints, continuing with intermissions till 8 o'clock (C. E. T., 5th), see K.

Although Cinnabaris, when taken in the stomach, is not digested, nor forms a constituent of our bodies, it does nevertheless as an alterative, wonderfully exhilarate the archæum, as long as it remains in the stomach (Ktz.).

*Symptoms of flatulence of the stomach, irregularity of the passages, pressing in the forehead, with a sensation of congestion, to which the prover had been subject for some time, have now nearly disappeared (Rt., 3d).

Dizziness and lightness in the head; soreness in the stomach, with tightness in the temples (Nd., 6th).

In the evening, pain in the head, increased to a heavy, stupefying ache, aggravated by thinking, reading and pressure. Tenderness in the epigastric region (A. J. B., 3d, 1st day).

Nausea, gaping and salivation, disappear on ceasing to triturate, but the heat and swelling of the face continue (3d, L.).

Nausea in the morning at 11 o'clock, the 3d day (B.).

Nausea alleviated by windy eructation (B.).

Rising nausea in the afternoon, soon after taking the medicine (B.).

Nausea in the evening, and then a pressure on the sternum upwards, like from water-brash (B.).

Slight nausea and salivation (3d, L.).

Drowsiness after supper, with nausea and water-brash, a burning from the breast upwards (B.).

Drawing sensation in the mouth, continued from 8 A. M. to 2 P. M., when it was modified by a continued tendency to hawk and spit, with an unusually large flow of saliva and mucus, also, a sensation of warmth under the sternum, and sense as if the secretions were flowing from the stomach and all the mucous surfaces, as well as from salivary glands (6th, C. E. T., 1st day).

Inclination to vomit, immediately (H.).

Nausea at 9 o'clock in the evening, then bilious vomiting, with much choking, and swelled face (2d day, B.).

Green vomiting, with violent choking, more in the night than in the morning (B.).

Anxiety about the heart, and vomiting (Geoffroy, Mat. Medica, Leipsic, 1760, vol. 1st, page 360).

Hypochondria and Abdomen.

An increased flow of saliva the second day; the same day, from 4 to 5 o'clock P. M., a severe pain, extending from the cartilage of the seventh rib, at its junction with the sternum, to the right hypochondriac region under the inferior border of the tenth rib (J. C. R., 30th).

In the morning, on rising, shooting pain in the right lobe of the liver (C. Hg., 3d).

Nausea, with occasional throbbing in the left hypochondrium; abdomen distended, stools hard, and too large (A. J. B., 6th).

Soon after taking the 6th dilution, *aching and somewhat sharp pain in the left hypochondrium, in front, over a space as large as may be covered by the hands,* worse in moving about in the open air. *Pain soon extending around the lower border of the ribs behind, and to region of left kidney, where it seems dull, and somewhat oppressive* (all felt, and disappeared in four hours). Soon after this, appearing in *the right hypochondrium in front, and extending around to back, and region of right kidney, where the pain is of the same character as the left kidney.* The dull pressive pain is felt in one and then in the other region of the kidney, alternately.

The pains intermit in severity, and those in the hypochondria are relieved by bending forward (H. R.).

He had, also, pains of short duration in the right hypochondrium, in middle of left breast, in front, in left kidney, and in occiput; itching over the body at times. In the evening, sticking pain in the region of the *left side* of fifth and sixth dorsal vertebræ; a sore spot which he felt on the third day after second trituration, on the right side of seventh and eighth rib, as large as a wafer, with a sore pain in and around it, continues; during the day, there were pains at a corresponding spot on the left side, of the same character, but without a sore spot. These last pains, which commenced on the 5th of January, were felt occasionally, until the 27th (H. R., 2d).

The prover remarks, that of all the pains which he experienced during his proving, the most severe were those in the hypochondria and kidneys (H. R.).

In four hours after taking the medicine, a sharp steady pain in the forehead, mostly in the right orbital region; soon after felt a sharp throbbing in the left hypochondrium, in the region of the spleen, and six hours afterwards he felt a dull aching pain in the bones of the fore-arms and legs (A. J. B., 3d).

Pain in the upper part of the left and right lung; an inward soreness over the heart, extending along the left arm on taking a long breath. Mucus which is thrown up, tastes like old tallow mixed with coffee. Pain under the lower point of the sternum, extending to the left side under the short ribs (J. H. H., 6th).

*In diseases of the spleen (melancholy?) (Ktz.).

Pinching in the abdomen the second day (B.).

Pinching in abdomen above and across the colon, with frequent emissions of flatulence of a fœtid odor, afterwards a passage the first day (C. Hg.).

Drawing pain in the abdomen for three hours in the forenoon, at 10½ o'clock (B.).

*Griping colic (Ktz.).

Some griping in the bowels, the only symptom with a man, who often took the 3d trit. (B.).

Pain in the forehead. Sticking in the chest, just beneath the sternum. Griping pain in the bowels (J. M. R., 6th).

(After eating pickled oysters and drinking cold water, pain in the left side of the abdomen, and much belching, without relief.) (C. Hg.)

Pain in the lower part of the abdomen, attended with diarrhœa, and also flatulence after taking the first dose (colic from eating boiled cabbage) (J. H. H., 6th).

During the first day and second night after taking the medicine, he was troubled with aching pains in the thighs, soreness in the umbilical region, obliging him to turn during the night as well as during the day. A weak sensation in the left eye, the same day (A. L., 6th).

Pains in the head in the forenoon, with a disposition to fall asleep while trying to listen to lectures several times, notwithstanding his making a great effort to keep awake. Constrictive feeling in the umbilical region, urine tinged yellow (A. J. B., 3d, 3d day).

Shooting pain in the bowels at intervals during the day. Flashes of heat, confined to the abdomen, with great flatulence, more in the forenoon, and less in the afternoon and evening (J. L. M., $\frac{1}{10}$, 1st day).

Pain in the bowels before each evacuation (J. L. M., 2d day).

Three or four hours after taking the medicine in the morning, his abdomen, below the transverse colon, felt hot, his tongue is covered with a white fur, and there is a beating, burning, in both temples, which he felt all day (S. A., 2d).

Six hours after taking the 2d trit., a rumbling through his abdomen below the transverse colon, lasting about one hour and a half (S. A.)

Upon lying down at night, there were rumblings in the abdomen, and pains passing from the epigastric to the pubic region. There was also, nausea and uneasiness in the stomach (J. P. D., 3d).

Chilliness in the warm room; an uneasy, indescribable feeling in the abdomen (A. J. B., 1st day, 3d).

Sensation as if the abdomen was too large, and wishes to have everything loose about his bowels; numb pressing pain in the eyes; numb feeling in the elbow, as if the ulnar nerve was compressed; also numbness in the knee-joints; hands cold; pain in the forehead; sticking in the chest, just beneath the sternum; griping pain in the bowels. The pulse, which was at 12 o'clock A.M., from 44 to 52, rose at 4 o'clock to 80 (J. M. R., 6th).

Slight inclination for stool in the forenoon, but no evacuation the first day (C. Hg.).

After taking daily the 3d trit. and during the first days he is costive; after a week the bowels are loose (B.).

The seventh and eighth day no passage; the ninth a regular evacuation after violent straining, preceded by much wind; afterwards prolapsus of the rectum, with pain until evening (C. Hg.).

Has been disposed to costiveness during the whole time of taking the medicine (H. R, 6th and 2d).

Constipation; only one passage a week (Nd., 1st).

Nausea, with occasional throbbing in the left hypochondrium; abdomen distended; stools hard and too large (A. J. B., 6th).

Pain on the seventh rib of each side in a spot as large as a quarter of a dollar; more on the left side. Violent constipation, lasting all the time he took the medicine, and for a long time after ceasing to take any. Bleeding piles for two days; violent itching in the anus, worse at night in bed; a whitish furred tongue in the morning (J. H. H., 6th).

Soft scanty stools twice a day, preceded by pinching; less afterwards (H.).

Unusual drowsiness in the morning; in the afternoon two passages of the bowels, the last one with straining (Nd., 5th).

Two passages daily (H.).

(Diarrhœa after eating cheese; afterwards great lassitude, the 4th day) (C. Hg.).

The second day thinner stools than usual (C. Hg.).

* Bloody dysentery (Ktz.).

Slight flatulency, with a sensation as if there was to follow a large evacuation, in the forenoon (C. Hg.).

In the evening a sensation of approaching looseness of the bowels (H. R., 2d, 1st day).

In the morning, after rising, a loose passage, with burning in the anus, preceded by griping (Nd., 3d).

Little pimples around the anus, with burning and itching; thin stools and tenesmus (B.).

After the afternoon stool, sensation of formication in the anus, as if from a large worm, 1st day (C. Hg.).

After dinner he had a feeling of weight in the lower part of the rectum, and a sensation like aching (H. R., 2d, 9th day).

* Less protrusion of the anus during the stool the first day (C. Hg.).

Urinary Organs.

Increased urination (3d, L.).

Frequent and increased emission of watery urine; also two or three times in the night (4th, L.).

A great increase of the flow of urine and saliva, lasting one hour, with shooting pain on the left side of the head, from the occiput to the forehead; flow of tears (Nd., 6th).

Increased urination (C. Hg., 3d).

Diminished secretion in the night (1st day, C. Hg.).

Scanty urine the second and third day (C. Hg.).

Film on the urine (3d, L.).

Flaky sediment in the urine (3d, L.).

Turbid urine (J. M. R., 6th).

Pain as if from a sore in the urethra when urinating, although the urethra is painless on pressure (H.).

Itching in the urethra in the afternoon (Nd., 3d).

Sensation as if there was a raw spot in the centre of the urethra, which woke him up two nights in succession (J. H, H., 6th).

* Gonorrhœa of very long standing, with much pain during urination, and soreness; the discharge is of a yellowish green color (Berens).

Male Genital Organs.

A heat apparently proceeding from the genital organs, which, however, are not hot; in the summer the eighth day (C. Hg.).

Sudden and violent twitching pain through the right testicle, and in the spermatic cord in the evening (1st day; C. Hg.).

Twitching in the penis (H.).

The penis is swollen (H.).

Redness and swelling of the prepuce, having the appearance of a sore, with painful itching (H.).

(Small warts on the prepuce in different places, which bleed on being touched) (H.).

Sycosis (Noack and Trinks).

Itching pain behind the corona glandis, from which exudes matter of a disagreeably sweet smell (H.).

Violent itching of the corona glandis, with a profuse secretion of pus; the itching was so violent as to cause him to rub it, which only eased it for a short time, when it returned with tenfold violence; two small red spots made their appearance on each side of the glans, secreting a large quantity of lardaceous matter. It had the appearance, according to his opinion, of herpes preputialis (J. H. H., 6th).

Blenorrhœa of the glans penis (Noack and Trinks).

Tearing stitches in the glans penis (H.).

Small shining red points on the glans penis (H.).

In the evening burning pricking itching on the extremity of the glans penis, which disappears on rubbing, but soon returns again with greater force (H.).

* It is used externally in syphilis (Ktz.).

Strong erections during the night in bed (H.).

Strong erections after midnight, towards morning (Nd., 3d ; 3d day).

The seventh day, in the morning, a very violent erection, almost amounting to priapism (C. Hg.).

Profuse sweating between the thighs ; violent erections in the evening. After finishing the medicine, all desire for an embrace is lost, which was not the case before he took the medicine (J. H. H., 6th).

A still more aggravated morbid state of mind, fretfulness ; also sexual excitement at the least provocation (4th day, Rt., 30th).

In the afternoon sexual excitement, as if he were to have an emission, but was able to combat the feeling (2d day, Rt., 3d).

Strong sexual desires, with much appetite (H.).

Increase of sexual desires, and prolonged orgasm during the coitus (C. Hg.).

For two mornings an almost irresistible sexual desire the seventh and eighth day (C. Hg.).

Frequently a spiritual sexual desire, with no inclination for its gratification first and third day (C. Hg.).

Sudden paroxysms of spiritual erotomania third day (C. Hg.).

A pollution of a copious quantity of inodorous semen the eighth day (C. Hg.).

From the seventeenth to the twenty-third almost daily a pollution (C. Hg.).

On Tuesday night he took forty glob. On Wednesday night sixty glob. of 30th. On Thursday night five gr. of $\frac{1}{10}$, and on Friday night ten gr. of $\frac{1}{10}$, with no perceptible effect until Saturday, when there was increased sexual desire with erections, which continued during the night, terminating by an emission of semen (J. C. R.).

Female Sexual Organs.

Catamenia appear a day too early. Observed several times (B.).

*A few days before the appearance of the catamenia, and during its continuance ; tearing pain in the forehead ; sensation of weakness in the eyes ; rending pain in the spine ; tearing pains and cramps in the bowels, with diarrhœa ; also great prostration (B.).

Leucorrhœa, causing during its discharge a pressing in the vagina (H.).

*Uterine difficulties, which cannot be relieved by opiates (Ktz.).

Nasal Mucous Membranes, Cough, and Chest.

Symptoms of cold in the head, with lameness of the thighs ; much mucus, in lumps of a dirty yellow color, in the posterior nares during the whole week (A. L., 6th).

Symptoms of cold in the head ; fulness of the head ; discharge of much mucus from the nostrils ; aching pain in the small of the back and legs (A. L., 3d ; 3d day).

A great deal of cold in the head (H.).

A good deal of mucus at the posterior nares, which comes away in lumps (D. W., 6th; 2d day).

Flow of mucus from the right nostril, lasting for three days (J. H H., 6th).

Cough, from tickling in the throat, the third day (B.).

Dryness in the mouth; burning in throat and the whole breast, with general weakness, tickling in the throat, and disposition to cough (14th, C. Hg.).

Cough, which seems to proceed neither from the breast nor from the larynx, but from the upper part of the throat, in the morning of the second day (C. Hg.).

(On lying down she has to cough continually; less on sitting up; single paroxysms of cough, perfectly dry) (H.).

(Every evening hoarseness, with croup-like cough) (J. H. H., 6th).

Hoarseness of the voice in the morning, going off in two or three hours (J. L. M., 2d).

Much yawning (14th, B.).

In the forenoon, while riding in the open air, very frequent slight yawning, with chilliness. As soon as he enters a warm room it disappears, during warm autumn weather (C. Hg.).

Chest somewhat oppressed; larynx asthmatic, in the morning of second day (C. Hg.).

After conversation a pressure in the upper and central part of the chest, which renders breathing laborious; he is obliged to bend forward, in order to inhale sufficient air; the forenoon (C. Hg.).

The chest often seems contracted, as though pressed upon; he is obliged to stretch himself, in order to breathe easily; the first and eighth day, only during the day and particularly in the forenoon (C. Hg.).

He awakes suddenly after midnight as if from a dream, as if he has no breath; a state resembling nightmare (H.).

Half an hour after taking the medicine, dyspnœa with heat, the same morning violent pains in all the limbs, commencing in the points of the fingers, and worse in the left side; at the same time weakness, burning in the throat and breast; dryness of the mouth and cough, incited by tickling in the throat (i 4, Fr. Husmann).

At five o'clock in the afternoon pressing pain in the centre of the chest, similar to a cramp of the stomach, to which she formerly had been subject. The pain extends to the throat and between the shoulders, and lasted until night. The spot was still sensitive on the following day (B.).

Sticking pain in the chest, just beneath the sternum (J. M. R., 6th).

Pain in the upper part of the left and right lung; an inward soreness over the heart, extending along the left arm, and on taking a long breath. Mucus, which is thrown up, tastes like old tallow mixed with coffee. Pain under the lower point of the sternum, extending to the left side under the short ribs (J. H. H., 6th).

From 4 to 5 o'clock P.M., after taking the medicine (30th dil.) the previous evening, a severe pain, extending from the cartilage of the seventh rib, at its junction with the sternum, to the right hypochondrium under the inferior border of the tenth rib. After two more doses of the 30th, and two of $\frac{1}{10}$, in four nights, and then again one of the 30th, he had on the 6th day occasional pains in the left side of the chest between the cartilages of the fifth and sixth ribs, and without another dose on the seventh day; in the evening again a return of the pains in the left side of the chest in the region of the heart, of a sharp cutting character, producing a difficulty of getting breath while they continued. On the eighth day, forenoon, again a return of the sharp cutting pain in the region of the heart, followed by wandering pains throughout the whole chest (J. C. R.).

Pain on the seventh rib of each side, in a spot as large as a quarter of a dollar, more on the left side (J. H. H., 6th).

An increase of the flow of saliva, and a pain running near the ensiform cartilage, from the seventh rib on the right side diagonally through the chest (Nd., 30th).

The fourth day, after 2d trit., itching on the body and canthi, and a spot on the right side on one of the ribs (7th or 8th) as large as a wafer, very sore to touch, with occasionally a sore pain in and around it, which continues for three or four days.

During the fifth day there were pains at a corresponding spot on the left side of the same character as the pain connected with the other, but without a sore spot.

On the fifth day, after 2d in the morning, there were also pains of short duration in the right hypochondrium, in middle of left breast in front, in the left kidney, and also in occiput (H. R.).

(In the evening nervous trembling of the heart with anxiety, to which she had formerly been subject, again returns) (Nd., 6th).

Within ten minutes after taking 14th, a very severe pain in the heart, as if it was twisted around (C. Hg.).

Soreness under the right breast, near the last true rib, particularly on drawing breath (Nd., 1st).

(A stitch about the eighth rib, particularly on taking a long breath, occasionally on the fourth day) (Nd., 3d).

At five o'clock A.M, a peculiar agreeable sensation of exhilaration, with fulness, extending from all sides of the chest, particularly the thorax, towards the stomach and heart, accompanied or followed by a similar sensation in all the joints, continuing with intermissions till eight o'clock* (C. E. T., 2d day; 5th).

Back and Kidneys.

On turning the head, pain in the right side of the neck, below the sterno-cleido-mastoideus muscle. Pain in the back part of the neck when the head is thrown back, extending to the occiput. The muscles of the back part of the neck seem as if contracted (J. H. H., 6th).

* Considering the previous state of the prover, these symptoms may probably be considered curative.

Eruption on posterior cervical region, and soreness from the right ear into the middle of posterior cervical region, as if the glands were affected, second day. This soreness increased on the third day, and was very severe in the evening. It continued until seventh day, but gradually decreased in severity (Rt., 6th).

About 4 A. M., the fifth day after taking second, he was awakened by a dull sticking pain in the region of left kidney, which lasted but a short time; afterwards tossing about and sleeplessness for an hour; after rising from bed, a fulness and pressure in the occiput and back of the neck, continuing with much severity till about noon, after which, the symptoms somewhat abated; heaviness and sleepiness during the day; pains of short duration in the right hypochondrium, in middle of left breast, in front of left kidney, occiput; itching over the body at times. The pains experienced in the hypochondria and kidneys were most severe.

In the evening of the same day, sticking pain in the region of the left side of the fifth and sixth dorsal vertebræ; the sore spot on right side, felt two days previously on one of the ribs (seventh and eighth), as large as a wafer, and sore to touch, with occasionally a sore pain in and around it, continues; during the day there were pains at a corresponding spot on the left side, of the same character as the pain connected with the other, but without a *sore* spot.

The sixth day after 2d trit., occasionally a sticking pain on the right side of the same dorsal vertebræ (fifth or sixth); pain sometimes in the left side of occiput (organ of amativeness), itching of eyelids and of various parts of the body; sore spot in the right side continues. The pains on the side of the fifth and sixth dorsal vertebræ have been occasionally felt until the eighth day (H. R.).

In ten minutes after taking the 3d trit. at night, he felt a warm glow through his legs, which was soon succeeded by a dull pain in the left arm just above the elbow, and by occasional darting pains in the lower extremities. There was also a dull pain in the lower dorsal portion of the spine, continuing only for a short time. A space about the size of a quarter dollar, just above and between the supra-orbital ridges, felt as though pressed upon by a cold metallic body, while within the cranium underneath, there seemed to be more warmth than usual (J. P. D.).

The third night, after taking the 3d trit., he had restless sleep, with many dreams, and feels tired in the morning, with aching across the small of back, and limbs. This pain continued the fourth, fifth, and sixth day. Again, all the seventh night and next day, he had severe aching and drawing pains in the back, from the region of the kidneys to sacrum, and in the thighs and legs. Drawing up the legs affords relief. The eighth day, also, slight pains in the back and legs, but much better than the day before. All these symptoms from one dose of 3d (A. L.).

Soon after taking the sixth dilution, *an aching and somewhat sharp pain in the left hypochondrium, in front, over a space as large as may be covered by the hand, worse on moving about and in the open air.*

Pain soon extending around the lower border of the ribs behind, and to region of the left kidney, where it seems dull, and somewhat oppressive (all felt and disappeared in four hours). Soon after this, appearing in *right* hypochondrium in front, and extending around to the back, and region of right kidney, where the pain is of the same character as in the left kidney.

The dull pressive pain is felt in one and then in the other region of the kidney, alternately. The pains intermit in severity, and those in the hypochondria are relieved by bending forward (H. R.).

One hour after taking the sixth dil., rush of blood to the back part of the head, attended with violent itching and heat, extending to each ear, and behind the left ear; there came three hard lumps, one the size of a small shot, the other that of a buckshot, and the last a size larger. On the same night, he felt a sharp pain in the region of the kidneys, as if some one had driven a nail on each side of the vertebræ. More profuse discharge of clear water (J. H. H.).

General pain all over the back, down to the loins, worse after every dose of medicine, aggravated on drawing a long breath (J. H. H., 6th).

Sore feeling, extending from the small of the back around both sides, over the ossa ilii, worse on pressure (J. H. H., 6th).

Aching in the small of the back, as if bruised (Nd., 5th).

Shooting pain in the region of the loins and sacrum, increased by stooping, and during labor (B.).

Tearing pains in the back from above downwards at 11 o'clock in the evening and through the night, so that she could get no sleep; second day (B.).

Rending tearing pain in the side of the back, as if it was broken, particularly at night, upon the least motion in bed, and in the arm when writing; these pains are relieved by the warmth of the stove (H.).

Upper Extremities.

Pain in the left shoulder, between the clavicle and scapula, interiorly the first day (C. Hg.).

In the evening of the second day occasional shootings in the upper part of the left temple along temporal ridge; dulness in the whole head, especially in the forehead just over the eyes; lame sensation in the right shoulder-joint (H. R., 6th).

After taking the medicine in the morning towards 10 o'clock, a pressing pain in the right shoulder, as from a blow, which continued for half an hour, then pain in the abdomen (B.).

Sudden pain in the middle of the upper part of the right arm, as though it would fracture, the third day (C. Hg.).

Pressing gnawing pains in the upper part of the right arm, as if they were moving about in the bones to and fro in the forenoon of the fifth day (C. Hg.).

Violent shooting pains in the arms at times (H.).

Shooting pain in the muscles of the inner side of right os humeri early in the morning after rising the third day (B.).

Shooting pain on the outer side of the right fore-arm, from 4 o'clock P.M., until bed time (the 3d day, B.).

He was awakened several times from sleep by a severe pain in the right arm. It continued in the morning and during the day, at times very severe, commencing about the centre of the os humeri, and extending to the elbow and along the radius to its inferior extremity; the pain was of a heavy, aching character, deep-seated, and caused lameness and difficulty in moving the arm. In the forenoon he had also a return of the sharp-cutting pains in the region of the heart, followed by wandering pains throughout the whole chest (J. C. R., 3d day, 30th dil., and after several larger doses previously taken).

Sensation of lameness in the right arm, the eighth day; the day before, wandering pains as if in the bone and pressing in the muscles (C. Hg.).

In the evening numbness of the arm on which he lies and supports himself, until the 13th day (C. Hg.).

Four hours after taking the 3d trit. he felt a sharp steady pain in the forehead, mostly in the right orbital region; soon after felt a sharp throbbing in the left hypochondrium, in the region of the spleen, and in about ten hours after the above dose, at ten o'clock P.M., he felt a dull aching pain in the bones of the forearms and legs.

Taking three days afterwards another dose of the same trit., at 11 o'clock A.M., he felt in half an hour a sharp aching pain in the right supra-orbitary region, shooting backwards and downwards to the ear and side of the neck. Front of the head very hot; the pain is worse in the warm room, and on moving the eyes and scalp; chilliness in the warm room; an uneasy indescribable feeling in the abdomen; numbness of the left arm, from the elbow down to the end of the little finger. Next morning all the symptoms are better, but in the evening, at 8 P.M., the headache, which had increased at 10 o'clock the previous evening to a heavy, stupefying ache, aggravated by thinking, reading and pressure, returned with a numbness and heavy aching in the arms and knees and lower legs, without a new dose being taken that day. The pains are all aggravated in the evening; better in the open air, and after eating and sleeping (A. J. B.).

Dull aching in the bones of the forearms and legs; numbness of the left arm, from the elbow to the end of the little finger, passing off on using the arm, and returning again while at rest (A. J. B., 1st day; 6th).

Pain in the left side of the head, temple and supra-orbital ridge; sensation as if the abdomen was too large; he wishes to have everything loose about it; numb pressing pain in the eyes; numb feeling in the elbows, as if the ulnar nerve was compressed; also numbness in the knee-joints; hands cold (J. M. R., 6th; 1st day).

In ten minutes after taking the 3d trit. in the evening, he felt a warm glow through his legs, which was soon succeeded by a dull pain in the left arm just above the elbow, and by occasional darting pains in the lower extremities. There was also a dull pain in the lower dorsal vertebræ of the spine, continuing only for a short time. A space about the size of a quarter of a dollar just above and between the supra-orbital ridges, felt as though pressed upon by a cold metallic body; while within the cranium underneath, there seemed to be more warmth than usual. *A dull pain felt before in the left temple and side of the forehead disappeared—urgent desire to urinate (J. P. D.).

Pain along the left arm, particularly in the little finger, third finger and thumb. On supinating the forearm, the pain is worse at the elbow. It feels as if the "crazy bone" was struck. The least twitch causes the elbow and shoulder to crack. Itching in the palms of the right hand. Pain in the little finger of right hand. Itching in the joint of right hand. Pain in the little finger of right hand. Itching in the joint of right hand (J. H. H. 6th).

A constant pain in the left arm-joint when turning and straightening the arm, and when writing (J. H. H. 6th).

In about an hour after taking 30th, sharp darting pains like electric flashes passing from the first phalanx of the ring-finger of the right hand to the middle of the forearm, and from the lower extremity of the radius of the left arm up to the elbow (J. C. R.).

The first joint of the right index-finger red and hot, but painless; next morning chill, with perspiration under the arms; cannot get warm, even near a hot stove (3d L.).

Joint of the first finger of right hand is red and hot (4th L.).

Pain in the left thumb, as if pierced by splinters of glass; (six or eight weeks before he had wounded his thumb with glass) (the 3d day, C. Hg.).

In two hours after taking the medicine a fulness and general pressure in the whole head, as after taking cold, with dull aching pain in the region of benevolence; better in the open air; *great drowsiness and lassitude in the warm room.* Occasional shooting and prickling pain in the two middle fingers of left hand, better by firm pressure upon the thumb. The above symptoms continued about eight hours (C. L. M. 6th).

Lower Extremities.

During the first night after taking the 6th dilution, drawing, aching pains in the thighs from the hip-joints nearly down to the condyles, aggravated by moving, and accompanied with great lameness, experienced on getting up and attempting to walk; getting better after walking a short distance. The two following days symptoms of cold in the head, with lameness of the thighs (A. L.).

Two hours after taking the 6th dil. in the morning, on straining at stool, shooting aching pain on posterior side of right thigh, from the hip-joint to middle of os femoris.

After a new dose of the 6th in the evening, a day after taking the last dose, he was troubled next day and night with aching pains in the thighs, soreness in the umbilical region, obliging him to turn during the night as well as during the following day. Also violent itching and pricking in the inner side of the knee-joint, ever since he has commenced to take the medicine; worse in the night and the morning before getting up.

The 5th day violent itching on the inside of the thighs, knees and legs, worse at the knees, especially at night (A. L.).

From the 2d to the 5th day after the 3d trit., aching pains in the small of the back and legs, with uncommon tiredness and weakness, and on the fifth night and sixth day severe aching and drawing pains in the back, from the region of the kidneys to sacrum and in the thighs. Drawing up of the legs affords relief. The pains in the back and legs still continued in a slight degree on the 6th day (A. L).

Tearing pains from the right hip-bone to the great toe, commencing at 9 o'clock in the evening, lasting through the night, and only diminished in the morning after rising (B.).

At 10¼ P. M., after taking the 3d decimal trit. in the morning, pain and tired feeling in the right hip, and afterwards in the left. Tired feeling in all the joints of the lower extremities, better from rising and walking; sensation of having taken cold and general feeling as not being fit for any mental labor, depressed; melancholy, cynical, state of mind; nervous system excited.

On the fourth night itching, especially on the inside of the thighs (Rt.).

An eruption on the inner and lower part of the thigh, with itching (D. W. 6th, 2d day).

Fetid and excoriating perspiration between the thighs when walking (H.).

Profuse sweating between the thighs (J. H. H. 6th).

Tearing pain in the left thigh bone the whole day (3d L.).

Tearing in the right thigh bone (4th L.).

(Rheumatic) pain of right knee-joint, increasing for two weeks, aggravated during walking, but most violent when ascending stairs; it disappears during rest (4th L.).

Itching in the palm of the right hand. Pain in the little finger of right hand. Itching in the joint of right hand. Pain in the knee-joint, worse at noon, while walking. Drawing in all the muscles of the lower extremities on the under surface. Sore feeling on the ankle, attended with heat and itching over the whole leg (J. H. H. 6th).

Numb feeling in the elbows, as if the ulnar nerve was compressed, also numbness in the knee-joints (J. M. R. 6th, 1st day).

In the forenoon of 2d day after 1½ trit., head full, nervousness and irritability for a short time, also for a short time sticking pain in the back part of left knee-joint; in the afternoon a slight pain in right knee-joint, similar to the pain in the left one, with a creeping sensation above and below it, seemingly about the bone, lasting about an hour. The above pains in the knee-joints have been felt occasionally every day for four days (H. R.).

Frequent pain in the lower side of left knee, near the inner side of tibia, lameness and frequent stitches on walking, particularly the inner side of knee-joint (C. E. T. 5th, 2d day).

Awakened in the night by a painful twitching in the lower part of the leg (H.).

Lassitude in the lower part of the legs, more in the afternoon; after 5 days (B.).

In 10 hours after 3d. trit. a dull aching pain in the bones of the fore-arms and legs, and in four days a numbness and heavy aching in the arms, knees and lower legs (A. J. B.).

Dull aching in the bones of the forearms and legs (A. J. B. 6th, 1st day).

In 10 minutes after taking the 3d. trit. in the evening, he felt a warm glow through his legs, which was soon succeeded by a dull pain in the left arm-joint just above the elbow, and by occasional darting pains in the lower extremities (J. P. D.).

Pain in the *tendo achillis* and *os calcis* after walking (J. M. R. 6th.).

Pressing sensation in the foot as if it would fall asleep (H.).

(Rheumatic pain in the large toe.) (H.)

Cold feet day and night (B.).

Coldness in the joints; shuddering and drawing in the arms and legs (H.).

* Wandering gout (Ktz.).

Skin.

A red itching spot, as large as the end of the thumb, on the right side of the forehead (B.).

Red herpetic spots on the forehead, particularly over the right eyebrow (B.).

Redness of the skin like a chronic eruption (Nd. 1st.)

Two small red spots made their appearance on each side of the *glans penis*, secreting a large quantity of lardaceous matter. It had the appearance, according to his opinion, of herpes preputialis (J. H. H. 6th.)

A pricking itching on the anterior part of the neck, with swollen glands, and in front on the chest; red points make their appearance converging into round spots, full of hard granular pimples; the itching of the eruption increases on scratching it, finally the spots are painful (H.).

Rush of blood to the back part of the head, attended with violent itching and heat extending to each ear, and behind the left ear there came three hard lumps, one of the size of a small shot, the other of a buck-shot and the last a size larger (J. H. H. 6th.).

In the evening violent itching on both shoulders, on which red streaks appear after scratching; besides that, small red elevations are to be observed, the itching from which is almost insupportable. After going to bed it disappears (C. Hg. 1st day).

In the morning red papulous eruption, without itching, on both elbows, left one the worst (9th day, C Hg).

An eruption on the inner and lower part of the thigh with itching (D. W. 6th, 1st day).

From the first time he took the medicine, he felt as if pimples were to come out over his body, with a general uneasy sensation and itching (The prover had this feeling for some time, but now in an aggravated form (Rt. 30th & 3d).

* On the finger a red eruption, sometimes with pustules filled with yellow matter, the same under the right knee, with occasional itching (Nd. 3d).

* Chronic impetigo (in a man who had gonorrhea some twenty years ago) pustules and scabs on the upper lip immediately under the nose, right nostril also somewhat tumefied (Nd. 3d).

* Chronic impetigo in another man on the same spot as the above (Nd. 3d).

* Does well in scabies ferina (Ktz.).

* Small pox (Ktz).

* It especially purifies the blood (Ktz).

* It is useful in gangrenous ulcerations. Ebn. Dsschold.

A cut in shaving bleeds very little (C. Hg.).

Itching of the lids of both eyes (J. H. H.).

Shooting pains in the inner canthus of right eye, with a burning and itching (J. L. M.).

Itching on the body and canthi (H. R.).

Itching of eyelids and of various parts of the body (H. R.).

In the eyes for two days excessive itching of the inner canthi (C. E. T.).

From 9 to 12 o'clock, itching on the outer canthi, severe and frequent, with a sense of stiffness in the upper lids (C. E. T.).

Much itching in the left ear, from the 1st to the 4th day, scurfy eruption in the right external ear, between the helix and antihelix (C. Hg.).

Much itching in the right ear (C. Hg.).

Itching on the left side of the face (J. H. H.).

Itching of the nose with bleeding after blowing it. The blood is very dark. The itching is caused by pimples in the right nostril (J. H. H.).

Small spot on the left side of the tongue which itches (J. H. H.).

Itching on the palm of right hand. Itching in the joint of right hand (J. H. H.).

Violent itching on the inside of the thighs, knees and legs, worse at the knees, especially at night (A. L.).

An eruption on the inner and lower part of the thigh, with itching (D. W.).

Itching at night, especially on the inside of the thighs (Rt.).

Violent itching and pricking on the inner side of the knee-joint, ever since he commenced to take the medicine, worse in the night and in the morning before getting up (A. L.).

Sore feeling of the ankle, attended with heat and itching over the whole leg (J. H. H.).

Violent itching at the anus, worse at night in bed (J. H. H.).

Violent itching of the corona glandis, with a profuse secretion of pus (gonorrhea glandis), the itching was so violent as to cause him to rub it, which only eased it for a moment, to return with tenfold violence (J. H. H.).

Itching on various parts of the body, while walking in the open air (H. R.).

Itching over the body at times (H. R.).

Sleep.

After dinner an unconquerable desire for sleep. (For a long time he has not been in the habit of sleeping after dinner.) (3d L.)

Less desire to sleep after eating (3d day, C. Hg.).

Feeling excessively sleepy at 7 o'clock in the evening, she went to bed and slept well through the whole night (2d day, B.).

Great desire for sleep in the evening, for several days, in the case of several provers (B.).

Increased sleepiness in the evening (3d day, C. Hg.).

Great sleepiness in the evening (13th day, C. Hg.).

At 11 o'clock A.M., pains in the head return again with a disposition to fall asleep, while trying to listen to the lecture, notwithstanding his making a great effort to keep awake (3d A. J. B., 3d day).

Disposition to sleep during the day (J. H. H., 6th.).

A dull, heavy and sometimes a sleepy feeling during the day (A. L., 1st day, 3d.).

Weakness and sleepiness in the eyes about noon; could scarcely keep them open (A. L., 3d, 6th day).

Head full, heavy, with strong pulsations of the temporal arteries; great inclination to sleep during the day (H. R., 1½, 3d day).

A dull, heavy and, at times, a sleepy feeling during the day (A. L., 3d, 1st day).

Weakness and sleepiness in the eyes at noon; he could scarcely keep them open (A. L., 3d, 6th day).

Heaviness and sleepiness during the day (H. R., 5th day, 1½ trit.).

At 11 o'clock A.M., unusual drowsiness and heaviness over the eyes (Nd., 1st day, 5th).

Unusual drowsiness in the morning (Nd., 1st day, 3d).

Nightly sleeplessness without pain and fatigue; he feels strong in the morning as if he had no sleep necessary (H.).

Sleeps an hour only; after eight days (B.).

He awakes very early but feels too indolent to rise and falls asleep again (1st week, C. Hg.).

Awakes early (C. Hg.).

Loss of sleep during the forepart of the night. Restless and tossing about during the whole night with anxious dreams, which he is wholly unable to recall after waking (A. J. B., 6th, 2d night).

Nightly sleeplessness; hears the clock strike all night. He awakes up suddenly as from a dream (Nd., 1st).

Before going to bed took the 30th dil. Slept very well but had very vivid dreams, which he could not remember. After taking the same dilution the next night, he felt a drowsy sensation as if he would readily sleep. But on going to bed, at 12 o'clock, the drowsy sensation continued, with very strong desire to sleep; he could not sleep, however, on account of a very disagreeable nervous sensation which caused him to toss about in bed for an hour and a half. He did not sleep so well as the night before; his dreams were vivid and rather pleasing, but he could not bring them to his recollection. After taking the same dilution again the third night, he is again restless and has vivid dreams. On the fourth night he took 5 gr. of 3d trit. He felt no desire for sleep but sat up and read until half past 1 A.M. He did not sleep for half an hour after going to bed. He dreamed continually but not so vivid as before. On waking at 8 o'clock his throat is dry; he is thirsty; sensation as if he had not had a refreshing sleep (Rt.).

After retiring did not sleep for over an hour but tossed about; very nervous and mentally vexed (Rt., 6th.).

Restlessness and sleeplessness at night from a constant flow of ideas changing from one subject to another (J. C. R., 30th) (1st night).

First night after taking 6th dil.; restless, uneasy sleep; second night after, the same dil. Increased restlessness, with constant dreaming; seemed to dream before getting asleep (D. W.).

The 5th night after taking the 1½ trit.; tossing about and sleeplessness for an hour, after being awakened at 4 A.M., by a dull sticking pain in region of left kidney, which lasted but a short time (H. R.).

Sleep restless with vivid dreams, but he cannot remember them in the morning (J. M. R., 6th).

After taking the 6th dil, on going to bed, great restlessness at night; continual dreaming and waking. He would scarcely be lost in a drowse before he would be dreaming. Vivid dreams of studies and business.

The 2d night, after taking again the same dose; he had many dreams and waked up often.

The 3d day; the same dil., in the morning. In the night continued restlessness, and dreams that a lump is in his throat and right ear.

The 5th night; again the same dose. In addition to the restlessness and dreaming he woke up with a throbbing pain in the organ of conscientiousness, extending to forehead over the eye.

The 7th night, without a new dose, he had vivid dreams of the lectures, particularly the anatomical. He could not believe that he was not actually there.

After taking at bed-time the 3d trit., he had several dreams and woke up several times through the night.

The 3d night, without a new dose; restless sleep with many dreams (A. L.).*

* It will be perceived from this symptom, as well as several others, that the restlessness and sleeplessness so frequently experienced at night did not depend upon the medicine being taken at night. Cinnabaris evidently produces sleeplessness at night and sleepiness in day-time.

Dreams with much talking during the sleep, which is very restless (J. H. H., 6th).

Although accustomed to dream much, yet he had more troublesome dreams than usual. He awoke and started up several times without purpose: once with a heavy pain in the forehead. In one of his dreams he saw a spider as large as an ox (J. P. D., 3d, 1st night).

Dreams of the events of the day (2d day, B.).

Dreams of unimportant events, sometimes to be remembered, sometimes not (3d day, C. Hg.).

Vivid dreams of a sensual nature (Nd., 5th).

Frightful dreams the 3d day (B.).

Does not remember his dreams in the morning, but they occur to him long afterwards (3d day, C. Hg.).

Fever.

Feeling of coldness and sensation of inertia, drowsiness (Nd. 1st).

Chilliness in the warm room (A. J. B.).

Skin moist and cool; pulse 60 (A. J. B. 3d day).

Hands cold (J. M. R. 6th).

Chilliness in the morning, with perspiration under the arms; he cannot get warm, even near a hot stove (3d L.).

Front of the head very hot (A. J. B. 3d, 1st day).

A heat when in bed during the night, that seems to ascend from the stomach into the neck and head, disappearing after rising (H.).

Internal and external heat of the body during the whole night; chilliness in the morning on rising; gripings, thin passage, and continual weariness of the whole body after nine days (B.).

He cannot endure the heat of the sun in his room (1st day, C. Hg.).

Heat as from hot weather, mostly on the right side of the head, and on the breast and arms, but worse on the left arm (1st day, C. Hg.).

* Some use it as an amulet in inflammatory fevers (Ktz.).

Seems to lower the pulse in the forenoon and make it irregular. The pulse, which was at 12 o'clock A. M. from 44 to 52, rose at 4 o'clock P. M. to 80 (J. M. R. 6th).

Pulse at noon 60; in the evening 80 (D. W. 6th, 1st day).

Profuse sweating between the thighs. All the other symptoms are most violent at night in bed, but the sweating is worse at 12 o'clock in the day (J. H. H. 6th).

Though in itself not a sudorific, yet it possesses many virtues (Ktz.).

General Symptoms.

Sensation of lameness in all the limbs; he is indolent and sleepy (H.).

Pain in all the joints, with lameness during the day (D. W. 6th).

Weariness, no disposition to labor (2d day, B.).

Feels very languid; he would go to bed if he had the time (3d L.).

Great excitement to activity, alternating with lassitude; the weariness of the body is better after a short repose (4th day, C. Hg.).

Tired and prostrated, particularly before and after eating; better when riding in the open air, but only for a short time (the first 4 days, C. Hg.).

In the morning a sense of general prostration; great weakness of all the limbs. Feeling of depression, and weakness of the whole system as after a severe illness (A. J. B. 6th, 1st day).

Lassitude, weariness, feeling as if an attack of typhus fever were to come on (J. H. H. 6th).

Uncommon tiredness and weakness (A. L. 3d, 5th day).

Feeling of cold and sensation of inertia; drowsiness (Nd. 1st).

Great drowsiness and lassitude in the warm room (C. L. M. 6th, 1st day).

Nervousness and irritability about noon, for a short time (H. R. 1½, 2d day).

A peculiar nervous thrill pervading the whole frame, even to the fingers and toes, affecting especially the joints. Sense of languor and depression, as after excessive exhilaration or intoxication. The above sensation continued without intermission for three days (C. E. T. 5th).

Unusual irritability during the whole time since he took the medicine (D. W. 6th).

The next day after taking the 30th, general nervous, uneasy sensation (Rt.).

Characteristics and Conditions.

Pains all aggravated in the evening.

Feels better in the open air and after dinner (A. J. B.).

All the symptoms except the sweating are most violent at night in bed. The sweating is worse at 12 o'clock in the day (J. H. H.).

The headache is much worse after sleeping (Nd. 1st).

The pains intermit in severity, and those in the hypochondria are relieved by bending forward (H. R.).

The first and second day more symptoms during the day (C. Hg.).

Its action continued nine days (H.).

Many pains resemble the slow and great movement of an irresistible power (C. Hg.).

Cinnabaris has four times as many symptoms in the left arm as in the right, and two symptoms on the left side of the face and tongue, and one on the left breast, but none on the right side of those organs.

It has three symptoms on the right supra-orbital region, one on the right side of the head, nostril, shoulder-joint and thigh, but none on the other side of the same parts of the body.

The symptoms in the other parts of the body seem to be nearly equally balanced between the right and left side.

As it seems to produce sleeplessness at night and sleepiness in the day-time, it will probably become an important remedy for these two conditions, and in two cases, where the former symptom was present, it has been very beneficial.

5. *Therapeutic Use.*

With regard to the action of *Cinnabaris* there yet reigns doubt; some consider it as entirely powerless, and others as a virulent and deadly poison. According to Wibmer, there is more ground for the former than the latter opinion. (How does he know? He himself confesses, that farther experiments must clear up the point.) (*Wibmer, Wirkung der Arzneimittel und Gifte.*)

Pure Cinnabar is very highly prized on account of its marked effects in the worst diseases (Ktz.).

Although *Cinnabaris*, when taken into the stomach, is not digested, nor forms a constituent of our bodies, it does nevertheless as an alterative wonderfully exhilirate the archæum, as long as it remains in the stomach (Ktz. See C. E. T.).

Mercury in combination with sulphur, as in *Cinnabar*, has not the same power, nor does it cause, bound by this fetter, the same evils as without it (Ktz.).

Crato says, (Ep. 7) that the strongest constitution can hardly endure its effects (Ktz.).

Fernelius de Ven writes, that horrible effects had followed the use of Cinnabar. But in the case mentioned it is doubtful whether the painter suffered from the effects of the natural Cinnabar, or from the orpiment (Ktz.).

It is the most reliable antidote to poison (Ktz.).

It exalts the virtues of other medicines (Ktz.).

Furitiere says in his book it is a poison.

Native Cinnabar, as an impalpable powder, is almost a universal medicine—10 to 30, 40 gr., or a drachm, for 40—60 days, *taking it always at bed-time* (Lemery).

Cinnabar is seldom used inwardly but for horses (Pomet).

There is a great deal of danger in painting the face with it, and bad consequences may follow (Lemery).

There is a strengthening power attributed to it, and therefore it is given in all desperate cases (Ktz.).

Sometimes the best native cinnabar excites nausea; vomiting, anxieties, heat, burning, etc. (J. Hill).

Native Cinnabar will not produce salivation, but the artificial will, speedily and easily (Lemery).

Cinnabaris is an excellent anti-venereal, expels the pox and all foulness out of the whole body, with all its consequences; it sweetens the blood, takes away all manner of pains and aches in any part, all manner of swellings, ulcers and nocturnal pains. Kills worms (Lemery).

Specific for falling sickness, excellent for vertigoes, apoplexies, palsies, lethargies and all diseases of the head and brain (Lemery).

Cinnabar is used in epilepsies, vertigoes, madness and all spasmodic affections (J. Hill).

Internally *Cinnabaris* is seldom used, except that it is an ingredient of several *pulveres anti-eptilepticos* (Ktz.).

It possesses the power of alleviating pain, particularly in epilepsy (Ktz.).

The celebrated Sennert used it in the form of powders against epilepsy (Ktz.).

Crato, (ep. 137) doubts the magnetic power of Cinnabaris against epilepsy (Ktz.).

Cinnabaris does wonders externally, if tied on the pulse (in the case of a person of high rank, lying sick with the small pox, and who had spasms) (Ktz.).

Cinnabaris cured in the case of a somnambulist a fever induced by the effects of sweet marjoram, but produced at the same time the most terrible spasms.

Cinnabaris is beneficial in indolent ulcers (Ebn. Dsschold).

It is beneficial in mortification and malignant pustules.

It arrests hemorrhages.

It is good in all salves and plasters (Garde de Sundheyt Lubeck Steffen Arndes, 1510).

Cases.

J. C. Pain in the back of the neck shooting to occiput with stiffness and hard swelling of the glands at the back of the neck; these symptoms were relieved by *Cinnabaris* 12.

B. L., æt. 3, of pale complexion, had formerly eruptions on the scalp, which were cured by *Sulphur.* She now has a soreness on the scalp on touching, with a pain in the left side of the head, about the organ of conscientiousness. One or two doses of *Cinnab.* 12 permanently removed the above symptoms.

Mrs. D. Pain from back of neck to back of head, behind the ear, shooting to forehead; cured by *Cinnab.* 30.

Rev. O. Heaviness from one temple to the other to occiput, cured by *Cinnab.* 12.

Ten similar cases, characterized by pain from occiput to forehead, only varying in some slight symptoms, were all cured by *Cinnabaris* 12 and 30. The majority of these cases were cured by *Cinnab.* alone; a few required other remedies for their final removal.

Four other persons also received the remedy for similar symptoms, but they did not return, in order to report their cure.

The observation of "Schroeder" in his "*Arzneyschatz*," that *Cinnabaris* is a great "*Specificum cephalicum*" is no doubt correct.

12.—MERCURIUS - SULPHURICUS.

By C. Neidhard, of Philadelphia.

MERC - SULPH. Yellow Sulphate of Mercury, Turpeth mineral.

For the purpose of affording a comparison with the *Cinnabaris* we add two experiments by those efficient provers, Drs. Hamilton Ring and J. C. Raymond, with the Sulphate of Mercury.

First Proving; Second and Third Triturations.

Dr. Hamilton Ring.—The remedy was prepared by Dr. Hering. Each powder contained two grains of the third trituration.

11 a. m. Took first powder.

On the evening of the day on which the powder was taken an unusually comfortable feeling in the head and increased clearness and vivacity of the mind—for several days some diminution of appetite.

The same symptoms after the other powder, which was taken a week afterwards.

Second Proving; Second Trituration.

The same prover.—Two powders of the 2d trituration were taken as before.

12 m. About one hour after taking each powder he experienced a sense of considerable weakness and much confusion in the head and oppression over the eyes—continuing for several hours. He had no appetite for dinner on that day, and for several days his appetite was considerably less than usual.

Third Proving; Third and Second Triturations.

Dr. J. C. Raymond.—1851, Oct. 27th, 9 p.m. In usual health; (pulse 75 per minute) a powder of Sulph. of Mercur., 3d trit.

Oct. 28th. Passed a wakeful and restless night; vivid dreams of fires, exerting himself to extinguish them; viewing a person hung and another cut up, seeing the blood and mangled remains. At half-past

8 A.M., experienced a violent beating in the left arm, commencing above the elbow in the course of the brachial nerve and extending along the radial nerve to the wrist, followed by pain similar to that which is produced by a blow received upon the arm below the insertion of the deltoid muscle; the pain affected, principally, the radial side of the fore-arm, the thumb and index-finger; numbness of the fore-arm and hand, also of the right hand; icy coldness of the hands; blueness of the nails; frequent yawning, dulness and chilliness; creeping chills ascending the back, when they reached the neck a general shudder ensued; pulse accelerated, counting 90. A dull pain in the forehead followed the above symptoms, with burning in the face and ears and slight febrile sensations.

Oct. 29th. Wakefulness after midnight; dreams less troublesome than the preceding night; awoke in the morning, pain in the head under the coronal suture, during the forenoon it was confined to the right frontal region; the pains were dull, extending deep into the brain and were very unpleasant when exercising; they passed off in the afternoon. Observed no other symptoms.

Oct. 31st. 9 P.M. Took second powder, 3*d trit. Sulph-merc.*

Nov. 1st. Wakefulness and dreams after midnight.

Nov. 2d. Chills from 12 M., to half past 1 P.M., with the same train of symptoms as those on the 27th Oct., except the beating sensation in the left arm. The pulse numbered 94.

Nov. 3d. Passed a restless night; vivid dreams of fires; the tongue is thickly coated white, inclining to yellow at the base, the papillæ are enlarged and their red points project through the coating on the tongue; a pasty insipid taste in the mouth. Pulse 70.

Nov. 4th. Tongue cleaner than it was yesterday. Chills with nausea from 10 A.M. to 2 P.M., with the same symptoms as those already described on 27th of Oct. The restless nights continued with slight chills on Nov. 6th.

Nov. 7th. Took a powder of 2d trit., 2 gr.

Nov. 8th. He recorded similar symptoms to those of Oct. 27th, but they were more severe, and there was also pain and lameness of the knees, noticed particularly when walking.

Nov. 9th. No symptoms.

Nov. 10th. Chills, slighter than those on the 8th.

Nov. 13th. Took 2d trit.; chills followed every other day until the 20th, with a similarity of symptoms to those already described. While taking the 3*d trit.* the urine was increased in quantity; the stools were softer and voided earlier in the morning than usual.

The 2*d trit.* produced hard, scanty and delayed stools. During the whole proving there was violent itching of the hairy scalp.

13.—COLOCYNTHIS.

By Dr. Watzke, of Vienna.*

COLOC. Colocynth, Cucumis, Colocynthis. Bitter apple. The bitter Cucumber. *Ger.* Koloquinte. *Fr.* Coloquinte.

INTRODUCTION.

There are homœopathic physicians who behold in the Hahnemannian Materia Medica a masterpiece absolutely perfect and neither needing nor admitting of improvements. Gross and Gouillon have quite recently declared,† "*that in its present state it is free from faults and needs no reformation.*" We regret that, in this respect, we are entirely of a different opinion from our respected colleagues. We hold that science has a right to demand this reform at our hands; we see in it, the highest desideratum of Homœopathy, the fundamental principle of its progress and development and the missing element, the obtaining of which will secure the scientific appreciation of our opponents.

While we thus openly, in the face of friends and foes, acknowledge our pharmacognostic deficiencies, we desire in the most earnest manner to deprecate the supposition that we undervalue or mistrust the provings of Hahnemann. We call in question neither the conscientiousness, the earnest truthfulness, the comprehensiveness, and the acumen of the observer, nor the accuracy of the experiments themselves; on the contrary, we are deeply convinced that nothing will conduce to place the merit of Hahnemann upon a loftier basis and to set his genius and observing power in a stronger light, than those very subsequent provings which must furnish the materials for a physiological construction of our Materia Medica.

It is high time we began to be ashamed of stretching our indolent limbs, and lolling lazily upon the couch prepared for us by the

* This valuable essay, from the pen of Dr. Watzke, of Vienna, is the first of the reprovings undertaken by the Austrian Association which was published. It appeared in the first number of the "*Oesterreichische Zeitschrift für Homœopathie*," from which we have translated it in full. An abridgement of it was published by Dr. Irvine, of Leeds, in the Appendix to the "*British Journal of Homœopathy*," but we have thought that the entire production would be an acceptable addition to our literature.—Ed.

† Allg. hom. Zeit. 25, No. 7. Arch. für hom. Heilk. 20. Heft 3, § 1.

laborious toil of the Master; let us muster up courage to tread bravely in his foot-steps, and pursue, with untiring patience, the path he has opened up to us. If, like him, we will devote half a life to the proving of drugs; if, with the same tireless zeal, industry and self-sacrifice, we will continue to experiment as he did, we shall soon become aware of the infinite affluence of observation and experience, the colossal piles of the most careful experiments which constitute the immovable basis of such provings as those of *nux vomica*, *belladonna*, *pulsatilla*, *bryonia*, *aconite*, *rhus*, and *mercury;* we shall then see the reason why those collections of symptoms, which to others seemed like chaotic fragments, or hieroglyphical mysteries, presented to Hahnemann, of necessity, a physiological picture of the greatest symmetry and order, and simply because he was himself the experimenter, or at least the exclusive director of the trials.

What is it then that calls for revision and reform in a work which we thus laud to the skies?

The necessity of a revision of our *Materia Medica* has reference less to its matter than its form. So far as *we* are concerned, it rests upon the fact, that the materials of our provings have been transmitted to us not in any natural, physiological order, but solely and *exclusively* as an artificial fragmentary index. The master-builder was mistaken in supposing that his disciples, who made incomplete experiments, or none at all, would inherit his own wisdom, and in thinking that those who were not familiar with the whole, would nevertheless, like himself, have a perfect conception of the value and significance of the separate parts.

The *unfortunate* schema, in which Hahnemann has delivered to us his results, leaves us in entire ignorance as to the mode and manner in which his experiments were made. *He has given us simply the answers to the problem; he should also have shown us the process by which the answers were obtained.**

We are entirely ignorant whether the symptom which is followed by this or that name, was the result of one or several experiments; nay, we do not even know that the same name always indicates that the symptom was observed in the same individual.† We are seldom in-

* We may seriously entertain a doubt as to the justice of this reproach against Hahnemann. When we reflect upon the entire novelty of his results, upon their absolute rejection by the world of science, and more than all upon their great bulk and upon the fact, if we may believe the tradition, that their publication at all, was due to the gratitude of a patient, we may well excuse the intelligent caution that submitted the results in an accessible shape without the monstrous burden of the literal provings. The original manuscrip s, however, from which the *Materia Medica Pura* was compiled, are understood to be in existence; and now that Homœopathy numbers her priests by thousands, and her votaries by the million, no more acceptable offering could be made than the literal reproduction of the original provings of Hahnemann and his disciples.—J. W. M.

† The name in question is sometimes used generically; thus, *Gross*, *Stapf*, and others affixed their own names to all the symptoms which they had collected from perhaps half a dozen provers.—Watzke.

formed of the size of the dose, or its form, or of the time and frequency of its administration. We consequently generally learn as little of the development, duration, course and termination of the drug-sickness, as of the appearance and disappearance of the individual symptoms. We have no means of discriminating between transitory and accidental phenomena, and those which are necessary and essential. We remain wholly, or almost wholly uncertain as to the centre and periphery of drug-action and its primary or secondary effects, as to its sympathies, synergies and antagonisms, and the extent and importance of the medicinal disease. We are kept in ignorance of the relation of the symptoms to the predisposing and occasional (medicinal) causes, and get no glimpse of the degree of intensity with which the drug acts upon the healthy organism in general, and upon individual systems and organs in particular.

We have called Hahnemann's schema "unfortunate," because, instead of presenting us with a clear picture of drug-diseases, it gives us only a monstrous agglomeration of symptoms, directed more to the memory than to the understanding; because it not only greatly increases the difficulties of acquiring a knowledge of the *Materia Medica* and the employment of the homœopathic practice by his disciples, but throws an almost insurmountable obstacle in the way of the conversion of sceptical physicians of other schools, and most unfortunate of all, not unfrequently deters the most energetic minds from its study, thus depriving the new school of the assistance of those best calculated to become its leaders and chief supports.

We give this free utterance to our sentiments, in the firm conviction that they are shared by the great majority of our colleagues, and that the work of reformation, which we have thus courageously begun, will find sympathy and support from many quarters. The noble example of Hahnemann shows what may be accomplished by *one* powerful will; and though we have set the physiological construction of his *Materia Medica* before us as our life-long task, still we are not guilty of the ridiculous presumption of supposing that we have the herculean arms that can singly bring the gigantic undertaking to a successful completion. As regards the reprovings, the most laborious part of the work, we are already surrounded by no inconsiderable number of zealous, able and sympathising friends.

May we succeed in so accomplishing our object, *that our exertions shall prove of lasting service, not to a system, but to science—not to the partizans of Homœopathy or Allopathy, but to the practical physician, and shall serve as a lasting proof that the advancement and perfection of* SPECIFIC PHARMAKODYNAMICS, *and the improvement of* PRACTICAL THERAPEUTICS *are essentially identical!*

CHAPTER I.

Names, Description, and Chemical Composition of Colocynth.

There is uncertainty enough in the nomenclature of Colocynth. LOBEL and BAUHIN long since complained of this difficulty, and in spite of all the efforts of the philologists, the derivation and original meaning of the word remain to this day a mystery.* The number of synonymes used by botanists and physicians is so enormous, that the reader is frequently left in doubt, especially among the writers of the middle ages, as to what name conceals the author's reference to Colocynth.

DIOSCORIDES and GALEN called it simply Κολοκύνθισ—the diminutive of κολοκύνθη, here at once indicating contempt and its inappropriateness as food. Hence some have derived it from κόλον, κύων, quasi, dogs' food! SCRIBONIUS LARGUS and BAUHIN translate it *Cucurbitula*, a little gourd. The κολοκύνθη ἀιγοσ, which DIOSCORIDES considers as a synonyme of *Colocynth* with the barbarian *Thymbre*, *Antogenes*, and *Tutastra*, according to CORNARIUS, and others, means κολοκύνθη ἀγριοσ; there is, therefore, no *Cucurbita caprina*. **HIPPOCRATES** and SCRIBONIUS LARGUS write, according to FŒSIUS (tautologically), κολοκύνθισ ἀγρια, and not as SCHULZE and others, κολοκύνθη ἀγρια. The latter is not at all the true, legitimate Colocynth, but one of the similar varieties of Gourds with hard, woody, pear-shaped fruit (low German, *Regelsbeeren*, *Gichtbeeren*) and juicy pulp, difficult to dry—the *Colocynthis Germanica*, *Colocynthis altera*, Trag.; *Colocynthis pyriformis*, Lobel.; *Colocynthis fœmina*, Dodon.; *Pseudocolocynthis pyrifor-*

* MARTINIUS and LEMERY derive it from the Greek: παρά τὴν κοιλὶαν ὂυ τον κῶλον κινεῖν, κνῆθειν, κύειν; *quod ventrem, alvum, intestina movcat, atterat, turbat;* DUVERGIE and RATIER repeat the derivation with a little modification; KRAUS does the same, and writes it "Koloquynthe"; while SCHULZE makes himself merry over it. It is probable, according to KALTSCHMIDT's Comparative Dictionary, that *Colocynth*, the Portuguese *Calabas*, the Spanish *Calabaza*, the later Latin *Calebassus*, the Arabic *Charaba*, as well as *Cucurbita*, *Cucumer*, ἀγγουριον, *Gurke*, *Kürbis*, *Cucumber*, *Gourd*, are all derived from the same, still undiscovered, Sanscrit root.

The worst of the matter is, that the learned are not agreed as to what was meant among the Greeks by κολοκύνθη. BAUHIN thinks it included the *round* fruits in our present family of *Cucurbitaceæ;* while those which were *longish* were called in different provinces σικύη, σικυώνη, σικυωνια, and most commonly σίκυος. MARCELLUS again maintains exactly the reverse of this. DIERBACH holds the antiquarian exegesis of the Cucurbitaceæ to be a very difficult matter, and translates κολοκυνθη by "Gurke" (Cucumber, Gherkin); GRIMM does the same, while PASSOW renders it by "Kürbis" (Gourd, Pumpkin). (*Grimm's Hippoc.*, B. 2, § 138).—*Watzke.*

mis, Eyst.; *Cucurbita vulgaris*, *canina*, *sylvestris*, *barbara*, *marina*, aliorum; σομφοσ Plinii.*

Whether HIPPOCRATES always intends the Colocynth by σικυώνη (*Cucumerulus*, Bauh.) is by no means as certain as *Galen* takes it; for, according to DODONÆUS (Stirp. hist. V. 2, 7), the expression is as often used to denote the *Elaterium* σικυος ἄγριος, *Cucumer sylvestris*. That the "uncut, small, round gourds σίκυη ἄτμητος τῶν μικρῶν και στρογγυλῶν," which HIPPOCRATES (*De Coxend.*) prescribes in enemata against Coxalgia from taking cold, is (according to DIERBACH) the *Elaterium*, and not our *Colocynth* (as GALEN thinks it is) becomes extremely probable from the fact that HIPPOCRATES (περὶ γυν. φυς. and περὶ ἐπικυης) prescribes the finely triturated pulp of the κολοκύνθις ἄγρια kneaded with honey, *together with* σίκυης ἐντεριώνη (*Cucumeris agrestis medulla*) as an anal suppository for purging the bile, and as a vaginal application in cases inclined to abort, and recommends the injection of an infusion of the same in wine and milk into the vagina in uterine ulceration.

Among other Greek authorities, Colocynth is known as σικύα πίκρα; among the Arabians as *Chandel*, *Kandel*, *Haanthal*, *Handal*, and (with the article) *Alhandal*. TRAGUS heads his chapter on Colocynth with the caption "*Colocynthis vera*"; LOBELIUS with "*Cucurbitula amara cathartica*"; DODONÆUS calls it *Colocynthis prima*, *Colocynthis mas*, and *Anguria sylvestris*; others again, *Cucurbita deserti*, *Cucurbita Alexandrina*, *Cucurbita Prophetæ Elisæi*, *Melo agrestis*. The medical poets bestowed upon it the fanciful titles of *sal* and *fel terræ*, *nex*, *pestis plantarum*, *mors in olla*.†

Botanically, the Colocynth is known as *Cucumis Colocynthis* (*Monœcia*, *Monadelphia Linn.*), *Citrullus Colocynthis* and *Colocynthis officinalis* (Schrader), and is related to the water-melon (*Citrullus vulgaris*)—the bitterest and one of the pleasantest of fruits! It is an annual plant, with a thick fleshy root, stem herbaceous, procumbent, clinging to neighboring objects by means of numerous filiform tendrils, fleshy, fragile, angular, branched, hispid; leaves alternate, ovate, pointed, five or more lobed, clothed on both sides with short, blunt, somewhat recurved hairs; flowers axillary, solitary, stalked, monophyllous, campanulate, yellow.

It grows wild at the Cape of Good Hope, in Japan, Arabia, Nubia, Syria, Asia Minor, Cyprus, in the islands of the Ægean Sea, and in Southern Spain.

* These latter appellations are found also among the synonymes of the *Elaterium* and *Bryonia!* *Hardouin* corrects σομφος into σπογγος.—*Watzke.*

† The young man of Elisha (2 *Kings*, c. iv. v. 38,) evidently not a very skilful botanist, in the time of the dearth gathered his lapful of wild gourds, and shred them into the pot of pottage preparing for the sons of the prophets. But while they were eating, they perceived the bitter taste, and cried out "O thou man of God, there is death in the pot!" These gourds were probably not Colocynth-apples, but the fruit of the *Cucumis Prophetarum*, which grows abundantly in Palestine, and greatly resembles the common gourd (Oken's *Naturgeschichte*, 3, 827).—*Watzke.*

The only part hitherto used in medicine almost without exception is the fruit—*pepones, fructus, poma colocynthidis*—(*Ger.*) *Koloquinten*—, *Purgier-*, *Purgierparadies äpfel*—; (Holl.) *Quintappel*; (Eng.) *Bitter apple.* They are globose, first green, then yellow, as large as an orange, and are covered by a smooth leathery rind destitute of hair. The fruit comes to us dried and deprived of its outer rind, and is covered with a thin, whitish-yellow skin which contains a very light, spongy, white, dry pulp (*pulpa colocynthidis*, σικυώνης σπόγγος (Hipp.) κολοκυνθίδος τὸ ἔντον (Gal.) *Colocynth-pulp*), containing numerous ovoid, hard, smooth, yellowish-white seeds, and having an extremely bitter, acrid, repulsive taste and a sweetish, nauseous smell The moderate-sized, externally full, perfectly dry specimens are the best.* The well-washed seeds are tasteless, the skin is mucilaginous, the kernel oily.

Meisner, Vauquelin and Braconnot have given us analyses of the Colocynth pulp.

Meisner.	
Bitter matter (Colocynthin)	14.4
Extractive	10.
Bitter fixed oil . . .	4.2
Resin insoluble in ether .	13.2
Gum	9.5
Bassorin	3.
Gummy extract . .	17.
Vegetable jelly . . .	0.6
Phosphate of lime and magnesia	5.7
Ligneous fibre . . .	19.2
Water	5.
Colocynth Pulp . .	101.8

Braconnot.	
Bitter matter (Colocynthin) with some resin . .	41.4
Azotic matter . .	21.4
Resin	4.3
Deliquescent salt of potash not soluble in alcohol .	7.1
Vegetable jelly . . .	18.6
Acetate of potash . .	5.7
Watery Extract of Colocynth	98.5

Vauquelin found in the Colocynth pulp a peculiar principle, *Colocynthin;* besides this he found oily matter, extractive, resin insoluble in ether, gum and various salts. The watery extract of Colocynth is a yellowish viscous liquid, which foams when shaken, like a solution of gum, and does not pass through filtering paper. Murray says that the alcoholic tincture will not filter, but we have not found this true with our tincture and our filtering paper.

CHAPTER II.

Ante-Hahnemannian medicinal Employment of Colocynth.

This remedy is as ancient as medicine itself; it was known to Hippocrates, Dioscorides, Galen and Pliny, was highly esteemed and frequently employed by the Arabians and the physicians of the middle

* The Arabian caution never to employ in medicine a Colocynth apple which was the solitary fruit upon the plant, is in more than one respect ridiculous. Mesue and Avicenna have also male and female Colocynth-mannikins!—*Watzke.*

ages, slighted by the moderns, and latterly consigned to the great lumber-room of obsolete drugs,—the medicinal *Hôpital des Invalides!* Some of the old Latins speak of it with as much enthusiasm and seem to have relied upon it with as much faith as you will find among the fashionable adherents of *Sal-ammoniac*, *Iodine*, *Calomel*, and the other remedies in vogue in our own day. Ettmüller declares that it formed with *scammony* and *helleborus niger*, a triumvirate that was capable of doing wonders!* It was frequently esteemed the *ancora sacra* in obstinate, long-standing cases which had even resisted the efficacy of *Agaricus* and *Turpeth mineral*, a fact of no small significance.

It seems to have been most in use among the Arabians. They recommended it in a great number of the most various affections of the brain, nerves, muscles, joints, lungs, thorax, kidneys and bladder; against chronic headache, obstinate hemicrania, chronic vertigo, weakened mental faculties, melancholy, apoplexy, epilepsy, delirium, paralyses, chronic spasms, articular pains, rheuma, podagra, lachrymation, angina pectoris, asthma, chronic coughs, dropsy, but above all in coxalgia,† and mucous and flatulent colics. They administered the finely pulverized Colocynth as a snuff for jaundice, decoction of the pulp in clysters for colics; the fresh juice of the leaves as a salve for the itch and cutaneous eruptions; the green leaves themselves as a poultice to discuss or mature swollen glands, boils and abscesses. They used a decoction of the root as a specific against the bites of serpents and scorpion stings.‡ The oil was used against dandriff and the falling off of the hair; they dropped it into the ear to remove noises, rubbed it into the bellies of worm patients, filled aching decayed teeth with cotton moistened with it, fumigated other dental affections with the kernel of the seed, fastened loose teeth by bathing the mouth with Colocynth-vinegar, applied the ashes of the burnt rind to the painful anus, and sprinkled dwellings with a decoction of the drug to exterminate or keep away fleas and other vermin. (*Joan. Mesuæ op. Ven.* 1589. *De simpl.* c. IV. *Avicennæ, Arabum med. principis Canon med. Ven.* 1608, lib. II, c. 130).

This pretty nearly exhausts the therapeutical applications of Colocynth previous to Hahnemann. Very little of it is the exclusive production of Arabian genius; it was mostly derived from their Greek and Roman models and predecessors.

We have already stated that HIPPOCRATES used it, and in what cases. DIOSCORIDES§ prescribes it in *Coxalgia* (frictions with the fresh juice),

* Alas! that in so potent a triumvirate we should be left in ignorance which was the real wonder-worker.—*Watzke.*

† RHAZES cured many thousand ischialgias by means of Enemata of Colocynth and Saltpetre. Notwithstanding, he recommends a legion of other remedies in that affection! (*Ejusd. op. parv.. Ven.* 1510. *De sciatica passione.*)—*Watzke.*

‡ RHAZES cured his own son with the decoction of the root when he had been stung by a scorpion in four places (*Bauhini, Hist. plant. univ. Yverd.* 1561, tom. II, lib. II.)—*Watzke.*

§ *Comment. in Diosc. Ed. Kühn*, p. II. c. 161. *Fernel* too found frictions of the fresh juice very beneficial in *Coxalgia*. *Pliny* recommends, also, friction with the oil.—*Watzke.*

in paralyses, colics and toothache; SCRIBONIUS LARGUS (*De Compos. Med. Par.* 1528, §99) in lumbago, epilepsy and amenorrhœa. ARCHIGENES (*Oribasii collect.* lib. VIII. *Ven.* 1558, c. 46) considered it an excellent purge for feverish patients, *when the fever was mild and favorable, and came on with headache, great weakness, and terrible pains in the hip.* He administered it as a sort of oleo-watery infuso-decoction in combination with *veratrum* and *scammony*. PAULUS ÆGINETA (*Ejusdem opus divinum de re med. Basil.* 1532, p. 374) considers it as rather a *nervous* than a *sanguineous purgative* (!) He esteems it highly in headaches, depending upon an affection of the dura-mater, or of the scalp; in vertigo, hemicrania, epilepsy, apoplexy, trismus, chronic lachrymation, asthma, chronic cough, arthritic affections of the kidneys and bladder. In coxalgia he rubs in the fresh juice (*in op. c.* p. 425). PLINY (*Hist. Nat.*, tom. II., lib. XX. c. 3) and *Johannes Activarius* (*Ejusdem methodi med., Ven.* 1554, lib. IV. p. 215) recommend it in nearly the same affections. Besides this, they both recommend it highly in jaundice; the latter would have it used with great caution, but adds, nevertheless, "*Dantur autem scrupuli duo!*"

Colocynth and Agaricus were the principal ingredients in the famous *Hiera Pachii Antiochii* (*Hiera diacolocynthidos*, διασικυώνης) a secret remedy employed by the greatest physicians of antiquity: APPOLONIUS, ASCLEPIADES, ANDROMACHUS, THEMISON and RUFUS EPHESIUS, against the most severe and procrastinated disorders, podagra, gout, paralyses, epilepsies, tetanus, aphonia, cancer, &c.* (*Schulze.*)

Nothing new has been developed in relation to the use of Colocynth by the great majority of medical writers since the days of Greece and Rome, those of the most modern times not excepted. It only plays the same part as a component of still more piebald, still more wonderful mixtures.

It owes to PARACELSUS the honor of having been admitted into the company of jalap, scammony, and rhubarb in the famous *Extractum Catholicum* (*Schulze, diss. de Coloc. Halæ*, 1734), which was, as its name imports, a panacea.† BONETUS and TIMÆUS (*Casus med.*

* This *Hiera* was a precious composition, a dram of which contained two and a quarter grains of Colocynth. PHILENIDES, of Katana, transcribed it on his death-bed, and sent it to the Emperor Tiberius. SCRIBONIUS LARGUS says of the discoverer of this sacred mixture, which he extols to the skies: *Hieræ*, i. e. *sacræ confectionis nomen, ei propter duas causas tribuit; unum, ne ejus verum nomen dicendo ostenderet, quæ esset; alterum, quo magis sub hoc venerabili nominis specie commendaret medicamentum.*

We cannot refrain from adding the following expression of SCRIBONIUS LARGUS on the subject of the *Hiera*: *Illud vero* (says he, *Op. cit.* § 103) *supra omnium opinionem est, quod ad stomachicos evidenter convenit, quam sit virosissinum medicamentum adversus stomachum.* Had he only been able to draw a corollary from this proposition! He contented himself, however, in pretty much the same fashion as our opponents do at the present day: "*Sed videlicet in ejusmodi rebus, potentior usus ratione est.*"—*Watzke.*

† The receipt of the Catholic extract was, however, not a stereotype; it underwent various changes and combinations, depending upon the author who prescribed and the disease against which it was used. TRILLER substituted aloes and hellebore in place of rhubarb; HOFFMAN, gamboge and *flores Martis;* POTTER

et. obs. 1667, lib. IV, *cas.* 9 *et.* 34, *et in Epist.* lib. III, *Epist.* 40,) recommend Colocynth in menstrual difficulties, especially in deficient catamenia, in suppressed lochia and for the expulsion of a false conception or dead child; the former prescribes it as a uterine suppository, the latter in decoction *sub forma suffitus, insessus aut injectionis.** DODONÆUS (*Stirp. hist.* III, 2, 26) employed it especially in apoplexy, chronic vertigo, hemicrania, deafness and violent colic. He says, also, that Colocynth was used in conjunction with aloes and myrrh for the purpose of embalming. BAYRUS AND SCHENK (*Obs. med. Francof.* 1665, p. 424) drew teeth by means of it without pain and without an instrument.† TRAGUS (*Stirp. Germ. Arg.* 1552, c. 97) found it useful in colics, putrid fever and particularly in dropsy; LOBELIUS (*Stirp. adv. nov. Lond.* 1570 *in cap. de coloc.*), in apoplexy and coma, administered in clysters containing from a scruple to a dram; ETTMÜLLER (*Op. med. Gen.* 1736, tom I, p. 758) in intermittents,‡ mucous colic and epilepsy. It figures among the chief constituents in the drastic mixtures which Sydenham employed almost exclusively in the treatment of dropsies (*Op. omn. med. Pat.* 1725, p. 565). RIVERIUS (*Op. med. univ. Ven.* 1687, t. II. p. 198) praises it as an excellent purger of the brain (*ad cerebrum potenter expurgandum*) in all diseases not inflammatory. SENNERT (*Inst. med. Vittenb.* 1644, p. 958) used it in podagra, asthma, colic and chronic rheuma. VAN HELMONT considers it the best *anti-syphiliticum.*§ It was also used against Syphilis by ZACUTUS LUSITANUS (*Prax. med. admir. Lugd.* 1667, t. II, p. 93) and BONETUS (*Thesaur. med. pr. Gen.* 1694, t. III, p. 309). For greater certainty, the latter used it in a diaphoretic decoction with mercury. He also destroyed worms in the ear with the decoctoin of colocynth (*in op. cit.*, p. 1004). ZACUTUS also found the external application of the colocynth oil of great service in nervous pains and diseases arising from cold and dropping it in the ear, in pain and ringing in the ears.‖ He also says

myrrh, crocus and senna. In hypochondria it was prepared with *castor*, in renal affections with *amber*, and in loss of fluids with *merc-dulc.*, &c.—*Watzke.*

* *Bonetus* altogether condemns Colocynthine pessaries in absence or deficiency of labor pains; although they hasten the labor, there is risk of killing both mother and child.—*Watzke.*

† They scarified the gum for this purpose; caused the patient to hold a decoction of Colocynth in vinegar, in his mouth, and then seizing the tooth with the fingers, extracted it at once with ease and without the slightest pain!—*Watzke.*

‡ It formerly possessed sympathetic therapeutic virtues in intermittent fever. "*Mirum dictu*," says PLINY *op. cit*, "*colocynthidis semina, si fuerint pari numero adalligata, febres sanare dicuntur, quas Graeci periodicas vocant.*—*Watzke.*

§ Half a colocynth-apple was macerated over-night in a well stopped flask of wine, and the wine was drunk in the morning. This was repeated five or six times, and the patient kept at home fasting. (*Ettmüller, op. cit.*)

SYLVIUS DE LA BOE (*Prax. med. pp. Lugd.* 1764, art. 257,) declares colocynth to be the most admirable antidote to syphilis. HORNEMANN tells us that the inhabitants of Fez know no other remedy for Syphilis than salt and colocynth, and that they succeed in curing cases which are not inveterate (*Tagebuch einer Reise nach murjat*, &c., Wien. 1802, §§ 89, 102).—*Watzke.*

‖ The oil was prepared by filling an excavated colocynth apple with oil and then roasting it in hot ashes.—*Watzke.*

that when rubbed into the head, it prevents the hair from turning gray and colors it black. JUNCKER (*Consp. med. Hal.* 1734, p. 216,) prescribed colocynth in phlegmatic constitutions for asthmatic paroxysms, suppressed hæmorrhoids and obstinate toothache. CRANTZ has seen good results from its employment in lethargy and serous apoplexy; KARTHEUSER (*Fund. nat. med. Francof,* 1767, t. I, p. 600) in obstinate diseases of the mucous membranes. LIEUTAUD (*Syn. pr. med. Amst.* 1765, p. 655,) rubbed a mixture of the pulp with ox-gall into the abdomen of verminous patients.* DAHLBERG praises the admirable effects of colocynth in gout (*cum fermite venereo*), especially in that of the head and hip, in intolerable pains from the abuse of mercury, as well as in paralysis and algid fevers. FABRE cured a severe affection resulting from suppressed gonorrhœa with colocynth (*Murray, app. med.* t. I, p. 583). COLOMBIER (*Code de med. milit.* I. 5, p. 420,) relates that many soldiers cured themselves of gonorrhœa in a few days by eating a whole colocynth apple in one or two doses.

Among the moderns, VOGT (*Pharmakod, B.* 2, *Abth.* 1, S. 318), RICHTER (*Arzneim. B.* 2, and *spec. Th. B.* 7, § 511, and *B.* 3, S. 336), and BURDACH (*Arzneim B.* 3), have labored on the therapeutic chapter of Colocynth. They recommend it in paralyses (especially of the lower limbs, bladder and rectum); in mental affections (lunacy, mania, melancholy and imbecility) arising from atony of the ganglionic system; in chronic spasms and other nervous disorders (epilepsy, vertigo, coma, nervous headache); in hypochondria, jaundice, intermittents, menostasia, and chlorosis, from congestions and obstructions in the portal circulation, liver and spleen, as well as in the lymphatics and glands, from mucous accumulations in the digestive organs, suppressed hæmorrhoids, &c. These recommendations are not derived from their experience at the bed-side, but have for the most part a purely ideal origin; and even the illustrations drawn from the practice of cotemporaries have generally the air of being only pathological reminiscences from the days of the Arabians. We add these latter, and append to them such memorabilia concerning the drug as we have been able to find in modern times.

BANG found the decoction of Colocynth the best remedy against dropsy, the simple result of serous effusion. KRANNER also employed the decoction with success in dropsy. HUFELAND considered it the most powerful diuretic for heavy, sluggish constitutions. WRISBACH (*Kleinert's Rep.*, 4 *J.* 11, 85) had occasionally excellent effects in the dropsy of brandy drinkers, accompanied by disorganization of the liver, stomach and spleen. SCHLESIER lauds his *pilulæ hydrogogæ* (coloc., gamb. and croton oil) against the same affections. DÜHRSEN (*Kleinert's Rep.*, 1836, 2, 62) employed colocynth with great advantage in chronic ascites following scarlatina. BUCHHAVE found it efficacious in hydrothorax. HILLIER wrote a treatise, which we have unfortunately not been able to find, on the use of Colocynth in dropsies (*Leip.* 1821).

* MURRAY (*op. cit.*) does not consider colocynth as a specific against worms. Lumbrici did not die in a saturated infusion under from fourteen to twenty-four hours.—*Watzke.*

HEIM employed the tincture externally as a powerful discutient in cases of herpes (with *Tinct. Ant. sapon*) and in scrofulous swelling of the glands (with castor oil). CONRADI employs it (with oil and opium) in large inveterate hernias, in which the fæces collect and give rise to obstructions. BERENDS found frictions with the tincture or the application of a Colocynth plaster, useful in cases of obstruction from accumulated fæces (*Kleinert's Rep.*, 1836, 10, 169). SCHMUHR restored a man of 70 from a gastric apoplexy, after leeches, emetics, irritating enemata and foot-baths; not only was the principal trouble relieved, but also the previous sleeplessness, obstinate constipation and imperfect paralysis of the upper eyelids and tongue. NEUMANN thinks he has cured paralyses of the upper and lower extremities of the colon, cœcum and rectum in scrofulous individuals. This drug alone relieved a paralysis of the masticatory muscles and eyelids after an attack of gout, and another of the thigh after a violent attack of hæmorrhoids.*

CHAPTER III.

Decline and Fall of Colocynth.

Notwithstanding the extended list of authors, both ancient and modern, who have treated on the employment of Colocynth, it has long since lost its high position in the learned treatises of the Pharmacopæists. Its fall began with the insinuation, that it was a heroic remedy full of danger, and the administration of which demanded mature deliberation; that it should only be used in rare cases of the severest forms of chronic diseases; † a drug the artistic employment of which could only be learned from the greatest masters of therapeutics (*Geoffroy*, *Mat. Med. Venet.* 1742, *Art. Coloc.*). Some counselled, on this account, that its use should be limited to older physicians, the younger being forbidden to prescribe it.‡

At the present time, when we all have such unbounded faith in

* We are far from supposing that we have thus presented a perfect picture of the allopathic therapeutic employment of Colocynth. Such was neither our intention, nor would it be of essential service if done. We must confess that when we compare the time and labor which we have expended in turning over some half hundred old folios and quartos, and more modern Journals and Repertories, with the advantage gained, we are somewhat at a loss whether to be proud or ashamed of the foregoing chapter.—*Watzke.*

† TRILLER (*Thesaur. Med. Franc.* 1774, p. II, p. 203) calls Colocynth "*infamium medicaminum exemplar, remedium triste, ingratum, suspectum, dubium, violentum, imo pœne virulentum, atque hinc merito proscribendum ex officinis.*" C. HOFFMAN, on the other hand, declares it to be to severe diseases what a big wedge is to a big log. Lions are not to be caught in mouse-traps, and many a chronic malady is suffered to go uncured because the physician is afraid of his drugs (*Geoffroy*).—*Watzke.*

‡ From this it is easy to see that the older physicians of those times understood the secrets of medical tactics as well as their compeers of the present day. The only thing we could wish is that the legal age at which colocynth might have been prescribed had been stated in the diploma!—*Watzke.*

counter-irritation we are less afraid of colocynth than formerly; but, inasmuch as it has been thoroughly settled that there is no such thing as a specific, we no longer, of course, consider colocynth as such, but allow it to share its virtues with at least ten other drugs (drastic substitutives)! the necessary consequence of which is, that people have become indifferent to a remedy whose place is so easily supplied. So far has this gone that our venerated instructor *Hartmann* ranks colocynth among the *remedia superflua!* and the hypothetical indications given by Vogt, Richter and Burdach for the therapeutical use of Colocynth are of such a character that they will answer equally well for more than half a dozen of its pharmacological neighbors.*

This indifference of the moderns and the horror of the ancients have their origin in the same causes, the immoderately large, often absolutely poisonous doses in which the drug was administered, and especially in the dim notions they had of its action upon the healthy organism. They had learned, to be sure, from accidental cases of poisoning, that "it set the stomach, bowels, and whole body in an uproar, produced the most dreadful pains, corroded the intestines, excited hemorrhages from the anus," &c. (*Geoffroy op. cit.*) but this was only the dark side of the physiological picture. The medical world, with a full knowledge of the no less poisonous properties of *aloes, jalap, barytes, calomel* and *iodine*, continues to dispense them with a liberal hand, but has only eyes for the deadly qualities of colocynth.†

It is wonderful what combinations of drugs have been excogitated to tame the wild and savage fierceness of colocynth. One of the most common favorites was sulphuric acid; Ettmüller on the contrary (*op. cit.*) considers the alkalies as the best *corrigens*, declaring: *Acida enim castrant, non corrigunt cotocynthidem.* Hoffmann (*Op. omn.* tom. I, pars II, c. 5) thinks the same of the decoction. Others subjected it to a fermenting or rotting process. Wedel (*Exercit. med. phil.* XVIII) and Neumann (*in Prælect. chymico-pharm.* p. 797) have observed that the pernicious principle of Colocynth only derived new power from fermentation with must so highly recommended by Boulduccius (*in Comment. soc. scient. Paris*, 1701). Mucilaginous and aromatic remedies were considered by many as the best *corrigentia;* it was commonly combined with mint, balm, myrrh, and the like, when prescribed as an emmenagogue. The Arabian physicians frequently made use of astringents for this purpose, but Mercurialis and Rolfink condemn this method of correction altogether. The violence of pur-

* Mesue *the younger* says that nothing should deter one from using a remedy, which, *like colocynth*, could not be replaced by any other. Now-a-days, however, Colocynth, too, has its surrogate. The entire periodical literature of the Hippocratic school for the last ten years cannot probably produce ten instances of the successful therapeutical employment of Colocynth.—*Watzke.*

† However true these remarks may be in relation to Germany, they do not apply with equal force to England and America, where colocynth has for a number of years been quite a fashionable component in pills and extracts for the *regulation of the bowels.* Morrison's "Hygeian pills" were said to have contained it. —J. W. M.

gatives was only increased by the addition of bdellium and mastic, and Colocynth acquired in this way a *vis furiosa.* Urine had its advocates as the best softener of the violence of Colocynth; RIVERIUS (*Prax. med. univ. Venet.* 1687, tom. II, p. 198) and FREITAG say that the urinary infusion not only loses all its bitterness and becomes tasteless, but parts with so much of its poisonous essence that it can be administered by the dram. Others, more refined, objected to this vehicle as not exactly æsthetic, and substituted the *sp. roris majalis.* Others still macerated it in whey, water or wine; many corrected it with simple olive oil, but the most followed the example of DODONÆUS, who maintained that colocynth could only be corrected by other violent purgatives.* *Not a soul seems to have fallen upon the best and surest corrigens—smaller and less frequent doses! This seems to have been the egg of Columbus which Hahnemann succeeded in standing on end by the introduction of little doses.*

To the apparently instinctive recognition of the necessity of diminishing the effect of the excessive quantities of colocynth administered by the cotemporaneous exhibition of its antidotes, poor suffering human nature owes a variety of the most ingenious formulæ. We have already referred to the *Hiera* of PACHIUS ANTIOCHIUS and the catholic extract. The following were not less celebrated weapons in the hands of the great masters of Therapeutics.

1. *Pilulæ de duobus.*—Equal parts of scammony and colocynth with q. s. of essence of cloves. This was often used by SYDENHAM and other English physicians; FREIND thinks he has used it successfully in confluent small-pox! (*Comment. de febr. ad Hippoc.* c. VIII, p. 206.)

2. *Pilulæ Cochiæ.*† The cerebral pills of NICOLAI and ALMANSOR contained, besides colocynth, aloes, scammony, absinthium, mastic, &c., and were the most approved remedy against hemicrania.

3. *Pilulæ trium Diabolorum.* The three-devil pills were composed of *Trohisc-Alhand., Diacryd* aa. gr. IV. *Merc. dulc. gr.* VIII.; *M. ft. pil No.* 4, *pro dosi*—a notorious clap-specific!

4. *Pilulæ iliacæ* of RHAZES. *Colocynth* 10, *Scammony* 3, *Sagapenum* 10. DODONÆUS thinks it the pleasantest and mildest laxative (*Stirp. histor.* III, 2, 26); ROLFINK (*De purg. veget. tab.* p. 149) considers it one of Paracelsus' many hobbies.

5. *Confectio Hamech.* According to SCHULZE, a disgusting, ungrateful compound of purgatives, with a basis of colocynth, which was used

* Paradoxical as this assertion may appear, it is still not entirely destitute of foundation. The older physicians had doubtless already had some intimations of the mutual antidotal relations of purgatives. CELSUS says (Lib. II, c. 12), "*Medicamenta stomachum fere lædunt, ideoque omnibus catharticis Aloe miscenda est.*" DODONÆUS entirely rejects the *Trochisci Alhandal* formed of colocynth-pulp finely triturated with trigacanth, which, apart from the excessive doses (from six grains to two and four scruples), was, next to the tincture, the best, simplest, and most effective form in which the drug was commonly administered.—*Watzke.*

† *Cochos*, i. e. *Caput*, says an old commentator upon *Rhazes* (*Op. parv. Ven.* 1510). We do not find *cochos*, however, either in the Greek or Latin lexicon: it may perhaps be tautological—τα κοκκια, *grana rotunda, pilulæ.*—*Watzke.*

against psora, lepra, cancer, elephantiasis, tinea, old ulcers, and chronic gonorrhœa.*

6. *Extractum panchymagogum Crollii et Hartmanni.* This was composed of colocynth, mild mercury and many other (drastic) remedies, and was employed in syphilis and in the beginning of malignant fevers (with violent cerebral congestions, delirium and constipation).

7. *Spiritus vitæ aureus.* RULAND'S *Golden Spirit of Life*, and KYPER'S *Spiritus panchymagogus* were prepared from *Alhandal*—the first with malmsey, and the second with anise (*Mart. Rul. in suis secret. spagyr. a Hagedornio edit.* c. 31). They were both esteemed as panaceas.

8. EMERICH, the Capuchin's *polychrest extract*, contained, besides colocynth, nearly thirty different substances, including, of course, the usual drastics; whereupon TRILLER exclaims—*facinorosa societas, apage!*

Colocynth enters also into the composition of the *Hiera Rufi*, the *Pil. lucis* of Mesué, the *Pil. de Hermodactilis majores*, the *Pil. fœtidæ majores et minores*, the *Pil. cachecticæ Charas*, the *Pil. aperientes Stahlii* (with aloes, cinnamon and iron), the *Pil. hydragogæ* of Schlesier (with gamboge and croton oil), Janin's diuretic pills (a chaos of drugs which in grossness of conception falls little short of Emerich's polychrest, containing fourteen other purgatives), Morrison's pills (with aloes, jalap, gamboge, and rhubarb *aa.*), Halle's *elixir vitæ*, the *Elixir purgans Herlini*, the acoustic essence, Barbett's *Spiritus aurium*, the *Unguentum de Arthanita* (*Rad. Azar. Europ.*), the *Oleum contra vermes*, Habakuk's oil,† and in many other pharmaceutical compounds, which are now, thank Heaven, mostly forgotten.

CHAPTER IV.

Knowledge of the positive effects of Colocynth on the healthy Organism before Hahnemann.

The knowledge on the subject of the effects of Colocynth on the human body previous to Hahnemann was principally derived from a few cases of poisoning which chance had presented to the observation of STALPAART VAN DER WIEL, TULPIUS, HOYER, PLATER, HOFFMANN and others. We shall be pardoned the slight anachronism, if to these older cases we add, for convenience sake, a few of later occurrence.

* "*Ipsa* (*confectio*) *diffusa mole et formula non congruens sæculi moribus, quod doses exiguas amat et sectatur.*" Thus a century before Hahnemann—Schulze wrote his dissertation in 1734—the world of patients were already demanding homœopathic doses! This electuary, with the application of *dialthæa* to the soles, cured a constipation that had withstood every other remedy (*Fried. Hoffmann*, *opera omnia*, tom. I, pars II, c. 5, and *Schulze op. cit.*)—*Watzke.*

† This Habakuk was *Loew*, the Prague professor. (See *Triller*).—*Watzke.*

1. Stalpaart Van der Wiel (*Observ. cent. I, obs.* 41) relates the case of a young, vigorous tavern-keeper at the Hague, who being in want of a good laxative, bought a colocynth apple, crushed and ate it. Soon after, he was attacked with unutterable colic pains and had bloody stools, followed by such violent cramps that he was rolled up like a hedgehog. It was with difficulty that his life was saved by the persevering application of the appropriate remedies.

2. A lad of 17 took a decoction of colocynth. Immediately afterward appeared bloody stools, horrible anxiety and fainting, great prostration and death. (*Hoyer, Ephem. Nat. curios. dec. III, arv.* 7, *obs.* 178.)*

3. A poor man, suffering from habitual constipation, drank a decoction prepared from three apples, and was affected in consequence with such extreme colic and so dreadful a hemorrhage from the anus that he nearly died. He was saved by copious draughts of oil and oily enemata (*Nic. Tulpius, obs.* lib. IV. c. 25).

4. Plater relates two cases. The first (*Ejusd. obs.* lib. III, p. 839) was that of a young prince to whom his physician prescribed purging pills, but finding them ineffectual changed them for powdered colocynth pulp. The patient had innumerable bloody evacuations and severe colic, whereupon the frightened doctor took to his heels. The second case ended fatally (*l. c. p.* 640). A man accustomed to purges was in the habit of drinking wine in which a colocynth apple had been soaked over night. He had often done it without injury, but it finally brought on a mortal dysentery. †

5. Riedlinus, who manifests great dread of colocynth and declares (*Lineæ med.* 1696 *mens. Jul. obs.* 2) that he had only employed it once in his whole practice, saw violent vomiting ensue upon the administration of two grains to a robust, stout-built servant-girl. Böcler says that those who handle colocynth for a long time become affected with vomiting (*Hartmanni Mat. Med.* 1745, p. I, p. 335). Sachse saw vomiting induced by laying it upon the stomach (*Hufel. Jour.* 1811, *April*).

6. Michaelis (*Kleinert's Rep. Jahr.* 7, 10, 95) states that the extract of colocynth laid upon the bare skin of the epigastrium, produced diarrhœa.

7. Chretien noticed frequently increased evacuation of fæces and urine from the external application of colocynth upon the abdomen (*Univ. Lex. der Pr. Med. u. Chir. Leipz.* 1839. *Art. Jatroleptica*).

8. C. G. Neumann states that violent colic and frothy diarrhœa

* Hoyer refers in the same place to the case of a man who had been so powerfully purged by colocynth, that no other purgatives would subsequently affect him.—*Watzke.*

† The quotation from Celsus, given by Schulze in elucidation of this fact, is worthy of the attention of provers. "*Possunt quædam subesse corpori vel ex infirmitate ejus, vel ex aliquo affectu, quæ vel in alio non sunt, vel in hoc alias non fuerunt eaque per se non tanta, ut concitent morbum, tamen obnoxium magis aliis injuriis corpus efficiunt.*"—*Watzke.*

with blood were produced by frictions with tincture of colocynth ($\frac{1}{4}$) and castor oil ($\frac{3}{4}$) (*Bemerk, üb. die gebräuch. Arzneim. S.* 15).

9. Fordyce relates (*Fragm. Chir. et Med.* p. 66) that a woman who had taken an infusion of colocynth in beer, had suffered thirty years (?) from colic! Friederich Hoffmann (*Op. omn. Gen.* 1740, pars III, p. 332), observed the frequent sudden occurrence of a fatal inflammation of the intestines after the use of colocynth in ascites.

10. Joh. Moritz Hoffmann was fortunate enough to witness one of the best cases of this sort. We insert his fine description in his own words: "*Ex generosa familia nata matrona tenera, post acidularum Egranarum finitum potum ex recepto more a sordibus residuis repurgatura, pomum colocynthidis vini cyatho per noctem infundit et insequente matutino tempore ebibit. Ast pessimis suis rebus. Accedebat siquidem mox insignis cardialgia, superveniebant vomitus creberrimi et cum ventris torminibus atrocissimis dejectiones alvinæ, primo mucoso-serosæ, mox biliosæ, tandem cruentæ; sitis aderat clangosa atque superiorum et inferiorum artuum musculares fibræ in subsultus et motus agitabantur spasticos; febrili æstu totum corpus exardescebat; demum cum animi deliquiis extremorum frigus notabatur ut adeo terrore et metu perculsi, adstantes me advocare curarint*" (*Eph. Nat. cur. Cent. X. obs.* 30).

11. Scheel observed a similar case of poisoning (*Beiträge Mecklen. Aerzte zur Med. u. chir. von Hennemann,* 1830 B. 1, H. 2). A woman upwards of forty had for a long time been affected with rheumatic pains in the left shoulder and thigh. A tailor advised her to boil half a pound of colocynth (*gichtbeeren*) in a measure and a half of red wine, and to drink the strained liquor before going to bed. Fortunately she divided the liquid into two parts; for she had hardly swallowed the first half before she was seized with frightful pains in the gastric region, great anxiety, vertigo, fainting fits, and convulsions. Frequent vomiting set in, followed by no relief; then evacuations, first fluid and feculent, then almost pure blood with dreadful tenesmus; the quantity evacuated amounted to five measures, and was accompanied by pieces of the intestinal lining membrane from 2 to 3 '' square. The pain then became concentrated in the stomach and lower part of the rectum; the abdomen fell in; finally the tenesmus ceased and she fell gradually asleep. The most effectual remedies were *oleosa, mucilaginosa* and *opium.* The patient was obliged to keep her bed a long while from weakness and dyspepsia, but was at length wholly restored.

12. The following case related by Carron d'Annecy was not so fortunate (*Orfila's Toxicol. 2d Edit.* p. 34). A man, æt. 28, who suffered from bleeding piles and dyspeptic troubles, drank two glasses of a decoction of colocynth, and experienced colic, frequent stools, and some hours later, great heat in the bowels, dryness of the pharynx and unquenchable thirst. Dr. Carron found the patient with a small, accelerated pulse, tongue red, abdomen tense and very sensitive to the touch, especially in the umbilical region, bowels constipated. Vene-

section, emollient fomentations, enemata and poultices were of no service, and on the succeeding day the abdomen was still more painful and tympanitic. Another bleeding and warm bath, and in six hours afterwards the pains had increased, there were retention of urine, retraction of the testicles and priapism. A dozen leeches to the anus, cupping on the abdomen and saltpetre injections. On the third day the retention of urine diminished, but the other symptoms continued; the pulse was small and contracted, and hiccough, coldness of the extremities and clammy sweat on the head and chest came on. In the evening the pains ceased, the bowels sank and there was manifest fluctuation; the patient died in the night. *Post-mortem examination.* Intestines red with black spots, for the most part glued together with fibrine (false membrane); a whitish fluid had been effused into the abdomen filled with a quantity of white flocks; ulceration here and there in the villous coat of the stomach; traces of inflammation in the liver, kidneys and bladder.

13. Dr. Carron was also called to see a young washerwoman who had drunk a decoction of colocynth and suffered from violent colic in consequence. Baths, oily, mucilaginous drinks and opium soon restored her.

14. The same author gives the case of a cachectic baker who took a decoction of colocynth for a quartan fever. He was cured of his fever, but remained weak, debilitated and chlorotic-looking, and died in six months of paralysis (*Orfila, Toxicol, gener.* 3, *edit.* p. 695).

15. Orfila (*Op. cit.*) heard of a man who took three colocynth apples to cure himself of a gonorrhœa of several years' standing. Immediately afterwards he had violent colic pains in the epigastrium and free vomiting; in two hours, copious stools, giving way of the lower limbs, dimness of sight, deafness, vertigo and slight delirium. The symptoms gradually disappeared after drinking copiously of milk, which caused vomiting, and the application of leeches to the abdomen.

16. The most interesting and instructive case of poisoning by colocynth is related by Duvergie and Ratier (*Univers. Lex. der pr. Med. u. Chir. Art. Coloc.*). A man fifty-five years old, of strong constitution, took for a swelling on the right knee a small quantity of a liquid which he had received from a female quack, and which subsequently proved to be tincture of colocynth. He was shortly afterwards seized with nausea and vomiting, with a feeling of heat and burning in the epigastrium. Full of insane joy at this result, he took a second and third dose to increase the effect. Copious, exceedingly frequent stools now came on, and such intolerable pains in the whole abdomen and so violent a colic that he sprang out of bed and rolled himself on the floor. And so infatuated was he that in the midst of his greatest suffering he blessed the hand that had administered the poison and pressingly besought the bystanders to give him a fresh dose of it. Convulsions of the most violent character soon set in, and the patient died in the evening. *Post-mortem examination.* The meninges were found white and somewhat thicker than natural; the cerebral

mass tolerably firm, but neither presenting red points nor injected; a small quantity of rose-colored serum in the lateral ventricles and cranial cavity; the vessels at the base of the brain somewhat engorged with blood. Lungs perfectly normal; stomach and duodenum externally purple, small intestines rose-colored; the mucous membrane of the first was vividly reddened, full of erosions, loosened and very easily removed. Similar abnormal appearances were found in the lower half of the small intestines, but less decided, and the large intestine was but little colored either externally or internally. The whole intestinal tract was empty.

It cannot be denied that the occurrence of such tragic cases of colocynth-poisoning is not calculated to induce practitioners to prescribe the drug at the bedside. Doubtless the original diseases of the stomach and bowels for which these individuals took the colocynth, played no small part in contributing to the violence of the symptoms; but inasmuch as in this very violence, the peculiar characteristics of colocynth are strongly marked, that circumstance detracts but little from the value of these involuntary physiological experiments. We have only to desire that some of the relaters had been more accurate and circumstantial in their details, and above all that we had an account of the *post-mortem* appearances in all the fatal cases.

CHAPTER V.

Hahnemann's Proving of Colocynth.

Hahnemann proved the Colocynth on himself and on six of his pupils. If we may draw a probable conclusion from the known effects to the unknown cause, we might infer that Hahnemann, Stapf, Rückert, Langhammer and Gutmann experimented with rather small doses, and Hahnemann's son Frederic and Hornburg with larger. The pictures of drug disease are obscure and lustreless; the characteristics of colocynth (which we have indicated in italics) are for the most part only hinted at, seldom sharply displayed.

1. *Hahnemann's Proving.*

Hahnemann, in other cases the very model of a bold drug prover, seems rather to have slighted colocynth; his own proving presents but few symptoms.* Bilious regurgitations, grumbling in the abdomen, water in the mouth, desire to drink without thirst, insipid taste in the mouth after drinking, pressure in the scrobiculus; constant pressure

☞* We have omitted the symptoms which Hahnemann himself designated as doubtful in the first edition. Why he removed the sceptical brackets in the third, he does not inform us.—*Watzke.*

and *bruised pain through the whole bowels ; tearing and tension in the left side of the face ;* sticking, tensive pain between the shoulder blades, obliging to walk bent over; bruised pain in the small of the back; *drawing tension in the right thigh ;* paralytic pain in the knee; weakness of the legs; shorter breath (for some days); coldness of the body; vivid distressing dreams; impotence.*

It is very doubtful whether Hahnemann himself, not to speak of others, would have recognized the action of colocynth in such grey, misty shadows of subjective symptoms, had he not known the drug beforehand.

2.—*Stapf's Proving.*

Stapf's Proving is but little more characteristic. "*Metallic taste on the point of the tongue ;* scraping in the palate; fine sticking on the velum palati as if from a beard of grain; scraping and tickling in the larynx, causing a dry cough (after an hour); *colicky pain* and discharge of flatulence, *with some inflation of the abdomen ; empty feeling in the abdomen as if after a diarrhœa ;* vertigo when rapidly turning the head; *pressive headache along the sagittal suture aggravated by moving the head and stooping ;* itching sticking in the ear; compressive pain in both the large cervical muscles (sterno-cleido mastoids?) disappearing on motion."

3.—*Rückert's Proving.*

In Rückert's case, too, it is hard to discover an occasional glimpse of

* In the third edition, Hahnemann adds, among the "*symptoms observed upon himself,*" some thirty new ones. "The highest ill-humor, and peevishness; the roots of the hair are painful; excoriated pain in the eyelids; stinging burning under the upper eyelid; painful looseness of an inferior incisor; tasteless saliva in the mouth (Is not the saliva normally tasteless? *Ed. Œst. Zeit.*) *;* bitter taste in the mouth after drinking beer; pressing pain in the stomach; occasional violent inflation of the abdomen; bruised pain in the hypogastrium, worse when walking and when sitting bent over; flatulent colic towards midnight, pain in the groin as though a hernia were protruding and as if it were replaced on pressing on the spot (for half an hour); squeezing from the side of the hypogastrium towards the groin; cuttings and stitches in the bowels from accumulated flatulence; itching stitch in the rectum; blind piles with pain in the anus; tearing through the urethra and glans; itching in the right testicle; violent sexual impulse with erections—nocturnal attack of asthma, with slow heavy breathing inducing cough; pressing drawing in the arm-bones; cramp in the calves; tearing in the heels; unusual disposition of the muscles to cramp; stinging itching here and there in the evening in bed, preventing sleep; irresistible propensity to sleep and inclination to lie down; sleeplessness."

Hahnemann does not tell us whether he had made any new provings of colocynth, and as it is well known that many of the symptoms of his antipsoric remedies were derived from the sick, and as we see also that he puts the symptoms of those affections which were cured by colocynth side by side with those obtained from provings on the healthy, and finally, as these symptoms, if obtained from actual provings, are partly sufficiently established by other more reliable testimony and partly seem to present a picture foreign to the effects of colocynth as exhibited in our researches—for these reasons we have thought fit to surround them in our *pure* Materia Medica with the most conspicuous of sceptical brackets.—***Watzke.***

the characteristic symptoms of Colocynth:—"Slight pressure in the head; feeling of thirst in the pharynx; sensation of pressure in the gastric region and *feeling of hunger* especially after eating; cutting pressing and *transitory cutting in the epigastrium;* pressure on the chest and in the bowels especially when sitting bent over and in the evening, for six days; *excoriating cutting in the hypogastrium, commencing when walking and increased by every step* (after 5 d.); hard stool (after 5–6 d.); pressure with a dull stitch in the scrobiculus; dull stitches in the right chest during inspiration, after an hour, during expiration after six days; stitches under the false ribs and scapula; stitches (after 4 h.) and bruised pain (after 5 days) in the arms; sticking tearing and tearing sticking in the thigh;* tensive pressure on the tibia; tearing in the calves; pressive tearing in the ancle; feeling of warmth creeping over the whole body (after 2 h.); he feels unwell, *peevish and taciturn.*

4.—*F. Hahnemann's Proving.*

The symptoms of F. Hahnemann appear to be the result of more numerous and somewhat energetic provings—though few in number, they still sketch out the Colocynth picture in bold strokes.

Soon after the dose, *bitterness in the mouth and severe nausea,* the first lasting four hours, the other on one occasion two, on another eight hours; accompanied by *rough feeling on the tongue as if from sand.* In one experiment the nausea was followed by twice vomiting of food.

After the lapse of scarce an hour there came on with violent chilliness, vertigo and dulness in the head, *pain across the hips* and trembling of the feet (as if from fright); *dreadful colic extending from a little spot beneath the navel and spreading* (*after eating*) *over the whole abdomen obliging him to bend forward and double himself up.* In another proving, *the colic remained fixed in a single spot in the umbilical region; it was sticking, compelled him to bend forward, was much aggravated by straightening himself up* and lasted eighteen hours. *The colic became much less in both instances after greenish yellow diarrhœic stools,* in the first experiment fifteen in eighteen hours. It was also ameliorated by smoking tobacco.†

5.—*Langhammer's Proving.*

We give these symptoms in his own chronological order. "Dull stitch in the forehead; shuddering over the whole body with cold hands, the face and rest of the body being warm, without thirst; *noisy discharge of flatulence; frequent urging to urinate with scanty emission;*

* The timid prover generally recognizes dimly and with difficulty his doubtful symptoms, and hence hesitates and wavers in his choice of words to express them. A well developed drug disease gives the prover but little trouble in the selection of his descriptive terms.—*Watzke.*

† The potato was probably only accidentally connected with the violent colic and rapid evacuation which followed the eating of it (S. 87).—*Watzke.*

white tongue (in the morning as if after much smoking); *fluent coryza;* whistling inspiration; hiccough; pimples in the face; *violent headache* disappearing in the open air; tearing in the dorsum of the foot; *violent drawing in the right thumb;* tearing sticking in the whole body; itching in different parts now here now there; boring stitches in the temple; weakness with trembling of the legs and sweat over the whole body; pressive pain in the orifice of the urethra after urinating; *hacking cough when smoking;* sleep disturbed by voluptuous dreams; sweat on the legs early on waking; *disinclination to talk.*

A proving which comes exceedingly near to having no significance at all! There is but little sign of Colocynth in the whole of it.

6.—*Gutmann's Proving.*

Gutmann's proving presents us with an excellent but at the same time a *very anxious* prover. What a pity he only experimented with small doses! Our numerous experiments lead us to the opinion that many of the following symptomatic minutiæ are simply due to the strained attention of the prover.

"*Dulness of the head especially in the sinciput; tearing pain in the whole brain, aggravated by moving the upper eyelids; pressing headache in the sinciput aggravated by bending forward and by lying on the back* (lasting six hours); *burning pain in the cheeks,* skin of the forehead, scalp and eyelids; itching, burning and *cutting in the ball of the eye;* compression, crawling and cutting sticking in the ear; *thumping and digging pain from the middle to the root of the nose;* twitching in the muscles of the chin; tearing in the inner side of the cheek and on the point of the tongue; stitches in the fauces; foul taste; bitter taste after drinking beer; *tensive, griping colic, disappearing on pressure;* tension and boring in the groin; *digging and tearing in the umbilical region, aggravated by expiration and laughing;* hard stool; *sticking in the right loin only perceptible during inspiration, worst when lying on the back;* itching stitch in the anus; creeping and crawling on the chest and abdomen; griping and muscular twitchings in the right ribs; *excoriated pain in the left scapula;* prickling burning in the right upper arm; itching sticking in the bend of the elbow; tension in the forearm; *cramp in the palm so that he can scarcely open his fingers; pain in the right thigh, as if the psoas muscle were too short, only when walking;* needle-like stitches in the ham, on motion; pain in the varices of the leg; vibrations, sharp cutting, itching sticking in the calves; itching, boring stitch in the dorsum of the foot; *tearing in the right sole, worst when at rest;* somnolence; lascivious dreams; depression; disinclination to intellectual labor; *disinclination to talk.*

7.—*Hornburg's Proving.*

This is by far the best of the Hahnemannian provings. Like F. Hahnemann, he probably made repeated experiments and in none of his colleagues do we find the characteristic symptoms of Colocynth stand out so strongly pronounced.

"*Head dismal and dreary as if after a night of debauchery; drawing, one-sided headache* (after ½ h.); pressing and drawing behind the left ear; *pain in the left lower row of teeth, as if the nerve were dragged; empty eructations;* pressure in the stomach as if from a stone; empty, at another time full, feeling in the abdomen; sensation in the bowels as if from having caught cold or improper mixture of food; *growling, griping, cutting, cramping and plucking in the abdomen; increased constriction in the hypogastrium every ten or twelve minutes,* accompanied by an internal shuddering through the cheeks ascending from the abdomen; *pain in the whole abdomen and especially below the navel, as though the bowels were squeezed between stones occasionally so severe* that the blood rose into his face and head and *sweat broke out on these parts, with muscular distortion of the face and closing of the eyes. He could neither lie quietly nor sit and could only walk entirely bent over. The pains were ameliorated by pressure with the hand and by bending forward;* they also became less after violent exercise and turning around; *they disappeared entirely after a cup of coffee. Violent, frequently recurring inclination to stool which could only be resisted by the strongest efforts.* Stool, scanty, tough and mucous or copious, yellowish-brown, thin, frothy with a sourish putrid taste; accompanied by a feeling at the termination of the rectum as though the parts had been weakened by a chronic diarrhœa. The colic was relieved by the evacuation but soon returned. Rumbling of flatulence; *inclination to stool immediately after eating;* continuous pressure over the pubes *with frequent urgency to urinate and scanty emission. Drawing pain from the right side of the neck to a point over the scapula as though the nerves and vessels were rendered tense; stiffness and violent drawing pain of the left side of the neck and nape, aggravated by motion;* feeling of weight in the nape; sprained feeling behind the right scapula; burning pain in the right middle finger; tickling pressure in the left buttock; the left foot goes to sleep; decrease of the quickness of the pulse from the commencement to the tenth hour; then internal and external heat of the body; a great variety of dreams, voluptuous, with pollutions.

Postcript concerning some errors in the Hahnemannian provings. It was with the greatest astonishment that we perceived in the third edition of Colocynth (*Antips. Rem.* part 3, *Düsseld.* 1837) the name of Ægidi among those of the provers of Colocynth and the symptoms 22, 29, 75 and 114* referred to him and introduced among

* 22. Tearing digging through the brain, aggravated to an unbearable extent by moving the eyelids (*Compare Gutmann's proving*). 29. Stitches as if from knives in the right eyeball extending to the root of the nose. 75. Empty eructation causing palpitation and cramp in the pharynx and keeps up a constant inclination to choke and vomit. 114. Periodical attacks of frightful cutting in the abdomen extending from the renal region and drawing the thigh convulsively up to the abdomen, so that the patient had to assume the most bent position possible.—*Watzke.*

those resulting from provings upon the healthy organism. These are the preliminary symptoms of a disease which Ægidi cured with Colocynth! We shall subsequently allude to the case further.

Hahnemann also cites in addition to STALPAART, HOYER, TULPIUS, PLATER and HOFFMANN, whose observations we have introduced in the original in the foregoing chapter, ZACUTUS LUSITANUS, SCHENK, KÖLPIN and SALMUTH, as authorities upon the physiological effects of Colocynth.

The flux of ZACUTUS LUSITANUS (*Sympt.* 101, *first edit.*, to which we always refer because we consider it the best) is not the result of an experiment but a mere conjecture.* The verification of symptom 103 "Hæmorrhage from the anus some hours after death" cost us considerable trouble. Hahnemann cites SCHENK for it (*Obs. med. rar.*, lib. VII, obs. IV.); SCHENK cites CAMERARIUS (*In horto med. et phil.*) and *he* refers us to DODONÆUS (*Med. obs. exempl. rar. Lugd. Bat.* 1685, p. 22) where we are first informed that the symptom *was most probably derived from an apoplectic subject.* "*Monendum nonnullos colocynthidis manipulum—drachmam—decoctis ad enemata Apoplecticorum addere. Tale autem decoctum frequenter ad duo aut tria enemata sufficit. Excessus enim colocynthidis (in enemate) periculo non caret. Abradit enim hæc intestina et oscula aperit venarum. Memini ab enemate cui incocta fuerat colocynthidis drachma, hominem robustum non diu superfuisse et mox post mortem, aliquot deinde horis sanguinem copiosum per sedem effluxisse.*" Symptom 103 then should read thus, "Copious hæmorrhage from the anus appearing soon after death and continuing some hours." So far as we ourselves are concerned we should say that neither the death nor the flux of blood had any thing to do with the clyster. DIOSCORIDES also has observed anal hæmorrhages succeeding Colocynth injections (*Op. cit.*), but never in the healthy nor indeed in the dead.

Symptom 176 cited from KÖLPIN, "Itching of the skin with sweat immediately following;" 177, from the same, "Scabious eruption" (erroneously referred to *Hoffmann* in the third edition); and 144, "Abscesses under the shoulder and in other parts of the body" are of no value whatever on two grounds. First, because they were not observed in the well but on the sick, and second, because they would in all probability have equally manifested themselves as what are called critical phenomena, after the administration of any other drug proving to be the specific in the given case.† The same remark applies equally

* *Colocynthis per se sola offerri non debet, nam fauces et guttur vehementi incendio vexat, corpus inflammat, viscera dolore conturbat, abradit intestina, ora venarum aperit et dysenteriam molitur.* (*Zac. Lus. Op. Lugd.* 1667, tom. II, p. 93).—*Watzke.*

† That the reader may judge, we give KÖLPIN's case in full. A man, æt. 40, contracted a rheumatism in the nape in consequence of catching cold. Six months afterwards he presented the following case. "Upper and lower extremities unsusceptible of motion; obstinate constipation; discharge of urine at times involuntary, at times suppressed; the hypogastrium from the

to symptom 179 cited from SALMUTH, "Scaling off of the skin of the whole body."* The whole of these symptoms are to be purged from our *Materia Medica Pura!*

CHAPTER VI.

Martin's Proving of Colocynth and his Society for Provings in Jena.

MARTIN and his society, at least as far as their results are exhibited in *Noack* and *Trinks' Arzneimittellehre*, have not remarkably enlarged our knowledge of the action of Colocynth. The experimenters appear to have been somewhat too apprehensive and anxious; the symptoms obtained do not bear the impress of a drug-sickness but look rather like fragmentary and purely subjective phenomena. We designate by *the types*, whatever we seem to recognize in them as characteristic of Colocynth.

"Heaviness of the head; susceptibility to intoxication (from beer); dulness of the head; vertigo; transitory deafness with roaring in the ears (after eating); *aching in the forehead* (*with colic and urging to stool*); pressure over a spot in the *linea semicircularis;* burning in the head and face; painful drawing in the face, alternating with itching and

navel to the pubic region distended by a sometimes spherical, sometimes longish swelling. After purges, the swelling disappeared and the urine was discharged voluntarily, but on the other hand clonic convulsions of the lower limbs set in whenever the patient was raised or touched. After a fruitless employment of various remedies, twelve drops of tincture of Colocynth were given him every two hours. In a fortnight there was a manifestation of motor power in the lower limbs. At the end of five weeks there came on every afternoon troublesome itching with subsequent sweat, whereupon the power of the extremities increased (but still more in the evening than during the day). In the fourth month of the treatment the patient has an itchlike eruption, and as this disappeared, abscesses formed under the shoulders and in other parts of the body. During this time there was free motion of the limbs and the patient was perfectly well. The numbness and want of motive power lasted longest in the ends of the fingers.—(*Hufel. Jour.*, 3, 575).—*Watzke.*

* SALMUTH's case is as follows; (*Obs. med. Brunsv. Cent.* III). Robert Venthusen, a valet-de-chambre in Anhalt, became sick while a soldier at Rotterdam. A comrade had prescribed as a laxative an *Elixir* prepared from the pulp of a whole Colocynth apple. Besides the usual symptoms accompanying the accidental ingestion of the drug, there came on, not only bloody discharges from the anus but also from the mouth. These latter were violent, continuous, lasting several days and reducing the patient to such a state of debility that he had not strength to open his mouth and spit out the blood, but it was removed by the fingers of the bystanders. The physicians gave him up as lost and departed, but an old woman gave him common oil with beer to drink morning and evening and saved him in spite of the doctors. *During his convalescence the whole epidermis scaled off in pieces the size of a dollar;* it took him seven weeks to recover his strength and his skin.—*Watzke.*

accompanied by pain in a molar tooth; teeth on edge; canine hunger and heartburn afterwards in the throat; sour eructation; pressure in the stomach (after eating) with headache, indolence, gloomy ill-humor, flatulence and diarrhœa; rumbling in the stomach; great heat in the stomach; aching and pressing, constrictive dull-sticking pain in the scrobiculus; *colic with a feeling as if diarrhœa were coming on;* violent colics with restlessness and *benommenheit* (*? !*) *of the body* (*the pains diminished after a thin evacuation;* fluid evacuation followed by weakness, paleness and exhaustion; violent itching at the anus; *diminished secretion of urine; pollutions at night;* oppression (about the heart); constrictive pain in the fore-arm; *painful, constrictive pains in the hand* and from there towards the fore-arm, alternating with similar pains in the cheeks and abdomen; *painful drawing in the fore-arm and thigh* alternating with itching; little ulcers upon the skin, itching and burning; unusual burning of some slight cracks; great liveliness and sleeplessness; alternation of heat and coldness; frequent, momentary but ever recurring sweat and fainting vertigo, ameliorated by covering the eyes with the hand; clammy moisture on the head and chest; copious sweat smelling like urine on the head, hands, legs and feet; peculiar frame of mind which will allow no thought to be attentively considered."

CHAPTER VII.

Hechenberger's Kolocynthognostik.

Colocynth has in Dr. Hechenberger an ardent advocate and a stout defender, but a timid prover and a weak observer. His monograph* is one, the like of which, in spite of its deficiencies, we could desire to see multiplied among our opponents. *Noack* and *Trinks* rank him among the old school, but it seems to us not altogether justly—for he is a Homœopath, at least in respect to Colocynth, though a secret one and a particolored.

The symptoms observed and recorded by him are mostly confined to the intestinal functions. He seems to have exhausted the whole of his observing power in the how and the when of the alvine evacuations.

A single drop of the tincture administered morning and night, in a tablespoonful of water, seemed to have no effect upon persons not endued with special irritability, during the first five or six days. On persevering in the use, a copious strikingly brown, frequently black stool came on preceded by painless borborygmi. If the dose were still continued, the stools kept growing thinner, but always brown, with lively rumbling in the bowels. After three months' continuance of this

* *Kolocynthologie oder Beobachtungen über die vortrefflichen, viel zu wenig beachteten, Heilkräfte der Kolocynthis.*—Insb. 1840.

dose, Hechenberger had regularly a single soft stool in the evening of the same day.

A drop given early in the morning and repeated every two hours brought on diarrhœa in persons not torpid, by the afternoon and evening, but without colic or the usual inconveniences. From four to eight drops in a single dose in the morning occasioned slight diarrhœa the same afternoon, or at farthest the next morning, preceded by griping in the umbilical region.*

The further almost constant symptoms from the continued use of Colocynth were: *Striking increase of appetite* and thirst; *more copious secretion of urine*, the urine being often light-brown like beer, and becoming cloudy on cooling, a copious, sometimes sandy, sediment being deposited; *noisy discharge of a great deal of wind; gentle, painless renewal of the hæmorrhoidal flow, but leaving behind a peculiar burning around the anus and along the sacral region; menses more profuse and too early.*

A pregnant woman who had taken a tablespoonful of the tincture of Colocynth was attacked in five hours with dysenteric diarrhœa, bloody discharge and a severe burning pain along the sacral region. This was accompanied by violent swelling of the labia with feeling of bearing down and heat in the vagina. A little tincture of Opium in warm milk soon removed all the symptoms except the swelling of the vulva, which was unusually troublesome during the whole period of pregnancy.

Secondary torpidity of the *primæ viæ*, as a consequence of long continued use of Colocynth, was not observed by Hechenberger either in his own case or in that of others.

CHAPTER VIII.

The Vienna Provings.

We choose Jörg as our pattern in describing the results of the proving. Our reasons for so doing are apparent from our Introduction. We repeat, that we do not see that it is possible to understand aright the positive effects of a medicine when no insight is given into the development, succession, intensity, and duration of each case of medicinal disease, or into the character of the different symptoms, and that,

* In order to avoid anything out of the way in his practice that is to say, to avoid the reputation of being a Homœopath, Hechenberger ordinarily concealed the admirable effects of his Colocynth in a vegetable decoction (*Graswurzelabkochung*) from one to three drams of the tincture to the pound and administered a half or whole tablespoonful every two hours—a respectable dose, inasmuch as every tablespoonful contained from two to eight grains of the tincture. The mixture had to be preserved in water: it was omitted as soon as the least trace of griping was perceived. There was no perceptible effect for the first day, but on the continued use followed in the afternoon and finally in the forenoon also, griping boring and digging, especially in the flanks, and a soft diarrhœa in the evening or at night.—*Watzke.*

in fact, it is this deficiency in Hahnemann's Materia Medica that makes a revisal of it necessary. If it is said that the reading of individual cases of medicinal disease is equally a tax and a task, and that our Materia Medica will by this means grow to a huge mass of thick folios, and that, after all, an arrangement of the symptoms according to an artificial fixed plan will become necessary; we reply that we see this perfectly well, but know of no remedy. Let our colleagues who use this language console themselves with the reflection that it is at all events more easy and amusing to read such records of experiments than to make them on one's own body. The hyper-scrupulous particularity of *Koch*, who proved *Calcarea*, with his cloudy mornings, sunny days, and cool evenings, and the anxious observations of others on the changes of the moon and variations of the barometrical, thermometrical, and hygrometrical states of the atmosphere, will not be found in the records of our experiments. We have to come to the conclusion, from our trials with Colocynth and other medicines, that they are, if not of absolute, yet of so considerable an influence over the human frame as to be scarcely if at all affected by such causes.

Have we set to work in the proper manner? Was our mode and manner of experimenting the true Hahnemannic? Those will doubt it who think they have in the decillionth doses Hahnemann's secret of winning symptoms. We confess that the favourite maxim of so many provers of medicines—*to make themselves as little sick as possible, or if possible, not sick at all*—does not please us. (We regret to see it adopted by some of our colleagues, and these are those who send us subjective symptoms.) Our opinion is, that if our Materia Medica is to become what it must one day be, *a science, a systematic knowledge of the families, orders, and species of medicinal diseases*, it is not enough simply to experiment with doses barely sufficient to excite re-action; we ought rather to take doses so large and so long continued as to penetrate the system to a certain degree, and to exert a lasting effect on the various organs and their functions; nay, further, we must, at least in the case of the lower animals (fatal cases occurring to human beings affording a most important supplement), experiment in such a manner as gradually to accumulate the needful materials for an anatomy of medicinal diseases, until supplied with which the science of pharmacodynamics must remain imperfect.

Our association for the proving of Colocynth consisted of fifteen members, the results of whose experiments we give below in alphabetical order. We have only further to remark, that we used the tincture prepared as Hahnemann directs, and *that almost all of the provers were ignorant as to what medicine they were proving.*

8.—*Arneth's Proving with the Tincture.*

The proving of our colleague, Dr. Franz Hector Arneth, though one of the poorest in symptoms, is, in reference to the theory and practice of Homœopathy, one of the most interesting.

Arneth is 25 years of age, of choleric temperament, and strong constitution. In spite of vaccination when a child, he took the small-pox when 21 years of age, and got favorably through it. Since that time he has enjoyed uninterrupted good health.

Will he attribute it to our desire to meet the scepticism of our macroposological opponents in reference to the rarity and paradoxical character of his results, if we add to this physiological portrait drawn by himself, its psychological complement? We may say, then, that our colleague possesses as sound an understanding, as unprejudiced a spirit of observation, as much acumen, honorable feeling and devotion to the truth as the very best of our opponents.

1842, Nov. 1st. 1.30 A.M., *one drop;* 11 A.M., *five drops;* 9 P.M., *ten drops* tincture of Colocynth. He did not perceive the slightest result.

Nov. 2d. 6 A.M., *ten drops;* 11 A.M., *twelve drops;* 4.30 P.M., *twenty drops*, and two hours afterward *twenty-five drops*. No result.

Nov. 7th to 13th. *Ten drops* three times a day on the first, increasing the dose one drop every subsequent day. The result was equally fruitless, not the slightest trace of the effects of Colocynth appearing.

Nov. 14th and 15th. *Forty-five drops* twice a day on each day. From the 16th to the 23d he omitted the medicine and during this time he had, contrary to his usual habit, two pappy stools a day, with slight griping in the epigastric region.

Nov. 24th to 26th. The evacuations having become regular again on the 24th and 25th, he took at 1 P.M. of the 26th *fifty drops* of the tincture. Two pappy stools, one that evening, the other next morning, and abundant urination, were the only symptoms which he observed.

Nov. 27th. *Seventy drops*, taken at 11 A.M., increased the secretion of urine that day, and gave rise on the following day to griping in the epigastric region after each meal, worse towards evening, and pretty severe drawing pain in the left testicle, lasting about a quarter of an hour.

Nov. 29th. *Eighty drops* of the tincture at 2 P.M. Next morning a furuncular eruption made its appearance on the face, and on the 2d December another on the back. Both disappeared in a few days.

This concludes Dr. Arneth's experiments with the tincture, which he took pure and without a vehicle.

9.—*Arneth's Proving with the Dilutions.*

Dec. 7th. All traces of the former action of the medicine having disappeared for a long time, he took, morning and evening, *two tablespoonfuls of the third dilution* of the tincture of Colocynth, prepared in the proportion of 1 Colocynth to 100 distilled water, and had after it two pappy evacuations.

Dec. 8th. Next day *two tablespoonfuls of the third dilution*, shortly before going to bed; he had scarcely got into bed before he experienced in the epigastric region more violent griping than he had formerly felt from the mother tincture, but which did not bring on an evacuation.

Dec. 9th. He took, morning and evening, *two tablespoonfuls of the third dilution*, and had each time two pappy stools; he then passed to the second dilution of the tincture.

Dec. 10th to 14th. He daily took *two tablespoonfuls* about noon.

Dec. 11th. Towards evening, irritability of the larynx began, and the voice became rough and hoarse. Dec. 12th. Besides these symptoms, there was distressing dryness of the air-passages, and on the two next days a perceptible and disagreeable feeling of fatigue in the affected parts. *Each time after taking the medicine, he perceived a remarkable aggravation.* From the 10th onwards he had had two pappy evacuations daily.

Dec. 15th to 20th. The medicine was omitted until the foregoing symptoms had entirely disappeared.

Dec. 21st, 22d and 23d. He took, at noon and in the evening, *two tablespoonfuls of the second dilution* each time. Nothing occurred the first two days except the usual griping pains in the epigastric region, which also continued on the four following days, and the two daily pappy stools. On the night of the 23d, when lying in bed, drawing in the right shoulder.

Dec. 23d. In the afternoon, violent drawing pain in all the teeth of both jaws—a symptom which struck the prover the more, from his never having suffered from toothache before.

Dec. 24th. Besides the pain (drawing and tearing) in the teeth, which had lasted the whole day, he felt in the evening moderate tension in the region of the anterior superior spine of the ilium of the left side.

Dec. 25th. Next day this sensation, hitherto a tensive feeling confined to one point, changed into *a violent drawing, extending from the spine of the ilium to the inguinal region and the upper third of the inner surface of the thigh; it continued pretty violent all day*, and did not disappear till the 26th, with a very singular feeling of stiffness in the left great toe. The toothache had disappeared the preceding night.

Dec. 26th. *Two tablespoonfuls* in the evening; next day, at noon, *three*, and in the evening again, *two tablespoonfuls of the first dilution* of the tincture of Colocynth. On the 26th, before going to sleep, he noticed a slight prickling in the *conjunctiva palpebrarum* of the left eye. Next morning it was perceptibly inflamed;* here and there were indications of commencing ulceration, which continued to increase till four in the afternoon, when it was complete; next morning cicatrization had taken place.

"I should not," says Dr. Arneth, "have alluded to this catarrhal (?) inflammation of the conjunctiva, such occurrences, though with no

* We cannot sufficiently warn our friends who are proving drugs, against the use of *mere names*. The symptoms should be *accurately described*. We want the *species facti*, not the hypotheses of the prover. Arneth calls this series of symptoms a *catarrhal inflammation*. We see in it neither catarrh nor inflammation, but only fusion of conjunctival miliary tubercles, such as we frequently see upon the cornea of children. Others would see in it fragments of a scrofulous ophthalmia with phlyctenæ, others something else. Such little abscesses, however—ruptured phlyctenæ—commonly leave no cicatrices, at least none visible upon the conjunctiva.—*Watzke*.

tendency to ulceration, not being uncommon with me, did it not seem to me likely that the unusually rapid cicatrization was due to the medicine; and I am the more inclined to this opinion from a catarrhal ophthalmia running a precisely similar course, having been one of the first symptoms which I noticed in the beginning of November, immediately after the first doses of the mother tincture, but which I did not put down, because its occurring once did not seem a sufficient warrant to attributing to the medicine a malady not uncommon to me."

10.—*Arneth's Proving with Higher Dilutions.*

Arneth was now desirous of ascertaining whether still higher dilutions would affect him, and how. He first waited until he no longer perceived the slightest trace of the former operation of the drug, and as from Dec. 27th, when he took the last dose of the first dilution, to January 6 (1843), he experienced great inclination to diarrhœa and frequently had three stools a day, it was only on Jan. 9th that he began the proving.

Jan. 9th. On this and the two following days at noon *two tablespoonfuls of the fourth dilution.* Soon after taking the first dose he had *violent eructations* lasting about half an hour—a symptom he had not had from the tincture nor from the lower dilutions.

Jan. 10th. Drawing and tearing in the right shoulder-joint in the morning, lasting all day. Painful feeling of tension in the left patella in the evening.

Jan. 11th. The pain in the patella became so considerable that walking was painful; patella hot and somewhat swollen on undressing in the evening, with an indistinct pulsation in the swelling. Itching in the anus all day. Stools natural.

Jan. 12th. The symptoms all disappeared.

Arneth could discern no effects from repeated experiment *with the fifth dilution.*

Must we attribute the want of effect from large doses, while in the same individual, small doses produce symptoms, solely to an idiosyncracy of the prover? Had the large doses which preceded in this case excited a susceptibility for the smaller ones? Can it be that in *dilutions* of vegetable tinctures (perhaps exceptionally) a similar process takes place as is known to occur in the trituration of mercury, gold, platina and other substances, which are thus first rendered fit for absorption into the fluids and circulation of the economy, and for the development of their medicinal powers? Is it not shown by Arneth's provings that, in many cases, the cure of the patient depends *solely* upon the dilutions of the drug?

11.—*Böhm's first Proving with the Tincture.*

Dr. Jac. Karl Böhm, æt. 40, of choleric temperament, rather weak, small, pale and lean, subject to blennorrhœas of all sorts, accustomed to the greatest moderation, never affected with any serious illness but atoning for every error in diet by a violent fit of colic, and apparently a highly susceptible subject for the action of Colocynth, and a very cautious prover.

Nov. 15th and 17th. He took on each of these days, in the morning, fasting, *two drops of tincture of Colocynth*, and on the 19th *three drops*. There was no notable effect. A week later he took in the same manner *six drops*. Immediately after dinner on the same day, violent cutting in the hypogastrium, forcing him to stool, and a fluid evacuation.

12.—*Böhm's Second Proving.*

Dec. 3d. *Twelve drops* in the forenoon. Slight colic in the umbilical region, soon afterwards; little appetite at noon; violent eructation after eating, cutting in the hypogastrium, and a fluid stool, with rectal tenesmus. The cuttings in the abdomen and the tenesmus lasted all the afternoon and only disappeared entirely in the evening when he got warm in bed. He slept well and felt well on waking while in bed, but soon after rising, he had a fresh attack of the umbilical colic and frequent eructations. On going out he felt very weak, had little appetite at noon, a fluid stool after eating, with discharge of flatulence and painful feeling in the abdomen the whole afternoon, which was only removed as before when he got warm in bed. These symptoms were daily renewed from Dec. 5th to Dec. 13th, when he took *Cocc.* as an antidote, and all his troubles rapidly disappeared.

13.—*Böhm's Third Proving.*

Dec. 24th. Böhm had the courage to repeat his experiment by taking *one drop* of the tincture triturated with sugar of milk. He repeated the dose for the next three days without the slightest result.

14.—*Böhm's Fourth Proving.*

1843, Jan. 3d. Böhm began a new series of experiments. How long it was continued he does not state, nor does he give us the phenomena in detail, but sums them up generally thus: "As often as the dose exceeded three drops of the tincture, cutting in the umbilical region and tenesmus came on after eating, and there remained for several days increased sensitiveness of the whole abdomen and constipation.

Since the sensitive bowels of our colleague (at least so he thinks) often suffered from the same symptoms without the intervention of Colocynth, it remains doubtful whether the phenomena produced by his few and timid experiments owed anything to the drug which he took. The results of provings upon the diseased organism, however carefully they may have been conducted, have, alas! but a very problematical value.

15.—*Fleischmann's Proving with the Tincture.*

Dr. Wilhelm Fleischmann, æt. 41, of choleric temperament, tolerably strong constitution, suffering for several years from various forms of gout, began his experiments with *five drops* of the tincture. As this produced no effect, he took on the second day *ten* and on the third, *fifteen drops.* Violent griping in the umbilical region lasting all day, feeling of coldness in the abdomen, looseness of the bowels. These symptoms lasted with more or less intensity for several days, and he omitted the Colocynth for nearly three weeks in consequence. He then began again with *ten drops.* Besides the above mentioned very troublesome symptoms he now had during the first days *discharge of blood from the anus, which after more than a year, still continues in greater or less quantity daily, with violent sticking and burning pain in the small of the back and anus;* he concluded he would not subject his gouty body to any further experience with Colocynth. *Before this proving he had never had a discharge of blood from the anus.*

16.—*Fröhlich's Proving of the Tincture on Himself.*

Dr. Ernst Hilarius Fröhlich, æt. 32, of sanguineous temperament, light hair and blue eyes, had tinea capitis when young. Subsequently had and still suffers somewhat from small furuncles on the face and back, is inclined to a sub-inflammatory affection of the larynx with hoarseness, to constipation and swelling of the hæmorrhoidal vessels; he proved the Colocynth on himself, on two girls and on several rabbits.

1842, Nov. 21st. *Five drops of the tincture* in half a glass of water at 6 A.M. fasting. No result during the day. *Ten drops* in the evening with the same effect.

Nov. 22d. *Ten drops* this morning fasting. No traces of action during the forenoon, but at about half past one P.M., seven hours after the dose, umbilical colic, with painful stitches in the bladder, and subsequently alternately in the rectum, disappearing on the discharge of flatulence. This was accompanied by transient headache, feeling as if the temples were screwed into, with heaviness of the eyelids without sleepiness. These symptoms disappeared after a cup of black coffee taken after dinner, except an inconsiderable griping in the left flank. Copious discharge of clear, watery urine during the whole day, and one soft but not copious stool.

Nov. 23d and 24th. Fröhlich woke with a slight griping around the navel. *Twenty drops of the tincture.* Half an hour afterwards loud rumbling in the intestines, with discharge of inodorous flatulence; griping around the navel, increased by eating fruit; transient stitches in the upper jaw, frequently recurring in the left flank and along the external border of the left sole; cramplike drawing in the right calf. These symptoms lasted all day and did not diminish after taking black coffee. At 7 P.M. of the same day *twenty drops.* The night was quiet, but the whole of the next day, the 24th, which was foggy, he felt uncomfortably chilly and had continual griping about the navel. In the evening he was very weak, the small of the back and lower limbs were painful as if after a forced march, and a tearing sticking pain encircled the right internal malleolus.

Nov. 24th and 25th. Nevertheless on the evening of the same day (24th) he took *twenty drops* more, and on the following morning *twenty-five drops* of the tincture. An hour after the last dose an easily resisted inclination for stool, and subsequently a half watery, half solid evacuation. The ingestion of some beer (at 11 A.M.) caused violent griping in the stomach, coming on in paroxysms and only disappearing after dinner. No other symptoms. In the evening *forty drops*. This was followed by no symptoms except a violent constrictive pain in the umbilical region, lasting a quarter of an hour, and which waked him from sleep the following morning at 3 A.M.

Nov. 28th and 29th. Having been several days without medicine and without symptoms he took *forty drops* on each of these days in the morning, fasting. In the forenoon, griping around the navel; urging to stool easily resisted; after dinner with a little wine, the griping and urging increased, and an almost formed stool followed, accompanied by slight tenesmus. The colic and violent urging to stool however continued until towards 4 P.M., when a second scanty stool occurred, accompanied by some mucus.

Nov. 30th. Fröhlich concluded his experiments by taking *sixty drops* of the tincture in the morning fasting, and *forty drops* in the evening. The results were very trifling, notwithstanding the heroic doses. Colic and griping about the navel, somewhat increased after dinner, and ceasing an hour afterward. In the evening, painful lassitude in the small of the back and lower extremities; flying stitches in the humeri.

Dec. 1st. On the following morning, pain in the ancle coming on when walking in the street, as if from a false step, ceasing when at rest; feeling of stiffness in the hands, continuing longer.

Dec. 2d to 7th. Stitches in the ancle; tearing in the shoulder; a stitch, occasionally deep, in the left flank; feeling of weariness in the small of the back, and a viscid, soft, scanty stool every three days.

Is this slender amount of symptoms due to the peculiar unsusceptibility of our colleague to the action of Colocynth? Or was he too hasty in his proving, thus disturbing the normal formation of the Colocynth sickness and preventing the maturing of the commencing symptoms? Or, again, did he take too large or too small doses, or did he conclude the proving too soon? His usual manner of life was not altered during his experiment.

17.—*Fröhlich's Proving of the Third Dilution on Two Girls.*

Fröhlich prescribed the third dilution of Colocynth in pellets to a weaver upwards of fifty, who suffered from pain in the small of the back, with instructions to take five of them three times a day. The patient was much better on the following day and told Fröhlich with a smile that his two daughters and his son had also taken the pills. The whole three experienced symptoms similar to those of Colocynth, and Fröhlich engaged the daughters to continue the experiment and to watch their symptoms more closely, under the superintendence of their invalid brother. Both young women were intelligent, occupied in weaving, and lived after their usual fashion, except that they drank no coffee, wine, nor beer.

18.—*First Proving with the Third Dilution.*

Amalie Ph., 22 years old, a soft delicate brunette, had recovered from chlorosis six months before, but still menstruated scantily and looked pale.

1843, April 29th. *Took two pellets moistened with the third dilution of Colocynth.* Soon after the dose, *inodorous eructations and unusual discharge of flatulence;** subsequently, *drawing tearing pains in the whole abdomen and in the finger-joints of the left hand.*

May 1st. *Three pellets. Copious, inodorous eructations; drawing in the nape* and in the dorsal muscles.

May 3d. *Three pellets. Pain in the small of the back; tearing drawing in both thighs and in the left arm down to the finger-joints.*

May 5th. *Four pellets.* Drawing in the left hypochondrium; *tearing in the left calf as far as the heel.*

May 9th. *Six pellets. Stitches penetrating deep into the abdomen; tearing in the joints of the left hand.*

The symptoms developed during the further progress of this experiment with globules administered every three or four days until June 6th, were either precisely similar to those already related or in the highest degree analogous. They generally appeared in from six to seven hours after the dose, lasted from nine to ten hours, and even manifested themselves the subsequent day in feeble repetitions.

19.—*Second Proving with the Third Dilution.*

Caroline Ph., æt. 24, of a lively disposition, strong constitution, brown hair and grey eyes, took the same doses as her sister, and had in every respect similar symptoms. She had, however, more frequently than her sister, isolated deep stitches as if from a needle, sometimes in the left sometimes in the right flank, apparently connected with the ovaries. Neither of them experienced any other symptom connected with the genital system.

20.—*Gerstel's Proving.*

Dr. Heinrich Gerstel, æt. 38, phlegmatico-sanguineous temperament, stout, full-blooded constitution, the father of healthy children, had never been very sick since his sixth year, when he had the hooping-cough violently. He is rather disposed to dyspeptic difficulties, cramp in the stomach, and diarrhœa (after taking cold in the feet), besides slight rheumatism, frequent palpitations and moderate hæmorrhoidal

* The italics indicate those symptoms which we attribute with confidence to the Colocynth.—*Watzke.*

bleeding every four to eight weeks. He has also been affected for several years with a torpid sensibility of the whole right side of the body, appearing clearly only after mental emotions. This most scrupulous observer, and of all our provers the obtainer of the most copious symptoms, instituted six experiments.

21.—*First Proving with the Tincture.*

1842, Nov. 20th, 4.30 P.M. *Fifteen drops of the tincture* of Colocynth, an hour and a half after a moderate dinner. The following symptoms all appeared within an hour and a half, mostly when seated.

A few minutes after the dose, a slow stitch on the right side beneath the navel; soon afterward on the left side of the navel, colic only perceptible when walking, disappearing when standing still, and even on violent agitation (as in going down stairs), but immediately becoming very perceptible again on walking on a level; drawing in the upper teeth of the right side, with feeling as if the upper lip was swollen; constant ringing in the right ear; slight flatulent inflation of the epigastric region, with pulsation in the small of the back, ameliorated by the emission of flatulence; general hot flush, especially in the face, with sweat on the forehead; compressive squeezing around the middle of the left leg as if from a narrow ribbon; copious discharge of flatulence.

22.—*Second Proving with the Tincture.*

Nov. 22d. *Twenty-five drops of the tincture* in the morning fasting, after his normal evacuation.

Soon after the dose, rumbling in the abdomen and *deep seated pulsation in it* when lying down, not perceptible to the hand laid upon it; sticking in the pubic region; transitory tickling itching on the thigh, and the same repeatedly in the face, shoulders, flanks, as well as on the point of the glans, with urging to urinate. On rising up, empty eructations. *Feeling of numbness* longitudinally along the external side of the right calf as though in the track of a nerve. This feeling increased in extent as if the nerve were swollen in its periphery, passed gradually into a dull pressing constrictive sensation and slowly disappeared. Soon afterward, the same feeling on the dorsum of the first joint of the great toe of the same side, and a similar but weaker sensation under the nail of the left great toe. Constrictive pressing in the dorsum and ancle of the left foot and in the right upper arm. Repeated urging to urinate.

All these symptoms appeared in the course of an hour while quietly lying in bed. Half an hour later he perceived: griping in the hypogastrium, going off in a stitch towards the left pubic region, with rumbling and sensation of inflation; immediately afterward, dulness of the right side of the head, especially in the temple; numbness of the right fore-arm; dull stitches in the left leg; yawning; lassitude copious urination.

23.—*Third Proving with the Tincture.*

Nov. 23d. *Forty drops of the tincture* at 7 A.M., fasting.*

A tearing in the left side of the nape, which he had experienced yesterday before taking the Colocynth, and which was aggravated during the action of the drug and afterward entirely disappeared, becomes again excited. Sticking pressure in various parts of the body. Some swelling of the abdomen about the navel, accompanied by slight dulness of the head in the forehead and temples, and a return of the vexatious thought which he had forgotten, but which soon yielded to an unusual cheerfulness (curative effect? *Gerstel*). Sensitiveness of the incisor teeth; tickling itching on the right arm, disappearing on scratching; empty eructations; unusual thirst; burning in the urethra after urinating; burning and excoriated pain, with moisture, at the anus, as if after a diarrhœa, and stitches in the rectum.

24.—*Fourth Proving with the Tincture.*

Nov. 23d. *Twenty-three drops of the tincture* at 11 P.M., just before going to bed.

Immediately afterward, pain in the vertex and left eye, as if a nervous pressure (? *Ed. Oest. Zeit.*); colic with violent rumbling, as if from the bursting of large bubbles; copious discharge of flatulence; drawing twitching with dull throbbing in the left iliac region, and in the right loin over the crista ilii towards the buttock; pain as though pressure were made upon both eyeballs from above downwards; burning of the under lip; prickling in the end of the glans; feeling as if from an incipient catarrh; heat, especially in the upper part of the body.

He fell asleep about half an hour after the dose. Once when he awoke in the night, he felt an unusual warmth over the whole body, but especially in the lower limbs.

Nov. 24th. In the morning, soon after waking, sticking drawing pains, now here now there. The usual normal stool was soon followed by one of pappy consistence and subsequent burning in the anus, and at the same time prickling in the orifice of the urethra after urinating.

Towards noon, *colic appearing only when walking*, disappearing every time he stood still. The pain arising from the epigastric region extended when it became more severe upwards towards the chest, and became then constrictive; it was sensibly aggravated by every shock, violent hawking and the like. The bowels were painful on strong pressure on the abdomen, as if excoriated; unusual thirst; another pappy stool.

Soon after dinner, when walking in the open air, oozing at the anus and discharge of moisture from the rectum instead of the expected flatulence. The oozing continued the whole afternoon; at 6 P.M. another

* A quarter of an hour earlier, he had a slight fit of vexation, which, however, soon gave place to a peaceful state of mind. Breakfast an hour after the dose, as usual of cold uncooked milk; at noon, plain food and water, the prover's only beverage now as ever.—*Watzke.*

pappy stool, with much mucus, and subsequent burning at the anus. The sensitiveness of the abdomen continued all the evening, accompanied by thirst and early sleepiness while reading an interesting work. At night, very sound sleep.

Nov. 25. Dulness of the head early in the morning, especially in the frontal region, with unusual weakness of the memory; normal evacuation. The frontal headache returned in the forenoon when walking. Towards noon, after violent exercise, the colic in the epigastric region of yesterday returned, but less violent, accompanied by dull pain in the right temple, aggravated by treading and gloomy mood. Finally, violent feeling of heat rising from the abdomen towards the chest, ending in partial sweat upon the abdomen and chest, with prickling and oozing from the anus, and a very copious discharge of urine.

Nov. 26 and 27. Some slight intimations of colic were perceived, principally about noon, on both these days.

25.—*Fifth Proving with the Tincture.*

Dec. 8. *Sixty drops of the tincture* at 7 A.M. The weather was moist and cloudy; he had had for two days some catarrh, with swelling of the right *ala nasi.*

Immediately after the dose: transitory pressing in the right eyelid; moderate pinching in the epigastric region; nauseous, bitter taste; empty eructations (frequently returning); dryness of the throat and hard palate, as though the parts stuck together; sensation in the pharynx and soft palate, compounded of roughness and burning, continuing until afternoon; constant hemming; the mucus raised had the bitter taste of the drug. *Dulness of the left side of the head, with pressing, burning pain in the left orbit, temple and nose, on the* dorsum nasi *and in the superior teeth;* it seemed as if the eye and nose were swelling and becoming longer; (these symptoms were clearly marked and lasting.) Stitches above the right eye, accompanied by itching of the scalp; sensation of obstruction before the left ear; pressing outwards in the right side of the abdomen; clucking in the left buttock; urging to urinate.

Soon after breakfast; when walking rather rapidly: symptoms of vertigo; *dulness of the head in the frontal region; constriction and pressing in the left malar bone, extending into the left eye;* pleasant feeling of warmth in the abdomen, which constantly increases and ends in griping, but disappears again while walking, with sweat upon the chest and abdomen. *Burning upon the tip of the tongue, continuing for several hours.* Slight burning and moisture at the anus, as if after diarrhœa. A prickling stitch darts like an electrical spark from the point of the glans through the abdomen towards the left flank, where it was perceived, and vanished in the same moment.

Towards noon, when walking, symptoms of colic, with inflation of the abdomen (the clothes became too tight). Immediately after dinner, a pappy stool, with horripilation over the head and back; soon afterwards, (when lying down,) pain and rumbling in the abdomen, with urging to stool and horripilation over the whole body; half an hour later, a watery stool, with griping, followed by continued and almost irresistible tenesmus. He became exceedingly sensitive to the damp weather; his legs were unusually weak; it was hard work going up stairs. He was somewhat confused by the beer drunk in the evening; before midnight, during a restless dozing, voluptuous dreams and a pollution, during which he awoke; on waking, tearing in the left tibia and ancle. Sleep after midnight undisturbed.

Dec. 9. This morning, empty eructations; stool soft, pappy, leaving behind tickling in the rectum; subsequently, sensation of a ball as large as the fist rising up in the pharynx, with oppressed respiration. In the afternoon, continued sensitiveness, and griping and commotion in the abdomen for several hours. Another pappy stool after eating, with subsequent burning at the anus, and cramp in the left calf.

(Dec. 8 and 9. Fluent coryza, constant and uncommonly violent, with constant dropping from the nose, worse in the open air than in the room.)

Exceedingly increased sexual impulse for several days.

26.—*Sixth Proving with the Tincture.*

Dec. 26. *Eighty drops of the tincture* at 5.30 A. M., fasting.

Empty eructations, frequently repeated during the following symptoms and sometimes amounting almost to sobbing; *disgust, accompanied by scraping in the throat;* the disgust disappeared after drinking a glass of water, but the scraping continued. *Compressive sensation in the epigastrium, returning at short intermissions, and passing into a sharp pinching, accompanied by slight dulness of the sinciput; constant roaring and throbbing in both ears*, especially in the left; pulsation in the whole body, most perceptible in the back and left side of the chest; palpitations. Itching in different spots, especially on the left side of the body, which smart like burning points. Prickling in the region of the right cheek-bone, as though an eruption were coming out. Exceedingly painful sticking burning on the edge of the left upper eyelid. Sneezing. *Pressing and dull throbbing in the left temple*, with a similar sensation about the left shoulder-joint, with itching of the scalp; tooth-ache on the left side, roaring and feeling of obstruction in the left ear, regularly going and returning; the roaring soon changed to singing; the pressure on the temple grew gradually acute and cutting. Troublesome pressure in the left side of the nape, increased by turning, as in rheumatism. Drawing in the lower incisors. Twitching pain from the left lower molars into the left arm as far as the elbow.

Aching in the region of the left sacro-iliac commissure, accompanied by crawling in the whole left sole as though it were asleep; paralytic pressing in the whole of the left arm, and fine sticking in the skin of the back of the hand. *As the sensation (as if asleep) in the left foot began to decrease, the same feeling came on in the right.* This was accompanied by persistent pressing in the right malar bone and eye; heat and swelled feeling in the roots of the right lower teeth; a similar sensation of swelling in the arms. At the same time, *heaviness and stupor of the sinciput; intimations of vertigo and nausea; burning on the anterior surface of the tongue; urgency to urinate.*

All these symptoms came on in the course of an hour and a half, while seated and quietly employed.

Pain in the bowels immediately on taking only a few steps in the room, and excitement of the tooth-ache on the right side. Immediately thereafter, when seated, pressing inwards and dull throbbing in the right lumbar region, palpitations, feeling in the right foot as if asleep, pulsation in the left popliteal space, rumbling in the abdomen, flying pains in the left side of the epigastrium, burning at the anus. Subsequently, constant crawling and itching, compelling him to scratch, on the whole left side of the head; continuance of the tooth-ache on the right side; dulness in the forehead; feeling of warmth in the right ear; burning on the forepart of the tongue; burning and feeling of swelling of the under lip; scraping and burning in the throat and on the hard palate (as if from pepper); frequent erections.

Five hours after taking the dose, *urgent inclination to stool, almost irresistible; and, in quick succession, two abundant, first pappy, then fluid evacuations, with ulcerative pain in the bowels, ameliorated by bending forwards, aggravated by an upright position.* Frequent yawning; weariness of the thighs, especially perceptible when going up stairs; the legs feel as if asleep; *moisture at the anus and perinæum. The burning on the point of the tongue* continued, and a corresponding *burning pain was felt in the stomach*, even when eating.

Chills after eating, especially in the upper arms, as if at the commencement of a catarrh, and repeated yawning. *The pain in the stomach and tongue, and the eructations, continued all day and grew worse towards evening*, when another yellow, pappy stool took place, accompanied by colic. *The abdomen continued tender and inflated* even after the evacuation. Little appetite at noon, none in the evening. *Frequent urination.*

Dec. 27. In the morning, pressing spasmodic pain in the stomach, rising up into the throat; sensation as of a foreign body in the throat, as though he had to swallow over a lump; pappy, but otherwise normal stool.

The burning on the tongue, and the eructations, continued the whole day, but less intense than yesterday. The moisture in the perinæum continued during the forenoon. Absence of appetite in the evening, with sensitiveness of the borders of the tongue when eating. Nausea and malaise after eating, as though from indigestion. (*Puls.* was taken for this.) Sleep disturbed by frequent waking.

Dec. 28. No more pain in the stomach early; moderate appetite at noon. Burning on the tongue and in the stomach again, however, towards evening, without cause; empty eructations, with burning in the pharynx; twitching in the region of the fifth and sixth left ribs; pain in all the upper teeth; fine sticking and drawing, varying in intensity with aching in the left orbit, and burning as if from pepper in the mouth, especially on the hard palate.

Subsequently, sensation as of a hank in the stomach and pharynx; sobbing eructations; salt taste of the mucus hawked up; burning in the stomach; pressing in the abdomen; discharge of much flatulence; prickling and crawling on different parts of the body; feeling of numbness, swelling and heat in the left foot, which gradually encroaches upon the whole leg, with itching and tickling, and lasts for a considerable time. Pressing throbbing pain on the upper part of the inner side of the right leg, extending to the posterior side of the thigh upwards towards the ischium (when sitting and walking).

Dec. 31. The scalded feeling at the tip of the tongue, the gastric troubles, the occasional eructations, the diminished appetite and depression of spirits continued, with evening exacerbations during the 29th, 30th and 31st. To them was then added a frequently repeated throbbing, finally twitching pain in the right upper arm in the region of the insertion of the deltoid, whence it extended through the shoulder towards the upper teeth, and as far as the region of the temples and vertex. The pain was in the periosteum, and after it had frequently returned, the muscular parts of the arm there became painful, as if sore, to pressure.

Every exacerbation of the symptoms, without exception, began with the burning at the apex of the tongue. The gastric pains were always accompanied by pains in the face and teeth. It was particularly observed that the symptoms appeared in groups, and were aggravated in the evening and during rest.

27.—*Hausmann's Proving with the Tincture.*

Nov. 8. Dr. Franz Hausmann, one of our most resolute Colocynth provers, began his experiments with a dose of *thirty drops of the tincture.*

After the lapse of six hours, the symptoms appeared in the following order. Continual tensive pain in the bowels; it seems as if they were gathered together into a ball, had fallen down, and were lying like a heavy weight in the hypogastrium; it appears as if the anterior parietes of the abdomen were wanting, and the bowels were in danger of falling out. Occasional pressing at the anus, as though a quantity of fæces were about to be discharged, with the escape of only a little mucus. Diffusion of a genial warmth, which seemed to deprive the limbs of strength. Weakness of all the joints, especially of the knee and elbow. Disinclined to exertion of either body or mind, even to visiting his nearest friend. Pressing pain in the right hypochondrium, at the arch of the diaphragm, oppressing the respiration.

Nov. 10. Having had no symptoms on the 9th, Hausmann took *half a drachm of the tincture* on the 10th at 12½ P. M.

Half an hour afterwards, a violent pressure suddenly set in upon the bladder, which was full, but as rapidly passed off on the expulsion of considerable flatus in rapid succession, which drove before it some mucous fluid. These turns of flatus frequently returned in alternation with the following symptoms:

Movements as if from the breaking of large bubbles in various parts of the abdomen; frequent pressure at the anal sphincter, which ceased at once on the escape of the slightest quantity of wind or mucus; pressing and tension in the occiput, most sensible at the inferior lateral protuberances.

Nov. 11. A very slippery soft stool at about 11 A.M.; tensive pressure over the whole forehead on its evacuation. The same symptoms returned in the afternoon, succeeded by pressure upon the bladder, alternating with pressure upon the anal sphincter. Finally, entire relaxation of the most remarkable degree, for a whole hour, during which he was entirely unfitted for either bodily or mental labor. The spasmodic yawnings constantly return.

Nov. 12. Both the last mentioned symptoms were repeated about the middle of the forenoon. A sudden shock, from behind forwards, passed rapidly through the hepatic region, and then in the same direction through the head. Sensation at the anus, as if successive slippery bubbles were escaping. When walking, discharge of copious flatulence, causing the rectum to vibrate.*

Nov. 14. Hausmann took a *drachm of the tincture* in the forenoon.

At about half-past eleven, frequent eructations. At noon, a soft, fluid, rapidly discharged stool, after a continual gentle pressure and the passage of a quantity of slippery flatus. At one P.M., a pressive pain in the left side of the forehead, occasionally slightly vibrating; it was clearly traceable in an arch which defined the lateral and superior boundaries of the left frontal sinus.

Towards four P.M., first griping (drawing hither and thither) in the umbilical region, gradually subsiding again, then returning and rapidly passing into cutting as if from a large chisel, which was thrust deep into the epigastrium, thence passing in a curve backwards and downwards into the pelvis, and thence cutting its way upwards again.

At half-past four, the cutting in the hypogastrium several times took the direction from behind forwards and upwards, and was every time relieved by a forcible discharge of flatus. It was also relieved by straining and the consequent expulsion of a long train of slippery bubbles of wind, and a small quantity of bland mucus. It returned in the same fashion at intervals of from five to fifteen minutes. Finally, towards five P. M., after such an interval, a very painful expulsive pressure, and in a short time, a quantity of thin fæces passed involuntarily through the sphincter, at a single impulse. It was perfectly bland, causing not the slightest burning nor smarting at the anus, which was rather protected all about by the slippery mucus, of which a great portion of the passage

* We do not interfere with our colleague's mode of expression; it has at any rate the great merit that, besides its originality, it is exceedingly clear and concise.—*Ed. Oest. Zeit.*

consisted. The pains in the abdomen all disappeared with this discharge.

Towards 8 P.M., when in pleasant society, violent, long continued pressure in the lateral occipital protuberances.

At night a succession of light, imaginative, pleasant dreams. Waking after midnight, he perceived, as he lay on the right side, pressure and weight in the left side of the forehead, which felt otherwise well. The left eyelid lay thick and heavy upon the ball, which seemed as though squeezed from before and above. A slight throbbing like a pulse in the left hypochondrium, at the summit of the diaphragmatic arch.

Nov. 15. Shortly after rising, easy discharge of inodorous flatus, sometimes silent, at others noisy; head befogged; difficulty in collecting his thoughts; no inclination to search after and grasp objects of interest. A slight exertion in walking fatigued him, and produced a gentle perspiration, which made his limbs feel weak, and ended in sweat; if he stood still, the air, though far from raw, struck through him, in spite of his being warmly clothed, like a cold drizzle.

He had no further stool until the afternoon, when it was of its usual consistence, and passed easily and smoothly. (The same peculiarity attended the evacuations of the following days.) Long and close successions of smoothly discharged bubbles of inodorous gas passed the sphincter at longer or shorter intervals; a symptom which returned for several days.

Nov. 16. Towards noon, when walking, drawing and tension in the interior of the right knee-joint, disappearing and recurring several times; painful tension in the right shoulder on first walking, continuing and becoming worse from using the arm. At half-past twelve, tensive and pressing pain in both sides where the diaphragm is attached.

Nov. 17. Mist before the right eye early in the morning, lasting several hours, and not removed by rubbing it.

Nov. 18. Frequent, long continued and violent ringing in the ears; sexual impulse highly excited.

Nov. 19. At ten A.M., shimmering before the right eye, in the shape of a circle with rays, coming on a short time after getting up from writing. Previously, tension over the forehead while evacuating a very soft and smoothly passed stool. Tension over the chest under similar circumstances in the afternoon. Aching in the right eyeball in the evening, upward and outward, aggravated by rubbing it with the finger; it feels harder than usual there. This aching lasted some days.

28.—*Hausmann's further Proving with the Tincture.*

1843, June 7. Seven months after his previous experiments, Hausmann began again by taking *one hundred drops of a very concentrated tincture*, at about 1 P.M.

At six P.M., he experienced, when walking, an unpleasant sensation about the navel, as if after taking cold, with urging to stool, which he was obliged immediately to attend to, as the sphincter showed no resisting power. The discharge was thin, orange-colored and pappy. After walking for half an hour, a renewed and increased sensation about the navel, as though he had been chilled; more violent tenesmus, to which he was obliged hastily to give way, with a result similar to the former. On bending over to examine it, a warm perspiration broke out over his whole face, followed by a bitterish eructation from the stomach. On walking further, a warm moisture overspread the whole body, and he became weak; abdomen inflated and tense.

After a quarter of an hour, during which he was incessantly walking, the same unpleasant sensation was renewed below the navel, with still greater violence. It increased to a drawing cutting, which darted repeatedly from behind forwards and upwards in a curve to the navel. This ceased on the occurrence of urging to stool, which became exceedingly pressing, and the evacuation ran in a watery stream out of the sphincter, which seemed paralyzed; it contained part of the contents of the soup eaten at the noon meal, still undigested. There was then ineffectual urging, which, when repressed by an effort of the voluntary muscles, gave rise to a pressing tension in the lowest part of the abdominal parietes, and an acute pressure at the inferior angle of the right scapula, with tensive pain extending thence downwards. On the cessation of the long continued tenesmus, a free, protracted discharge took place, the sphincter standing wide open as if paralyzed; at the same time, burning in the orifice of the urethra on the passage of the last few drops. Frequent, for the most part empty, eructations on rising from the stool. The sitting posture was easy, and ameliorated all the pains.

After a considerable interval, during which he had remained for the most part seated, an urging to stool without the preceding colic, which, nevertheless, on the third or fourth repetition, took away all command of the sphincter.

A little before, (while seated,) a great, white, very bright light was seen at the side of and below the right eye; but as he turned his eyes rapidly sideways in order to examine it, it vanished.

Notwithstanding the occurrence of all these powerful effects of Colocynth upon the prover, his tongue remained constantly clean, and his inclination for food was not diminished, but rather increased.*

Dr. Hausmann is thirty years old, of a strong constitution, and sanguineous temperament. His health has never been interrupted for any length of time. Two attacks of fever, the consequence of violent mental exertion under unfavorable conditions, ceased in three days with the usual copious critical evacuations. He has twice spit blood after immoderate long continued exercise, but experienced no further evil con-

* In an appendix to his experiments, Hausmann states that he once took Colocynth in the evening, immediately before going to sleep. (He does not say how much he took.) In the morning early, on going out, the first colic pains came on, but disappeared after taking a cup of coffee. At the first step he took afterwards, however, so violent a tenesmus came on as instantly to deprive him of all power over the sphincter.—*Watzke.*

sequences. He has now been for a long time perfectly well in every part of his system.

29.—*Maschauer's Proving with the Tincture.*

Dr. Karl Maschauer, 28 years old, of a scrofulous constitution, delicate build, and phlegmatic temperament, showed but little sensibility to the action of of Colocynth, and experimented with doses far too small to affect so insensible a system.

1842, Nov. 7. He began by taking *five drops of the tincture* in the forenoon, in a little water. Two hours afterwards, he felt some constriction in the chest, and subsequently stitches in the upper part of the left half of the chest, especially when walking.

Nov. 8. *Five drops* in the forenoon, and a *similar quantity* five hours afterwards, but without result.

Nov. 9, 10. *Five drops* were taken morning and evening. Movements in the bowels, with oppression of the chest, came on each time two hours after the dose.

Nov. 11. *Ten drops* in the forenoon, caused, soon after taking them, constriction of the chest and empty eructations, which lasted almost the whole day.

Nov. 12, 13. *Fifteen drops* each day. In half an hour, empty eructations, and in two hours, griping in the abdomen, with discharge of flatulence both upward and downward, followed by a thin stool and relief of the pains. *Twenty drops* taken on the following day produced no other effect than violent eructation (immediately); griping and rumbling in the bowels (after four hours); and (two hours afterwards) two pappy stools, with discharge of flatulence.

30.—*Second Proving with the Tincture.*

Nov. 20. *Fifteen drops.* Constrictive sensation, with flying stitches in the chest, beginning soon after the dose, and troubling him all day, especially when walking.

Nov. 21. *Twenty drops.* Griping about the navel, with discharge of much flatulence (after five hours).

Nov. 22 to 25. *Twenty-five drops* every morning at eight o'clock. The few results obtained were the same as before. Oppression of the chest (soon after eating); six hours later, violent griping, rumbling and cutting around the navel, with discharge of flatulence, and after four hours more, a pappy stool.

Nov. 26. *Thirty drops*, taken in the forenoon, only sufficed to develop a few traces of a drug-disease, and principally subjectively, in the torpid organism of the prover. Violent griping and cutting about the navel (after six hours), increasing from hour to hour; the abdomen tense, inflated painfully, sensitive to the touch; some diminution of the pains after two watery stools; during the night, great restlessness and sensibility of the abdomen, so that he could scarcely bear the lightest pressure upon it. The sensibility of the abdomen continued the following day.

Nov. 28, 29. A similar dose was followed by similar symptoms, but in a less degree.

31.—*Third Proving with the First Dilution* (1-10).

Dec. 1 to 14. Maschauer made a third proving with the first (decimal) dilution, continuing it for fourteen days, but with no result. On the first day he took *five drops* and increased the dose each day by five more, without experiencing the slightest abnormal sensation.

The prover made no change in his very simple and regular course of living during the proving.

32.—*Puffer's Proving with the Third Dilution.*

The experiments of Dr. Franz Puffer, who is of a venous-lymphatic, phlegmatic-bilious temperament, forty years old, and one of our most timid provers, deserve mention, as we trust he will agree with us in saying, as they afford some evidence that the Colocynth will act, even in dilutions, upon a tender bowel.

He took for six days in succession, at about noon, four or *five drops of the third dilution of Colocynth tincture.*

Immediately after the dose, bitter taste in the mouth, and bitter eructations; an hour later, rumbling in the abdomen and excitement, as if diarrhœa were about to come on, with discharge, however, of only some fetid flatulence. The subsequent stool was hard and unsatisfactory. On one occasion, the evacuation, which began knotty and dry, ended in a diarrhœa. Sleep interrupted by lively dreams and frequent call to urinate; urine remarkably increased.

33.—*Reisinger's Proving of the Tincture.*

Dr. Edward Reisinger, 30 years old, strong, thick-set and phlegmatic, has enjoyed good health for a long period. His experiments present few improvements upon those of his two predecessors. He began with ten drops of the tincture, gradually increased the dose to twenty-five, and then declined again to the first trituration of the drug.

1843, Nov. 3, 4, 5. *Ten drops*, morning and evening. Stiffness of the right forearm, with painfulness of the extensors. On the evening of the 5th, no symptom. This feeling continued the next day.

Nov. 6. *Fifteen drops* in the morning. After five hours, griping and cutting in the umbilical region; discharge of fetid flatulence, and a soft evacuation. The colic did not cease after the evacuation, but became aggravated, and accompanied by a chilly feeling over the whole body.

Nov. 7, 8, 10, 11. *Fifteen drops* on the first day, and *twenty drops* on each of the subsequent days, were followed by nothing but eructations, griping and flatulence.

Nov. 12. *Twenty-five drops.* After five hours, violent rumbling, with very severe cutting in the left hypochondriac and umbilical region, and three very soft brown stools. The colic pains continued this time all day, and were not removed as on former occasions, after taking black coffee or warm soup.

Nov. 13. *Twenty drops*, in the morning. Toward noon, slight drawing in the right upper arm, remarkably increasing after dinner, and becoming almost painful, but decreasing again when walking in the open air. No remains of colic the next day.

Nov. 14. *Fifteen drops.* Drawing in the right upper arm the whole day; towards evening, slight griping and a pappy stool, with burning at the anus; feeling of coldness in the whole body, succeeded by heat without thirst. The drawing in the arm continued into the next forenoon.

Nov. 19, 20. *Five grains of the first trituration* (1 to 9). No symptom on the 19th, but on the 20th, *nausea, empty eructations and griping in the abdomen, with accompanying transitory head-ache in the left side of the forehead.*

We know not whether to regret that our colleague did not experiment with larger doses, or that he did not pursue so promising a proving with the smaller ones.

34.—*Rothansl's Proving with the Tincture.*

Dr. Joseph Rothansl's pharmacodynamic experiments with Colocynth were crowned with the success they deserved. He had to contend against an extreme insusceptibility to the action of the drug.

1842, Nov. 2, 3, 4. No result from *four, five and twelve drops of the tincture.*

Nov. 5. *Fourteen drops.* Pressing in the scrobiculus and constriction of the larynx, obliging him to swallow frequently.

Nov. 6. *Sixteen drops.* In addition to oppression of the chest and constriction of the larynx, which lasted all day, *pressing in the forehead and at the root of the nose*, as though a violent catarrh were coming on, continuing for three hours.

Nov. 7, 8, 9. *Eighteen drops* each day. On the last day, movements in the abdomen and *three pappy stools, with feeling of coldness in the whole body.*

Nov. 10, 11, 12. *Twenty drops*, with no visible traces of effect.

Nov. 19. On this day, however, after taking *fifteen drops*, violent *colic-like pains emanating from the umbilicus, with frequent discharges of flatulence, which afforded relief. The pains continued all night, and deprived him entirely of sleep.*

Nov. 20. Constriction of the larynx, disappearing in the open air (after half an hour); *sleepless the following night from cramp-like pres-*

sure in the scrobiculus and constriction of the stomach; this latter was so sensitive that he could not endure the pressure of the lightest covering.

Nov. 21. Towards morning, loud rumbling in the abdomen, eructations and discharges of flatulence, which relieve. *Fifteen drops* taken in the forenoon; tensive head-ache in the right temple; single, rapidly passing stitches in the left flank. In the afternoon, cutting and thumping in the abdomen; abundant discharge of flatulence, which affords relief; diarrhœic evacuation. (The stool was of the same consistence on the two following days.)

Nov. 24. *Twenty-five drops.* Aching in both temples, aggravated at first in the open air, then entirely disappearing; feeling of burning in the left foot along the tibia (when walking); constrictive pains about the navel, in the evening; constrictive pressure of the larynx.

Nov. 25. *Thirty drops.* Cutting in the abdomen immediately after eating; a diarrhœic stool, with tenesmus.

Nov. 26, 27. *Thirty-five drops* each day. The same symptoms continued. The last doses continued their effect over the three following days, producing *colic pains continuing all night between the 27th and the 28th, with the most excessive sensibility of the abdomen; general lassitude and painful weariness in the small of the back* on the 29th, *and pressing head-ache* on the morning of the 30th.

35.—*Second Proving with Small Doses of Tincture.*

Dec. 5, 6. *Three drops* of the tincture, with no result.

Dec. 7 to 19. With the exception of the 10th, 11th, 15th and 16th, he took *five drops* every day, with the following results:

Dec. 7. Great oppression of the chest before midnight, driving away sleep; restless sleep after midnight, with vivid, troublesome dreams.

Dec. 8. *Pressive head-ache, early, in the temples, and annoying twitching of the right upper eyelid;* the last symptom continued during the three following days. In the evening, movements in the abdomen, soon followed by a pappy stool; slight cramp in the stomach, at night,* rising along the œsophagus into the throat.

Dec. 9. Sudden, rapidly passing vertigo, with darkness before the eyes, in the evening, on sitting down.

Dec. 13. Rumbling in the abdomen and slight head-ache early in bed; at noon, *tensive pain in the left thumb, impeding its motion.*

Dec. 14. Heaviness in both knees; tearing in the left knee, disappearing when walking, in the evening.

Dec. 15. *Repeated tensive pain in the left thumb.*

Dec. 16. In the evening, considerable *head-ache, and unfitness for every occupation.*

Dec. 17. Eructations (immediately after taking it); noon and even-

* See note, *ante*, p. 311.

ing, slight colic after eating; extremely restless sleep, with vivid, nonsensical dreams; troublesome oppression of the chest.

Dec. 18. In the evening, *numbness of the limbs in the knees* when stooping down, so that it was somewhat troublesome to get up again; restless night, full of dreams.

Dec. 19. *Drawing pains in the right thigh as far down as the knee;* a symptom which continued with nearly equal intensity through the next three days (20th to 22d).

The intestinal canal was torpid during the whole time while he was taking from three to five drops, the evacuations were hard, and took place, contrary to his usual habit, only once in two or three days.

Dec. 23. *Ten drops* in the morning. Immediately after dinner,* rumbling in the abdomen, constrictive pain in the umbilical region, and a pappy stool; during the succeeding night, colicky pains, with discharge of flatulence.

Dec. 26. *Five drops* each morning, on the 26th, 27th and 28th. Cutting abdominal pains after dinner and supper.

Dec. 27. *Head-ache and sticking in the right patella*, commencing in the morning. In the evening, rumbling in the bowels, cutting around the navel, and two pappy stools.

Dec. 28. *The sticking in the patella, which was experienced yesterday, returned; it comes on when walking, and disappears on continuing to walk. Violent attacks of colic, the two succeeding nights.*

Distinct Colocynth symptoms were experienced by the prover, for four days after he took the last dose; on the 30th and 31st, in the after part of the day, sticking in the right patella; frequent griping in the abdomen; painful cramp in the stomach at night, relieved by eructations of wind; restless sleep; tossing about in bed.

1843, Jan. 1. Eructations early in the morning; soon afterwards, vomiting of a bitter-tasting, yellow, serous fluid; bitter eructations after dinner; in the evening, absence of appetite and thirst, violent head-ache, fluent catarrh and frequent sneezing. Pleasant night's rest.

Jan. 2. The prover was attacked with a regular angina, setting in with chills, head-ache and burning pain between the shoulders, and was not inclined to attribute either the symptoms or the catarrh of the preceding day to the Colocynth; he, therefore, took no further account of his sensations.

Our colleague, whom no one can easily accuse of too strong a pharmacological faith, or too earnest a lying-in-wait for symptoms, closes his memoranda with the following remarks, in which we heartily join:

"I took *four hundred and thirty-six drops* of Colocynth in the whole. My conclusion from the foregoing detail of symptoms, is, that its action

* From the fact that many provers experienced various and particularly abdominal symptoms immediately after dinner, we may with some probability infer a direct causal connection between Colocynth and the ingestion of food, but none between the remedy and the time of day. Most of the experimenters took the medicine between 7 and 9 A.M., and Colocynth generally requires from five to six hours to develop its action.—*Ed. Aust. Jour.*

is principally directed to the abdominal viscera, and specially to the intestinal canal. By far the msot prominent and troublesome symptom in my case was the colic, which never came on except at night. *The rheumatic pains in the limbs and joints are, however, so much the more important phenomena, and with greater certainty ascribable to the drug, inasmuch as I had never experienced the like, either before or since.* I am thirty-one years old, of an excitable temperameat and slender build; I have always enjoyed good health since passing through the usual diseases of childhood, except in 1832, when I had an attack of cholera, which kept me for several weeks in a dangerous condition. My manner of life is regular, and presents very rare departures from my usual course; my diet consists of a moderate amount of meat, and beer as a beverage."

36.—*Wachtel's Proving with the Tincture.*

Dr. Cajetan Wachtel, thirty odd years old, of a bilious-melancholic temperament and stout frame, has been uninterruptedly well for years; he is an excellent observer, and not the less so because he is perhaps a little timid as a prover.

1842, Nov. 16. *One drop of the tincture* taken in half a glass of water, an hour after a milk breakfast, produced no symptoms.

Nov. 17. *Two drops.* Dulness of the head for an hour.

Nov. 18. *Three drops.* No symptoms.

Nov. 19. *Four drops* in the morning. Griping around the navel for some minutes.

Nov. 20. *Five drops.* In the afternoon, twitching at the anus, and, soon after, two evacuations of the usual character.

Nov. 21. *Five drops,* with no special result beyond more copious urination than ordinary.

Nov. 22. On this day, and the 23d and 24th, *ten drops* each day. Soon after the dose, *pressing feeling in the orbits,* towards the root of the nose. In the afternoon, *feeling of heat in the nape,* burning and twitching in the rectum and at the anus; soon after, three fluid, mucous, but painless stools.

Nov. 23. Feeling of stiffness in the muscles of the nape, when moving the head; after dinner, flying stitches in the hepatic region and sacrum; in the evening, feeling of dryness in the eyes.

Nov. 24. In the forenoon, *urgency to urinate, with discharge of a great quantity of clear watery urine* (returning at pretty near hourly intervals). In the afternoon, *dulness of the head, with pressure in the orbits; feeling of coldness over the whole body,* especially in the knees, notwithstanding the room was warm enough; subsequently, ineffectual pressing in the rectum, soon followed by itching at the anus, and at the orifice of the urethra. In the evening, uneasiness and weakness of the whole body, especially of the lower limbs; *canine hunger,* with particular longing for bread and beer.

Nov. 25. *Fifteen drops,* and the dose was increased *five drops* each day, until the 29th. The symptoms observed were not very characteristic, and may be summarily stated. Dulness of the head; scraping in the throat; rumbling in the abdomen; constriction in the umbilical region; inflated abdomen; feeling of emptiness and soreness in the bowels; pappy stools with burning at the anus; itching in various parts of the body, obliging him to scratch; transitory stitches in the hepatic region, sacrum, dorsum of the right foot, foot-joint and left great toe.

37.—*Wachtel's Proving with the First Trituration* (1 to 9).

The first trituration of Colocynth (10 grains of the pulp to 90 of sugar of milk) yielded more abundant and more characteristic symptoms to this prover than the tincture.

Dec. 20. From this day to the 28th, he took *ten* grains every morning. No result on the 20th.

Dec. 21. Nothing but pressure in the forehead.

Dec. 22. *Increased secretion of the urine*, and towards evening *dulness of the head.*

Dec. 23. Transitory drawing sticking in the periosteum of both bones of the forearm.

Dec. 24. Scraping in the throat in the region of the uvula.

Dec. 25. Throat reddened and swallowing difficult.

Dec. 26. A true *angina* set in, for which the prover took *bell.*, and subsequently *lach.**

Jan. 3. After the throat affections had subsided, he began again with the former dose of *ten grains of the first trituration*, which he took regularly every day until the 15th. *Frequent urging to stool*, without any evacuation.

Jan. 4. The taste of Colocynth seemed, to-day, to be very disgustingly bitter, and continued all night. In the evening, *sticking drawing along the left tibia* into the ancle bones, accompanied by *burning pressure in the left eye;* these pains disappeared again in five or six minutes. Subsequently, *a very hard evacuation*, as if he were passing stones.

Jan. 5. Pressure in both temples, itching in various places in the skin, exciting constant restlessness, so that he can scarcely remain seated. At noon, beer tastes remarkably bitter. In the evening, when walking, *sensation as if all his strength was failing; feeling of emptiness in the stomach, and canine hunger.*† *No evacuation* the whole day.

Jan. 6. *Towards noon, a violent cutting pain, like an electric shock, darted through the whole abdomen to the anus.* Soon after, *urging to*

* Why did not the prover suffer this *apparently* drug-sickness to run its natural course? And instead of a barren *name*, why does he not give us an accurate description of its symptoms? Can it have been a pure accident, that three of our provers (ARNETH, ROTHANSL, and WACHTEL) were attacked with similar throat affections during their provings?—*Watzke.*

† Compare WACHTEL'S proving of Nov. 24, [*ante.* p. 331.]—*Watzke.*

stool without an evacuation, which appeared an hour afterwards in single pieces of a stony hardness. In the afternoon, flying stitches in the right side of the chest from before backwards. During the whole day, *sensation on the tongue as if it had been scalded with a hot fluid.**

Jan. 7. Towards 3 P.M., the feeling of weakness in the whole body returned, but without the subsequent voracious appetite. Towards evening, transitory drawing in the upper and lower limbs; single stitches, as if from needles, under the left *pectoralis. No stool.*

Jan. 8. The scalded tongue appeared again, but less severely.

Jan. 9. Drawing aching in the left foot. At noon, extreme sleepiness. After dinner, a sticking cutting pain in the right foot, as if a nail were driven through.

Jan. 10. Soreness of the skin on the vertex, as though the hair on this part were constantly dragged upwards.

Jan. 11. The feeling in the scalp continues, and is accompanied by a drawing, pressing pain in the occiput. Both symptoms disappeared towards evening.

Jan. 13. Drawing sticking in the joints of both feet, lasting for a minute, often recurring, and not interfering with walking. It becomes worse after coffee and wine, and is accompanied by boring pains in the bones of the lower limbs.

Jan. 14. The above described pains continued the whole day, with inconsiderable remissions, but in diminished intensity. The upper extremities were similarly affected in the afternoon.

Jan. 15. Pressive pain in the sacrum, diminished by movement.

While the last massive doses of his first proving had continued to act for two days only, and that in a very weak and scarce note-worthy degree (want of appetite, feeling of weakness in the stomach, frequent discharge of flatulence and absence of stool), WACHTEL continued to recognize clear and unmistakable drug-symptoms for a full fortnight after he took his last dose of the first trituration.

Jan. 16. The rheumatic-gouty† pains came on more violently than ever before, sometimes in the joints and sometimes in the bones of the upper and lower extremities, but did not last long. In the afternoon, a drawing aching came on in both shoulders.

Jan. 17. In the evening, in addition to the rheumatic gout of the day before, heat in the head and palpitations, which continued the next day in a less degree, and disappeared on the day after.

Jan. 20. In the forenoon, *feeling of repletion in the gastric region; rumbling in the abdomen, with great inflation; violent colic pains,* continuing for an hour, but disappearing after two evacuations, following each other in quick succession.

* "*I had this feeling in the pharynx also during my angina,* and am almost tempted to believe that it was caused by the Colocynth, and the more so, *as I never before had suffered from sore throat.*"—*Wachtel.*

† We repeat that a prover cannot commit a greater error than in recording his symptoms by means of the nomenclature of any nosological system, instead of describing them in definite and clear expressions.—*Ed. Aust. Jour.*

Jan 22. Night restless from *flying stitches in the hepatic region;* on the following day, *continuous pains in the left knee-joint, impeding walking.*

Feb. 1. Our colleague was still troubled by his rheumatic gout in the joints and long bones of both extremities, of greater or less intensity at different times.

38.—*Weinke's Proving with the Tincture.*

Dr. FRANZ KARL WEINKE, thirty years old, of a sanguineous temperament, irritable disposition and strong constitution, made several pretty energetic provings with Colocynth. He has an excellent appetite on taking a good deal of exercise in the open air, his feet perspire summer and winter, which he does all over from slight causes; subject to catarrhs, not strict in his diet, but capable of disposing of considerable quantities of wine and beer without injury. He is one of the provers who carried his experiments on to the production of a veritable drug-sickness.

1842, Nov. 19. *Twelve drops of the tincture* in water, at half-past ten, A.M., after a half hour's walk in the open air. *An hour afterwards, while writing, he perceived in the dorsum of the right foot,* more on the left side towards the great toe, *a painful pressure, with slight numbness of the right leg;* the whole was less perceptible when walking, and spontaneously disappeared after a quarter of an hour. *Fifteen drops* were taken at a quarter after ten, in the same forenoon. In the afternoon, towards 3 o'clock, he had a pappy evacuation, followed by slight, intermitting griping, accompanied by a feeling of having taken cold in the umbilical region, and rumbling in the bowels. Subsequently, transitory stitches in the left side of the chest; moderate flatulency. At 7 P. M., *a semi-fluid stool, accompanied by a perfect storm of flatulence, and followed by considerable discharge of wind. The unpleasant feeling, such as is experienced from catching cold at night in the bowels and feet, and having a diarrhœa in the morning in consequence, continued the whole afternoon.*

Nov. 23. *Twenty drops of the tincture* taken at half-past ten A. M. In half an hour, rumbling in the abdomen, feeling as of taking cold in the same, and two semi-fluid stools. In the afternoon, lassitude, notwithstanding which, excited sexual impulse.

Nov. 30. *Sixty drops of the tincture* in half a glass of water, at about half-past ten, A. M. Shortly afterwards, transitory stitches in the left half of the chest; feeling as of taking cold, and slight rumbling in the abdomen. At a quarter before twelve, *pressure in the dorsum of the right foot,* extending towards the left to the great toe. At noon, *an enormous appetite.* At 2, P. M., *sudden tenesmus, soon followed by a copious pappy evacuation, succeeded by griping,* and sensation as if taking cold in the abdomen,* sleepiness, disinclination to study. At 4, P. M., another *diarrhœic stool,* with subsequent flatulence, and disa-

* The evacuations were followed, in most of the provings, not by an aggravation, but by an amelioration of the abdominal symptoms.—*Ed. Aust. Jour.*

greeable though not a very remarkable or excessive feeling of general debility.

As Weinke was exceedingly inconvenienced by the very marked action of Colocynth upon his lower extremities, especially when walking, he discontinued the experiment. The symptoms which he experienced during the three following weeks may be summed up as follows: Heavy sleep, full of dreams; dulness in the morning, with late waking and dislike to get up; *heaviness of the lower limbs; increase in size of both feet*, so that all his boots were too small in the instep. A constant dull-pressing, cramp-like pain, as if in the periosteum, *on the dorsum of the right foot*, in the scaphoid and internal cuneiform bones; the skin was not discolored nor tense over the painful spot; *a swelling on the right edge of the tarsus, soft, pale, painless, clearly circumscribed, and as large as a pigeon's egg, appearing like a common lymphatic tumor. The same pains in the left foot as in the right, and in the same spot*, (sometimes, also, in the second joint of the great toe,) but less severe, and accompanied by no swelling.

These symptoms were somewhat ameliorated while walking, but were always perceived in the evening, after considerable exertion, and then connected with indescribable weariness in the lower extremities. As long as these phenomena lasted, the bowels were sluggish, acting only every other day, but not particularly hard; constant flatulency, urine apparently rather diminished. Black coffee never removed the above detailed symptoms. The circumscribed swelling on the foot was still present after the lapse of six months.

39.—*Würstl's First Proving with the Tincture.*

The three provings of our colleague, Dr. J. P. Würstl, lose a little of their positive value in one point of view, from the fact that he had formerly frequently experienced the same symptoms, gouty-rheumatic pains, toothache, diarrhœa, &c., as he suffered while taking the Colocynth; but, on the other hand, they are a little remarkable from the fact that the drug proved a specific for those ailments, which have never since troubled him in the least. He is 39 years old, of a sanguineous temperament, and of tolerably strong constitution.

1842, Nov. 1. *One drop of the tincture* in the evening; soon after which, much flatulence, with tension of the abdomen.

Nov. 2 and 3. *One drop morning and evening.* Violent pain in a hollow tooth; feeling of coldness in the stomach; rumbling in the bowels; great looseness.

Nov. 4. *Two drops* morning and evening. Fulness in the abdomen; discharge of much flatulence.

Nov. 5. *Two drops* in the morning. Sudden sticking pain in the forehead, towards the nose; frequent sneezings, with dryness in the nose. The sticking ceased after a quarter of an hour, and the whole head became dull for an hour.

Nov. 6 to 11. *Three drops* night and morning the first two days, *four drops* the next two, and *five drops* the last two. Stiffness in the left knee when sitting, disappearing when walking, yet frequently recurring; discharge of a great deal of offensive flatulence.

Nov. 11 to 13. *Six drops* on the first two days, morning and evening; on the third day in the morning only. Dulness and heaviness of the head, with feeling as if a catarrh were coming on; slight vertigo in the evening.

Nov. 14. *Seven drops* in the morning; *eight drops* in the evening. Frequently recurring vertigo, with dulness of the head. *All the symptoms came on, generally, half an hour after taking the drug, and disappeared after from six to seven hours.*

Nov. 15. No more medicine; the symptoms however continued. Sudden cramp-pain in the right great toe, in the evening, extending towards the metatarsus; waking accidentally in the night, he found the whole right foot, especially the metatarsus, swollen; this continued the whole of the next day, but was only painful when stepping on it or making strong pressure.

Nov. 17. The pain and swelling notably diminished; he can tread now with care, but the affection did not disappear until the 19th.

40.—*Second Proving with the Tincture.*

Nov. 25. *Six drops* in the morning. Pressive headache in the frontal region, after half an hour; tension in the abdomen; discharge of much flatulence; two stools; copious urine.

Nov. 26. *Six drops.* More violent headache than yesterday, after one hour; cramp-pain in the second toe of the right foot, extending towards the metatarsus, after two hours. The headache returned frequently the next day, but never remained long at a time.

Nov. 28. *Eight drops* in the morning. Great tension in the abdomen, with violent rumbling; copious urine; threatening of cramp-pain, alternately in the right second toe, and in both knees, with feeling of stiffness.

Nov. 29. *Eight drops.* Dulness of the head, with transitory attacks of vertigo, frequently recurring in the course of the day.

Nov. 30, Dec. 1. *Ten drops* in the morning of each day. Violent pressing over the forehead, from the temples towards the nose, with feeling of dryness in the latter, after half an hour; pain in the right second toe and knees, alternately appearing and disappearing for almost four hours. The pain in the lower extremities disappeared after drinking beer; the headache was aggravated.

The headache, and pains in the knees and foot, came on daily at about 8 A. M., until Dec. 3, and continued until afternoon, when a soft stool took place. On the 4th they were weaker and not so often, but he had frequent attacks of vertigo; he was not perfectly well until the 8th. During the whole time of this proving, he felt very weak and relaxed, and the sexual impulse was remarkably diminished.

41.—*Third Proving with the Tincture.*

Dec. 8 to 10. *Three, four, and six drops*, taken in the morning, produced not the slightest effect.

Dec. 11. *Seven drops ;* pain and stiffness in the knee manifested themselves slightly, with much rumbling in the abdomen and frequent eructations.

Dec. 12. *Eight drops* produced violent griping in the umbilical region, troublesome cramp-pain in the knee and calves, ineffectual urging to stool, and copious urine.

Dec. 13. *Nine drops.* Drawing and feeling of stiffness alternating between the right and left knee, frequently recurring (after half an hour); at the same time, rapidly passing stiffness in the hip-joint; griping and rumbling in the bowels the whole forenoon, more painful when walking than when at rest; much flatulence, and two, almost fluid, yellowish stools in the afternoon ; great debility and weariness.

Dec. 14. *Ten drops* in the morning, caused the pains in the lower extremities to increase until noon, so as to be frequently troublesome in walking. Constant pinching in the abdomen around the navel; frequent eructations ; inclination to vomit; frequent urging to urinate, with scanty emission ; stitches along the urethra. All these symptoms disappeared in the afternoon.

The drawing pains in both knees were perceptible for several hours on the three following days.

During the succeeding week, the prover took occasional doses of *five drops*, at two days interval, and perceived slight intimations of drawing and stiffness in the knees, soon disappearing, especially on walking; feeling of looseness in the bowels, and somewhat increased discharge of urine.

Since this last proving, our colleague, to his own great astonishment, finds himself perfectly relieved of all the pains which formerly annoyed him so frequently, and has continued for the past year stronger and more healthy than ever before.

42.—*Wurm's Proving with the Tincture.*

Dr. FRANZ WURM, æt. 36, sanguineous temperament, athletic build, perfectly healthy for years past, one of our most assiduous and careful provers, made three experiments with colocynth; the first, with the strong tincture, of which he took the enormous quantity of *six hundred and forty-one drops in the course of five weeks ;* the second, with the first trituration of the marc; and the third, with the first dilution of the tincture.

1842, Nov. 8, 9, 10. *One, two, and four drops of the mother tincture* were taken, with no result except that, on the next day,

Nov. 11, his usual stool was absent; *six drops* at 10 A. M., were followed by dulness of the head, most severe after dinner, nearly disappearing towards evening; feeling in the afternoon as if he should have a stool; frequently recurring tearing in the right metatarsus, towards the great toe joint, in the evening; frequent urination.

Nov. 12. *Eight drops* half an hour after his accustomed stool. Another stool at 4 P. M., with slight subsequent burning at the anus.

Nov. 19, 20. *Ten and fifteen drops* produced no other effect than a quantity of inodorous flatulence.

Nov. 22. *Twenty-five drops.* Violent urging to evacuate the bowels (after five hours), demanding instant attention. Copious fæcal diarrhœa, accompanied by great discharge of wind.

Nov. 23. *Thirty drops* in the morning. Little appetite at dinner, although the food tasted well; insipid taste in the mouth after dinner for an hour and a half; pretty violent pressing pain in the left little finger about 6 P. M., particularly towards the middle joint, soon disappearing; then the same pain in all the right toe-joints, except those of the great toe, lasting eight minutes.

Nov. 24. *Forty drops* in the morning. Movements in the bowels, soon after dinner, followed by an abundant soft stool, succeeded by griping in the abdomen, particularly in the vesical region; a thin diarrhœic stool at 4 P. M., whereupon the colic remitted.

Nov. 25, 26. *Twenty and thirty drops* produced almost a repetition of the same scene, except that the colic was more violent, and lasted longer.

Nov. 27. *Forty drops* in the forenoon. He continued perfectly well, and had no evacuation all day; slept badly the following night, was often aroused by vivid dreams, and every time found himself in a perspiration.

Nov. 28. *Fifty drops* at 9½ A. M. Pressing in the posterior joint of the left great toe, as if the boot were too tight, only perceived when quietly seated, disappearing when walking about; throbbing in the same spot, likewise vanishing on motion; heaviness of the feet, most troublesome tn the forenoon, as though he had made a great journey on foot; constant sensation in both feet when sitting, especially in the left, as if they were going to sleep. Itching, inducing scratching in various places, most frequently on the scalp. Movements in the hypogastrium after dinner, disappearing after a soft evacuation.

Nov. 29. Heaviness in the feet, early, after waking, diminishing after getting up, and going off on going about. A hard, unsatisfactory evacuation at about 5 P.M., discharged with difficulty. Many and vivid dreams during the succeeding night; he woke almost every half-hour. At the same time, another unpleasant symptom was discovered; the prepuce was drawn back, and, as it were, slightly constricted behind the glans. Every time he brought it forwards, he found it again drawn back at his next waking.

Nov. 30. *Forty drops* at 8½ A.M., and *twenty drops* at 5 P.M. Aching in the hypogastrium soon after dinner, ameliorated by the discharge of abundant fetid flatulence, and disappearing after the subsequent stool, at about 4 P.M. *Sensation of violent pressure in the left temple, continuing the whole afternoon* (migraine?), better while seated, worse when standing and walking, but especially when urinating. Night's rest interrupted by vivid dreams and frequent waking, when he always found himself upon his back.

Dec. 1, 2. *No medicine.* Frequently repeated aching in an upper hollow tooth; drawing in the right ancle towards the internal side; rapidly passing sensation of pressure in different parts of the body, especially in the posterior joint of the right middle finger and right great toe; an unsatisfactory stool.

Dec. 3. *Fifty drops* in the forenoon; after six hours, griping, four fingers below the navel; discharge of abundant flatus. Colic very violent in paroxysms, obliging him to bend forwards. It continued two hours, and only ceased after the evacuation of a soft stool. He felt very weak and debilitated in the evening before going to sleep.

Dec. 4. The same feeling of weariness and lassitude on waking the next morning, but it soon disappeared on moving about; no evacuation the whole day; frequent urination; itching in various spots on the body; feeling of pressure in the joints.

Dec. 5. *Sixty drops* at 8½ A.M. Dulness of the head, most perceptible in the right frontal region, continuing the whole day. Violent griping pains in the abdomen at 2½ P.M., worst at about three fingers below the navel, obliging him to bend over, and disappearing after a pappy stool at 5 P.M. Sensation as if the left foot would go to sleep, in the evening when sitting. The lassitude, the itching in various spots, and the feeling of pressure in the joints, as yesterday.

Dec. 6. With the exception of drawing in the calf and thigh, and absence of an evacuation, no symptoms.

Dec. 7, 8, 9. *Fifty, forty, and thirty-five drops,* taken in the forenoon, produced almost identical phenomena: dulness of the head, discharge of abundant flatus after dinner, colic, pappy stools, followed by disappearance of the abdominal troubles, frequent urination, feeling of pressure and heaviness in the small of the back. On the 9th, in addition, transitory drawing in various joints of the upper and lower limbs, especially of the fingers and toes, disappearing instantaneously on motion, and as rapidly recurring in rest.

Dec. 10, 11. This last symptom troubled him also quite often the two following days, on which he took no medicine.

Dec. 12. *Forty drops.* Movements in the abdomen at 5 P.M., followed by a soft stool.

Dec. 13. On getting out of bed, drawing in the left popliteal region, as if the tendons were too short; dulness of the head; fluent coryza; pressive drawing in the joints of the toes and fingers, as well as in the right knee-joint. The joint difficulties continued the whole day, but did not remain long in one place.

Dec. 14. *Forty-five drops* in the forenoon. Urging to stool, and a soft evacuation after dinner; continuance of the coryza; oppression of the chest in the evening; feeling of rawness in the throat, and cough; frequent urination.

Flying drawing in the posterior joint of the left thumb

and right great toe, in the right knee, and on the left side of the neck, especially when turning the head; coryza less; roughness in throat, and oppression of the chest, the same.

The pains in the joints returned for several days, but less frequently and less violent. On the 17th, in the evening, he had besides, for several hours, violent pressure in the small of the back, and the left foot felt as if it were going to sleep. On the 18th, in the evening, sprained feeling in all the toes of the left foot when going up stairs.

43. *Wurm's Proving with the First* (*centesimal*) *Trituration.*

Dec. 19. *Twelve grains* taken at noon. Pressing in several of the finger and toe joints, especially during rest.*

Dec. 20, 21. *Twenty-four and forty grains.* No symptoms, except that on the 22d he perceived burning in the orifice of the urethra after urinating, lasting an hour.

Dec. 22, 23. *Fifty grains*, taken in the forenoon of the first day and morning of the second, produced no other effect than dulness of the head, unsatisfactory stool, with burning and sticking in the anus, and burning in the urethra after urinating.

44.—*Wurm's Proving with the First* (5 *to* 100) *Trituration.*

Dec. 24. *Twenty grains*, at 9 A. M., produced several unmistakable Colocynth-symptoms. *Cramp on the middle of the left thigh* (after three hours); *discharge of fetid flatus after dinner, and movements in the hypogastrium, both symptoms disappearing after an evacuation.* Pressing in some of the toes, and in the calves in the afternoon. Towards 5 P.M., universal lassitude, with chills, violent thirst and accelerated pulse; this febrile excitement lasted for about half an hour. It was very singular that, during its continuance, he could not, without difficulty, get rid of the idea that he was not in his own room, but in another. He felt perfectly well in the evening.

Dec. 25. The usual morning stool was absent. The sensations of pressure, and drawing in the posterior joint of the right great toe and ancle and knee-joints, as well as in the left hip, returned in short paroxysms, especially when walking around. At 7 P.M., when walking, *cramp-like drawing in the inner side of the right thigh throughout its whole length;* he felt very much debilitated, but only when at rest. On the next day, he felt perfectly well, except that he had no stool.

Dec. 27, 28. *Thirty and forty grains* developed a succession of symptoms, which continued for twelve days. Discharge of much flatus; two unsatisfactory stools. Tension and stiffness in the left knee on getting out of bed on the morning of the 28th; pressure in the posterior joint of the right great toe in the evening.

Dec. 29. Transitory drawing in the left trochanter, followed by drawing

* Apparently a remaining effect of the last 45 drops of the tincture.—*Ed. Oest. Zeit.*

pressing in the left metatarsus, and when this ceased, drawing in the teeth (forenoon); pressure in the middle of the left thigh, drawing in right elbow-joint, pressure in the posterior joint of the right great toe, when moving about, lasting all the evening; with this, cold feeling in both upper arms, as if after taking cold, returning for several evenings in succession; no stool all day.

Dec. 30. A hard, unsatisfactory stool in the morning; violent itching on the abdomen in the umbilical region in the evening for half an hour; followed by *drawing in the inner side of the left thigh as far as the flank.*

Dec. 31. A stool in the morning and another after dinner, hard and unsatisfactory; pressing on the posterior joint of the right great toe, lasting nearly all day, most perceptible during rest; *drawing in the external condyle of the right femur*, in the elbow, fingers, toes, but especially in the knees, on motion.

Jan. 1, 2. The drawing and pressure in the joints returned on these two days, but less violently and less frequently.

Jan. 3. Three small boils appeared on the left side of the neck with burning pains, and a larger one at the lower angle of the left scapula. *Drawing on the inner side of the left thigh* in the evening.

Jan. 4. Drawing in the right knee-joint in the forenoon, and on this ceasing, *drawing in the right thigh.* Constant burning pain in the boils.

Jan. 5, 6. Two pappy stools a day in the forenoon.

Jan. 7. *Drawing in the inner side of the left thigh, the whole afternoon.*

Jan. 8. On the next day he was perfectly well.

45.—*Wurm's Proving with the First (decimal) Trituration.*

Jan. 15 to 19. He took *fifteen grains* on the morning of the 15th, and *thirty grains* on the 16th, 18th, and 19th, and satisfactorily proved the efficacy of such doses; the results, however, are but a few morbid phenomena. *Movements in the abdomen; discharge of much flatulence; more frequent urination; disturbances in relation to the character and time of the stools which were either absent, or instead* of coming, as normally, in the morning, *appeared in the afternoon and were either too soft (diarrhœic), or too hard and unsatisfactory.*

46.—*Wurm's Proving with the First dilution of the Tincture.*

Jan. 21 and 24. *Ten drops* every morning produced no effect, except that he was waked on the 23d at about 4 A.M., by a violent pressing-throbbing headache in the forehead. Although the pain went off on sitting up and moving his head, still his head was very dull all the forenoon.

47.—*Watzke's Proving with the Tincture.*

1842, Nov. 3. I began my experiments with Colocynth when convalescing from an *isthmitis*, with *a single drop* of the tincture taken in a spoonful of water at 8 A.M., after a breakfast of bread and milk. With the exception of slight sensation of nausea towards noon, I perceived nothing; it seemed to have no effect upon the still remaining soreness of the throat. During the succeeding night, excellent refreshing sleep, with pleasant dreams.

Nov. 4. *Four drops* on a piece of sugar, at 7, A.M. The head seemed a little affected soon after the dose. Towards 9 A.M., much rumbling in the abdomen; at noon, the same intimations of nausea as yesterday; restless at night, and had horrible, exciting dreams.

Nov. 5. *Seven drops* in a few spoonfuls of water, at 7 A.M. Towards 10 A.M., *sensation of inflation in the umbilical region, with compression in the throat and nausea.* These symptoms lasted the whole day, and became worse some hours after dinner. Towards evening, disgust before eating, and inclination to vomit.

Nov. 6. No medicine and no symptoms, except occasional slight drawings in the shoulder-blades.

Nov. 7. *Fifteen drops* in a little water, at 8 A. M. This was followed by frequent eructations of breakfast. Towards noon, *movements in the abdomen, and two brown, thin, almost watery, painless stools, one following the other in rapid succession.* No other symptoms.

Nov. 8 to 11. No medicine; *constant sensitiveness of the abdomen in the umbilical region;* frequently repeated long stitches in the left chest and left knee; *several pappy stools a day.*

Nov. 12. *Twenty drops* in the morning, soon after breakfast. In the forenoon, *acute pain in the umbilical region, increased by walking;* subsequently, transitory drawing in the right shoulder; towards evening, stitches in the left side, cutting short the breathing; drawing in the scalp; *painful pressure in the eye-balls, especially when bending over;* frequently returning stitches in the right elbow and fore-arm. *During the whole day, borborygmi and empty eructations.*

Nov. 14. *Ninety-five drops* in half a glass of water, early in the morning, fasting. The disagreeable, bitter taste of the drug remained for several minutes in the mouth. Half an hour afterwards, (immediately after breakfast,) rising of a bitter, white, frothy liquid; *Violent pain in the umbilical region the whole forenoon, without intermission; it was situated in a spot about the size of the hand, and was a bruised pain, aggravated by walking but not by pressure, and becoming more tolerable after eructations of air. At times, twitching stitches from the umbilical region towards the loins and spine; intimations of nausea; urging to stool* (which, however, was under control). Towards 11 o'clock, constant burning pain in a spot on the right side of the chest; feeling of roughness in the throat; pressure in both temples; *smarting in the eyes; painfulness of the eye-ball;* excited, irritable state of temper; taciturnity.

The pain in the abdomen became worse after dinner, gnawing and boring, and obliged me to sit down or lie and bend forwards; violent tenesmus came on at first, with pappy, copious, strong-smelling stools, which, an hour later, were watery, scanty, yellow, and almost inodorous. Twitching pains in the dorsum of both feet towards the tibia, when walking in the street. The colic diminished somewhat after taking black coffee, at 4 P.M., but became much more painful again after supper,* accompanied by dulness of the head *and aching in the sinciput, aggravated by bending forwards.* Restless sleep at night, vivid dreams, frequent waking, apparently produced by the continual painfulness of the umbilical region.

Nov. 15. No medicine. In the forenoon, occasional sticking pains in the right chest; two pappy, yellow, painless stools. In the evening, *painfulness of the whole head and eyes, very much aggravated by bending forwards; constant colic, with urging to stool,* which was, however, subject to control. Night very restless; *umbilical region unintermittingly painful;* profuse perspiration towards morning.

Nov. 16. *Colic again more violent, gnawing after moving about,* in the forenoon; somewhat diminished towards noon, but not entirely intermitting during the remainder of the day. Frequent pressure and oppression of the chest in the afternoon; dull stitches in the chest and sides. *Sensitiveness of the head* during the whole day, as though it were compressed, *especially in the sinciput* and temples, with painfulness of the eye-balls, aggravated by bending forwards; better in the open air.

Nov. 17. After a quiet night, I was waked in the morning by griping in the bowels, and tenesmus, notwithstanding which, the stool that followed was perfectly normal. The griping disappeared after drinking black coffee, but returned in the course of the forenoon, accompanied by rumbling and movements in the abdomen; the sensitiveness of the head of yesterday, the pressing in the temples, and the painfulness of the eye-balls, came on again. Bruised pain in the right middle finger, at noon; after dinner, a yellow, diarrhœic stool, without tenesmus or pain. In the evening, painfulness of the umbilical region, stitches in the back; spots on the anterior part of the thorax, that were sore and painful, as if bruised.

The following is a condensed statement of the results of the next ten days, until the 28th Nov.: "I am not yet free from the effects of the drug taken during my last proving of the 14th. I am constantly annoyed by a feeling of compression, of a hank in the umbilical region, sometimes more, sometimes less. At times, especially towards morning, it increases to a piercing or cutting pain. I generally wake in the morning with colic and tenesmus, and have every day several thin pappy stools. I have frequent attacks of the painfulness and aching in the sinciput and eye-balls, and the dull stitches in the flank, interrupting

* Unquestionably because the anodyne effect of the coffee had continued until then.—*Ed. Oest. Zeit.*

the respiration. *Since the 24th, I have perspired very profusely over the whole body, every night towards morning, and my urine presents a very striking similarity in appearance to that in dropsy after scarlatina. It is of a faint flesh-color, deposits a light-brown, flocky, unequal, translucent sediment, and upon the vessel, small, hard, and solid reddish crystals, which adhere so strongly that they are not easily removed by water.* The urine passed during the day is somewhat lighter colored than that made towards evening, night and morning.

"The umbilical pains were much alleviated, and the head difficulties entirely disappeared, on the appearance of the night-sweats and flesh-colored urine. These are, then, unquestionable phenomena, on the occurrence of which, my medicinal disease, already become chronic, and resembling a congestion (hyperæmia, inflammation) of the small intestines more than anything, was happily brought to an end. Thus we have a *drug-crisis*, or lusis!"

Dec. 1. "The above described urine was present also on the 29th and 30th of November. To-day, the water is bright again, but of a somewhat deep wine-yellow, and contains a transparent cloud. Every abdominal symptom has disappeared."

Dec. 4. "The morning sweats, and cloudy reddish urine, with brown, flocky, mucous sediment, have returned for two days past; the pressing, sometimes gnawing pains in the umbilical region come on, particularly in the morning, fasting; movements and rumbling in the bowels are often observed. On the evening of the 3d, I had a gnawing, pressing pain in the inner ball of the left foot, and, subsequently, painful stitches in the cardiac region on going to bed."

Dec. 10. "Since the 5th, several little boils have been developing themselves on the ulnar side of both hands, and a stye on the left eye, which followed the usual course to suppuration—perhaps accidental phenomena, though I have not been previously troubled with such symptoms. All the abnormal manifestations have now disappeared, excepting a tension, a feeling of pressure in the region of the navel."

While I thought that the effects of the drug had long since vanished, I was taken by surprise on the 18th, at 7 A.M., while writing, *with exceedingly painful long stitches in the right metacarpus, frequently repeated in the course of a few minutes, and somewhat embarrassing the operation of opening the hand and stretching the fingers.* The stitches came both during rest and motion; a symptom which I had never had before. At 8 P.M., while reading, the same symptoms recurred, only the pain was more continuous, the stitches more intense and longer. The same symptoms were repeatedly perceived at different times on the following days.

After I had no longer for several days observed the slightest trace of the drug-action, and the process, *after a duration of five weeks*, was unquestionably at an end, I undertook a new experiment *with the triturated pulp.*

48.—*Watzke's Proving with the Third (decimal) Trituration.*

Dec. 26, 28. *Ten grains of the third (decimal) trituration* were taken fasting on the morning of each day. The transitory sticking, drawing, twitching, itching, burning, and smarting, which I subsequently observed in different parts of the body, now here and now there, do not seem to me to stand in the relation of cause and effect with the drug taken.*

49.—*Watzke's Proving with the First (decimal) Trituration.*

1843, Jan. 10. *Ten grains of the first trituration* were followed by intense bitter taste in the month for some minutes; three hours later, griping in the abdomen, especially about the navel, with easily repressed tenesmus (continuing nearly two hours); a diarrhœic stool after dinner, without colic or tenesmus; during the next days, especially in the forenoon, frequent intimations of abdominal pains, weakness, nausea rising from the stomach; also irritable disposition, and a strongly-marked aversion to the drug.

Jan. 14. *One grain*, taken at 8 A.M., produced merely transitory griping in the bowels. Having taken *two grains*, four hours afterwards, I had painful griping and movements in the gastric region (continuing for a long while), followed by a soft, almost diarrhœic stool. Towards evening, pressive pain in several places on the thorax, in the hepatic region, and over the heart, impeding respiration (continuing for several hours.)

Jan. 15. Long stitches on the inner side of the left thigh, from the ischiatic tuberosity towards the knee, in the forenoon, when walking (frequently repeated for several minutes); towards noon, griping about the umbilicus, and sensitiveness of the abdominal integuments, aggravated by external pressure.

50.—*Watzke's Proving with the Tincture applied Externally.*

The experiments which I instituted in December, 1843, by rubbing in the tincture on the abdomen, did not, unfortunately, lead to the development of a medicinal disease, as I was in hopes they would.

Ten, twenty, thirty, and forty drops produced very slight symptoms of Colocynth-action, such as transitory griping colic; several small soft evacuations a day, with frequent inclination to stool; clucking in the inner side of the groin.

* On the other hand, *ten grains* of the same trituration, taken subsequently, on the morning of Jan. 22, produced unmistakable Colocynth-symptoms. Movements in the abdomen, frequently repeated during the day; on the following morning, constant, violent smarting on the middle of the tongue at the apex, as though the part were sore (*See* GERSTEL'S *Proving, ante, p.* 321); drawing, sticking pain on the external side of the thigh, when waking.

Can it be that the deep-seated action of the 95 drops of the tincture, taken five weeks previously, was too recent, and that the organism was too deeply affected by it, to respond to the impression of a dose, relatively so weak as a few grains of the third attenuation?—*Watzke.*

Fifty drops, rubbed in towards midnight, produced an unusually noisy discharge of much flatus in the morning, movements in the bowels, sensitiveness of the abdominal integuments, repeated inclination to stool, which, however, was easily resisted.

One hundred drops caused sensibility around the anus, with freqent urging to stool, which was *unsatisfactory and diarrhœic*, but painless; clucking in a spot below the navel; painfulness of the abdominal integuments (particularly when walking); griping in the abdomen and frequent urination, with an apparently increased flow.

The same symptoms returned with more intensity and annoyance on repeating the same application the next day. The tenesmus, hardly indulged before it again returned, became also ineffectual, or produced only a slight diarrhœic discharge. On the evening of the same day, painfulness of the whole head, most troublesome in the frontal region, aggravated by bowing or turning the head, with incapacity for intellectual exertion—a symptom which I had experienced six months before, during my proving of *Colocynthin* hereafter referred to. It then troubled me for a long time, and, although it now disappeared after a few hours' continuance, still the violence with which it attacked me frightened me from further prosecuting my experiments with the external application of the tincture.

I am forty years old, of a sanguineous-bilious temperament, small in stature, and of a strong constitution, with no special predisposition to any disease. I have never been seriously unwell, with the exception of the usual exanthemata during childhood, and some acute congestive attacks of the head and throat during subsequent years.

Experiments with Colocynthin.

Description.—Colocynthin is a brown or pale-yellow, translucent, uncrystallizable, brittle substance, with a conchoidal fracture. Its taste is extraordinarily bitter; it leaves, after burning, a black, very voluminous charcoal; it is soluble in water, alcohol, and ether.* Chlorine precipitates the watery solution; acids and deliquescent salts produce a greasy precipitate, insoluble in water. The solution of Colocynthin is precipitated also by tincture of galls, proto-sulphate of iron, and sulphate of copper, but not by corrosive sublimate, nitrate of silver, or acetate of lead. The caustic alkalies do not cause a precipitate; it is not easily destroyed by nitric acid, as it decomposes it.

The most simple mode of preparing it, according to Vauquelin, is to exhaust the pulp, freed from the kernel, by water, and evaporate the solution, when the Colocynthin separates in oily drops, which become solid on cooling. Braconnot recommends exhausting the watery extract with alcohol, evaporating the filtrate, and treating with a little

* According to Pfaff, (*Syst. Mat. Med.* III., 170,) sulphuric ether takes up nothing.—*Watzke.*

water, when the Colocynthin remains behind.* We have used both preparations in our experiments, and detected no difference in their effects.

According to PFAFF (*loc. cit.*), *Colocynthin* stands nearly related, in its chemical properties, to *bryonin*. Others are of the opinion that a further and more exact examination of these two substances would lead to the conclusion that they were modifications of one and the same base—a theory, by the by, which, notwithstanding the botanical and pharmacodynamic affinities of *Bryonia* and *Colocynth*, deserves to be ranked among the dreams of the alchymists, as a pure impossibility.

Our object in proving the *Colocynthin* was to ascertain whether the medicinal power of Colocynth was solely due to its presence (as PFAFF declares), whether Colocynth and Colocynthin were identical in their effects upon the human organism, or whether the latter stood in a similar pathogenetic relation to Colocynth that Quinine does to China. How far we have accomplished our purpose, our colleagues can judge from the results of both provings herewith submitted to them.

Besides myself, Colocynthin was tried by Dr. GERSTEL upon himself, and by Dr. FRÖHLICH upon two rabbits. These latter experiments will be found in the next chapter.

51.—*Gerstel's proving of Colocynthin, Sixth (decimal) Dilution.*

1843, May 28. Dr. GERSTEL began with *twenty drops* of the sixth decimal dilution (prepared with distilled water), taken fasting at 7 A.M. He perceived nothing abnormal, except a slight intimation of dulness of the head, and a gentle feeling of warmth in the abdomen, as if from a congestion of the bowels (!) followed by a copious discharge of flatus in the afternoon.

May 29. *Thirty drops* on this day, and *twenty drops* on June 3, produced no striking phenomena.

52.—*Gerstel's Proving of Colocynthin, Fifth (decimal) Dilution.*

June 4. *Forty drops* taken in the morning, fasting. Soon after the dose, slight dulness in the sinciput; formication of the eyelids, and crawling in the lower incisors on the left side; pressure in the temple; prickling and metallic taste on the point of the tongue. These symptoms soon disappeared, and there were no others during the day. During the night of the sixth, he had a pollution—a very unusual occurrence with him.

June 6. *Fifty drops* in the morning, fasting. Four painless, pappy stools during the day; sensations of tenesmus in the urethra and rectum after urinating.

June 7. *Fifty drops* in the morning, fasting. Soon after the dose, pain in a hollow molar, and drawing in the incisors, with sensation of

* *Handw. d. Chem.* von LIEBIG, POGGENDORF und WÖHLER, Art. *Kolocynthin*, and PFAFF, *loc. cit.*—*Watzke.*

swelling of the left cheek; tickling in the left external ear, with burning of the tip; dulness in the left side of the head, especially in the temporal region; painfulness of the whole left side of the face; paralytic weakness of the right fore-arm while writing; tearing in the left shoulder; prickling in the left calf and sole; tickling in the rectum; crawling in the penis, with sexual desire. In the course of the forenoon, weakness of the legs, transitory heartburn, and feeling of moisture at the anus.

June 8. *Fifty drops* produced not the slightest effect, (a fact which throws considerable doubt upon the numerous phenomena observed the preceding day. Is it not possible that such almost purely subjective alterations of sensation might be, for the most part, the effect of the prover's imagination, or of his overstrained attention to his own feelings? *Ed. Oest. Zeit.*)

53.—*Gerstel's proving of Colocynthin, Fourth (decimal) Dilution.*

June 20. *Thirty drops* of the fourth dilution produced no symptoms.

June 21. *Sixty drops*, with no better result.

June 22. *One hundred drops*, taken in the morning, gave rise to clear manifestations of Colocynth. *Intimations of colic, with inflation in the umbilical region; pressing pain in both soles, with feeling as if they were swollen**; *frequent urination. The same dose repeated in the evening* before going to bed, manifested itself in an unmistakable manner, by *slight colic some fingers below the navel* (after six hours) and palpitation, but particularly by *pulsation in the scrobiculus*, accompanied by prickling stitches on the back, in the neighborhood of the middle thoracic vertebræ.

54.—*Gerstel's Proving of Colocynthin, Third (decimal) Dilution.*

June 24. *Fifty drops of the third dilution* in the morning, fasting, left behind a persistent, earthy, bitter taste upon the tongue, and a decided feeling of heat in the stomach, as if from hot water. *Eighty drops*, taken in the evening of the same day, produced the same earthy, bitter taste; sharp inpressing pain in some spots on the nape, as if from a sprain, aggravated by movement, the spot itself being sensitive to pressure from without; at the same time, short hacking cough, excited by a tickling in the throat; vivid dreams at night; continual burning pressure in the stomach up into the œsophagus during the following forenoon.

55.—*Gerstel's Proving of Colocynthin, Second (decimal) Dilution.*

June 27. *Twenty drops of the second dilution* taken in the morning, fasting. Soon after the dose, seizure of the whole head; slight pains here and there in the left leg and arm; congestion towards the genital

* Compare WEINKE's proving, *ante*, p. 334.

organs, especially the scrotum, with feeling of heat and persistent burning in a small spot upon the same, without erections; stitches in the region of the lowest dorsal vertebræ; pain in the right great toe, accompanied by a dull, not easily described feeling, as of heat on various places on the right thigh, especially on the posterior side in the course of the sciatic nerve; at the same time, a similar sensation in the external ball of the little toe of the same side. Some hours later, pressure in the left cheek-bone and left great toe; burning in the posterior wall of the pharynx; colic pains, with inflation of the abdomen. All these symptoms were developed when seated, lasted for almost two hours, and disappeared entirely on walking.

June 28. *Forty drops of the second dilution* were taken, but the prover remarks that, taking a long and fatiguing walk immediately after the medicine, he did not pay the requisite attention to the symptoms that might have been caused by the dose.*

June 29. *Sixty drops of the second dilution,* taken early, fasting, upon sugar of milk, caused a persistent, disgusting, bitter taste in the mouth; soon after, burning sticking, and sensation of warmth on the dorsum of the right foot; pressing-digging pain in the external side of the second toe of the left foot; cramp-pain in the muscles of the left wrist; feeling of pressure and swelling in the under eyelids; slight intimations of colic, drawing from the hypogastrium to the hepatic region; accompanied by shuddering in the scrotum (?), with erections, and pain in the buttock.

Watzke's Provings of Colocynthin.

In reference to my slender experiments with Colocynthin, I must premise that, in the beginning of the year 1843, I had commenced some trials with massive doses of common salt, and continued them until the end of April. The obstinate, deep-seated effects of that drug, however, continued for several weeks after I had taken the last dose. The irregularity of the stools, both in respect to time, repetition, and character, which I had observed during the whole proving, continued far into May; the characteristic painful tension on the flexor side of the joints, especially of the groins and knee, also frequently returned. My appetite continued somewhat slight, my sleep was disturbed, and I felt for several weeks uncommonly dull, depressed, and debilitated.

Previous to my first experiment with the Colocynthin, I had suffered for eight or ten days from a peculiar, very troublesome, periodical spasm of the urethra and rectum. There frequently came on in the afternoon, but irregularly, sometimes several times in an hour, often at intervals of five or ten minutes, and again once in two, three, or four hours, sensibility of the urethra, not aggravated by external pressure, a constric-

* We are but little concerned about the loss to our *Materia Medica* of those symptoms which are not recorded through the insufficient watchfulness of the prover over his own sensations. Not only should the experimenter be on the look out for symptoms, but the symptoms should be such as to *compel* his attention.—*Ed. Oest. Zeit.*

tive pain in that canal, and in the rectum, with tenesmus of both passages The urine was clear and in sufficient quantity, and discharged without pain; with the emission of urine, the rectal tenesmus generally disappeared also. This latter could generally be controlled, but drove me several times a day to stool, which was soft, rather fluid, without preparatory griping, and not accompanied nor followed by tenesmus. *There was, besides, not the least discharge from the urethra, nor the slightest disorder in the genital system.*

56.—*Watzke's Proving of Colocynthin, Sixth (decimal) Dilution.*

1843. May 21, 22, and 23. My friend, Dr. Gerstel, having informed me that Colocynth had excited in him symptoms similar to those from which I was suffering, and having suggested that it would, perhaps, be serviceable in removing the troublesome effects of *natrum-muriaticum* which I have above related, I took twice each day *six drops of the sixth (decimal) dilution of Colocynthin.* With the exception that, on the morning of the 22d, I awoke with griping and movements in the abdomen, I noticed no trace of Colocynth-symptoms. The urinary and fæcal troubles were scarce any relieved.

57.—*Watzke's Proving of Colocynthin, Fifth (decimal) Dilution.*

May 24.—I proceeded, therefore, to the *fifth dilution*, of which I took two doses in the forenoon, of *six drops* each, and on the 25th, of *ten drops each.* On both days I had two scanty, fluid stools, with no tenesmus, and scarce perceptible colic, one at midday and the other in the evening.

May 26. In the morning, two soft, rapidly and easily discharged stools in quick succession, which strikingly recalled the evacuations during my former proving of Colocynth. No other symptoms. My stool and urine difficulties were not so prominent, and my appetite began to increase a little.

58.—*Watzke's Proving of Colocynthin, Fourth (decimal) Dilution.*

May 26, 28, and 31. At noon of the first day, *six drops of the fourth dilution*, and in the morning of the other two days, *ten drops* each time. In the afternoon of the 26th, some slight, rapid, brown, soft stools. In the evening I felt all over hotter than usual, and remarkably depressed, but nevertheless had an excellent appetite. I slept very restlessly the following night, had many and vivid dreams, and perspired profusely towards morning.

May 27. In the morning, great depression, dull headache in the frontal region, aching in the eye-balls, aggravated by straining the sight, moving the eyes rapidly, and bowing the head, lasting all day. Several soft stools, rapidly and easily discharged.

May 28. All these symptoms continued, but much more mildly. A very striking symptom was a feeling of great stiffness and heaviness in the tibiæ. Towards evening, sticking, continuing for several minutes, in the epigastrium, which was tense and inflated. The urethral and rectal spasm, formerly so troublesome, and which had been somewhat mitigated for a day or two past, disappeared wholly on the 28th, and has not shown a trace of itself since.

59.—*Watzke's Proving of Colocynthin, Third (decimal) Dilution.*

June 7. For several days after the conclusion of my previous experiments with Colocynthin, which were finished on the 31st of May, I perceived transitory symptoms of Colocynth, such as pinching and movements in the umbilical region, sticking in the epigastrium, several soft, easily and rapidly passing stools a day, painfulness in the frontal region, and aching in the eye-balls. Towards the evening of June 7th, painful tension in the right inguinal region, and drawing along the spermatic cord into the right testicle, which was somewhat sensitive. I slept well during the night.

June 8. In the morning, the sensibility of the testicle and the tension in the inguinal region were worse, and were aggravated by walking, bending over, and going up stairs. Appetite excellent; two soft, brown stools every day. In the evening, frequent urging to urinate. No perceptible swelling in the groin; the right testicle, however, and particularly the epididymis, was considerably swollen and painful to external touch.

June 9. After a quiet night, the swelling and sensitiveness of the testicle and tension in the groin were less, but became worse again towards noon after long going about, and were still further aggravated in the evening. Stitches now came on, when walking, from the small of the back to the groin, and a hard tread caused pain in the right testicle, so that at last I feared to move about. At the same time, the left testicle became sensitive also. The pain was much ameliorated by rest, and especially by bending over.

In order to satisfy myself whether these phenomena were the remaining results of my salt-proving, as I conjectured them to be, or were attributable to the Colocynthin, I took, at 8 P.M. of the 9th, *five drops of the third dilution.*

June 10. *Five drops of the third dilution,* taken in the morning. The troubles of the groin and testicle were already less perceptible, and on the next day (11th) had wholly disappeared, and did not return on this or following days, even after a great deal of exercise.

June 15, 16. *Ten drops of the third dilution* on the first day, and *sixteen drops* on the second. No symptoms, except slight pinching colic, and transitory, easily controlled, urging to stool.

60.—*Watzke's Proving of Colocynthin, Second (decimal) Dilution.*

June 18. *Ten drops of the second dilution,* on sugar, at 9 A.M. On going out after it, it appeared to me as though my vision were sharper than usual. Looking through my ordinary spectacles was rather straining; slight dulness of the head, sensibility in the temples and forehead, transitory attack of vertigo.

Three hours later, after violent pinching in the umbilical region, and strong, irresistible inclination to stool, a scanty brownish-red evacuation with painful tenesmus, lasting some ten minutes. Inclination to stool several times in the afternoon; fine stitches in the scrobiculus, and pinching in the bowels. Towards evening, unusual debility and depression, heat in the whole body, thirst, somewhat accelerated pulse; towards 11 P.M., a copious, thin, pappy evacuation, easily and rapidly discharged without tenesmus. Very restless sleep at night; at first, dry heat and tossing about; later, toward morning, sweat. In the morning, depression and weariness of the whole body, painful pressure in the eyeballs and temples, appetite somewhat less, pulse still over 90.

June 19. No medicine; great depression all day; heat, accelerated pulse; dull head- and eye-ache, increased thirst, no stool; urine clear; in the afternoon, and especially in the evening, aggravation of the symptoms; (I could hardly keep myself on my legs). In bed, painfulness and feeling of heat along the whole spine; chest somewhat painful and oppressed; at times, dry cough; frequently repeated stitches from the left axilla down to the elbow; pulse 100; sleep excessively restless; at first, dry heat, then some perspiration; uninterrupted, confused dreams.

June 20. In the morning, dulness of the head, painfulness of the eyeballs, debility—but in less degree than yesterday; great desire to lie down, requiring great exertion to get off the bed; increased temperature of the skin; pulse 92. The feeling of depression and debility increased towards noon; accompanied by painfulness of the whole head, especially of the temporal and frontal regions, scalp and eyeballs, aggravated by moving the eyes, straining the sight, or bending forwards; at times, stitches in the brain. There was a return also of the feeling of warmth and sensitiveness along the spine, the oppression of the chest, and dry cough. At the same time, feeling of roughness in the throat, repeated stitches in the scrobiculus, painfulness of the malleoli. No pain in swallowing, nor difficulty in taking a long inspiration; appetite somewhat less; much thirst; tongue moist, slightly coated; taste natural; no stool all day; urine fiery, becomes cloudy on standing, but deposits no sediment. Amelioration of all the symptoms in rest. Night good; I awoke several times and always found myself in a profuse perspiration.

June 21. On getting up at 4½ A.M., I felt myself much strengthened by sleep and the head scarce affected at all. Breakfast, cold bread and milk, relished highly. Urine less highly colored than yesterday, and taking a longer time to become cloudy. Stool soon after breakfast, formed and normal; an hour afterwards, a second diarrhœic evacuation. I felt very comfortable until towards noon; head somewhat heavy, but not painful; the cough, which was still occasionally excited by the roughness in the throat, caused no pain either in the chest or abdomen, and was accompanied by a whitish-yellow mucus, expectorated without difficulty. From half-past 11 A.M., I rode for an hour in the rail-cars, and while riding felt the pain in my head becoming more perceptible. The concussions of the cars became by degrees more painful, and on coming out, I was obliged to move slowly and to tread softly, as the contrary course seemed to make the brain shake about, as if loose, against the scull (in the median vertical region); this was accompanied by very severe sore pain, and as it lasted during the whole quarter of an hour's walk, put me in a very bad humor. The cough, which came on occasionally, produced violent stitches through the cerebellum. I perceived no decided pain in the spine, but noticed the former sensation of pressure and warmth.

Rest and dinner, meal-porridge, fricassed chicken and water, (eaten with much relish,) so far set aside these symptoms that I took my seat in the cars again with renewed good humor. But they returned during the ride, and still more on leaving the cars, in all their former severity. In addition, I was troubled the whole afternoon with a disagreeable feeling of chilliness, great debility, unusual want of temper, so that I could not bring myself to take notice of the stitches, tearings, pressings, crampings, and such little matters, which appeared and disappeared in various parts of the body, especially in the joints and external side of the thighs and upper arms; (what struck me most was a cramp pain in the penis which lasted several minutes, during which it seemed as if it were bent double). A cup of black coffee immediately relieved the symptoms, but they did not entirely disappear until I went to bed, which I was glad to do at 7 P.M. I slept uneasily, and perspired copiously, but felt pretty well when I awoke the next morning.

June 22. I coughed frequently during the early part of the morning, and raised without difficulty a thick, yellow mucus, but had no pain either in the throat, chest, or head. I was able to resume my usual morning ablution of the whole body with cold water with tolerable ease, though previous to yesterday I had omitted it altogether, and had only done it then with great repugnance and no great thoroughness. The morning urine was somewhat more highly colored, but deposited no sediment.

Notwithstanding I rode and walked much, the amelioration continued until towards 6 P.M. Heaviness and pain in the occiput and painfulness of the eyeballs then came on; on coughing occasionally, I perceived the previous exceedingly painful stitches darting through the cerebellum like lightning; a heavy tread also caused stitches to traverse the occiput. In addition, the chilliness, debility, and want of temper of yesterday appeared again, and, with the headache and pains in the eyes, continued to increase until 8 P.M., when I went to bed. There I began gradually to grow better, but I did not feel able to get up until after a cup of black coffee, which I took at about 9 o'clock, when I read and wrote a little. Profuse perspiration during the night.

June 24, 25, 26. A good deal of perspiration nights; felt well in the mornings; loose cough; excellent appetite for dinner; occasional pressure on the vertex in the evening; sensitiveness of the cerebellum (on rapidly turning the head).

June 29. Perfectly well, with the exception of an occasional cough, accompanied by scanty, easily raised expectoration.*

CHAPTER IX.

Experiments on Animals.

Provings upon the various races of domestic animals are the *sine qua non* of a rational homœopathic practice for the veterinary physician; they must constitute the foundation of their *Materia Medica.* They are of value for us, too, inasfar as they exhibit (*per analogiam*) the pathological changes which a fully developed drug sickness is capable of producing in the human body. They are the only source of such information to us in those cases in which accidental poisonings and the subsequent post-mortem examination have not revealed to us the actual changes which take place in man's organism.

The experiments which we have made upon animals with Colocynth have remained far behind our desires. We had flattered ourselves with the expectation of enlarging and perfecting our *Materia Medica* on the veterinary side also, by means of a satisfactory course of provings upon animals. But we found the plan attended by greater difficulties than we had imagined. Half of these arise from the position in which physicians in full practice are placed, and cannot be avoided; and could we expect by future provings to remove the other half, we could not but still perceive that the object could not as well be attained as by veterinary practitioners themselves.

So far as Colocynth is concerned, we have fortunately the necessary pathological information in the examinations which have been made of those who have died from poisonous doses (see *ante,* Chap. IV.) The veterinary physician, too, is spared much toilsome labor by the experiments of Viborg and Orfila, which, together with those of our colleague, Dr. Fröhlich, we proceed to relate.

* I would willingly join those who have never proved a drug upon their own bodies, and recognize in the above train of symptoms nothing more than an accidental acute bronchial catarrh. But, apart from the considerations that I am not in the least degree inclined to catarrh, having not been so affected for years, and that I cannot assign any of the usual causes for its appearance, the abdominal symptoms which accompanied its commencement presented the greatest possible similarity to those which attended my former proving of Colocynth. The headaches, however, which continued during the whole malady, were so violent and so prominent, that I have no hesitation in considering the disorder of the brain as the primary trouble, and the slight affection of the bronchial mucous membrane as merely secondary.—*Watzke.*

61.—*Viborg's Provings upon Animals.*

Viborg experimented (*Abhandlungen für Thierärzte*, b. 4) on different domestic animals.

A watery infusion of 2½ ounces of Colocynth-pulp was administered to a horse, with no other result than frequent urination, excited appetite, increased and well-digested stools. Five and a half ounces of the triturated powder produced the same effect.

Another horse was unaffected by from one to five-and-a-half ounces of the Colocynth apple. Six ounces produced (after 24 hours) copious discharge of loose stool with increased appetite; the pulse, however, was smaller and slower.

An infusion of two ounces, administered to a ram, caused (in 12 hours) violent diarrhœa, lasting two days; loss of appetite and debility. He was better on the third day. Half an ounce produced no effect upon a sheep; two ounces produced hard evacuation in another.

Two drams of the marc occasioned increased appetite and slight diarrhœa in a swine. Diarrhœa and violent vomiting were brought on in an old poodle by two drams.

62.—*Orfilas' Provings upon Dogs.*

Orfila (*Toxicol., sec. edit., p.* 34) instituted six experiments with Colocynth upon dogs.

1. A small, hungry dog took, at noon, a decoction of two drams of Colocynth, which was so diluted with water as to be colorless and tasteless. The œsophagus was tied, he endeavored to vomit, had vertigo after four hours, and died in the night. (From the Colocynth or the operation? *Ed. Oest. Zeit.*)

2. The œsophagus of a medium-sized dog was tied, after two ounces of extract had been administered to him. He soon after manifested violent efforts to vomit; in four hours his gait became unsteady and he fell. Two hours subsequently he gave scarce any signs of life, and suffered himself to be shoved about like a lifeless mass. Death in eleven hours after the dose.

In the stomach was found a part of the still undissolved extract; mucous membrane, dark red, with blackish red streaks; muscular coat, cherry red; intestines but little changed, except the rectum, the mucous lining of which was highly inflamed, and of a vivid red; lungs filled with blood, but crepitating; cerebral vessels turged with black blood; pia mater much injected.

3. An infusion of two ounces of Colocynth in wine was introduced into the stomach of a moderately large dog, and the œsophagus tied. He whined during the day, became weak, and had two copious stools. Death in 22 hours.

Mucous membrane of stomach, duodenum and ilium, reddened throughout its whole extent with dark red spots; jejunum and cœcum, and commencement of the colon almost normal; in the lower part of the colon, and in the rectum, blackish, elevated streaks were scattered upon a ground of a vivid red; lungs healthy.

4. An opening was made at 9 A.M., in the œsophagus of a medium-sized dog; two drams of finely-powdered Colocynth were inserted and a ligature applied. At 2 P.M., he had a fluid, blackish evacuation, whined a great deal, but showed no signs of vertigo or convulsions. At 8 P.M. he could no longer stand up, but lay like a lifeless mass; respiration somewhat accelerated and labored. He lay motionless on his side until he died at midnight.

The stomach was internally purple, and contained, besides food and Colocynth, a considerable quantity of fluid. At the bottom the membrane was blackish red, but otherwise of a bright red; the duodenum, ilium, cœcum, and a portion of the colon were intensely reddened; the rectum showed a number of bright red spots.

5. Two and a half drams of Colocynth were digested for six hours in five ounces of white wine, and the fluid introduced into the stomach of a dog at 11 A.M., the œsophagus being then tied. At 6 P.M., the animal passed two fluid stools, and whined violently; he died in the night. A Colocynth apple, which he had been made to swallow the day before, had been vomited up after being down an hour.

Mucous membrane of the rectum and lower part of the colon dark red, and the subjacent muscular tissue also inflamed; lungs, stomach, and other viscera not specially changed.

6. A wound was made in the inner side of the thigh of a dog, two drams of finely-powdered Colocynth inserted, and the lips brought together. The animal did not seem troubled on the second day, did not whine, and went about as usual, but died during the following night.

The mucous membrane of the rectum was very much altered; almost the whole surface was covered with blood-red spots; the rest of the digestive canal and the lungs were unaltered; the wounded leg exhibited an extensive inflammation with infiltration of blood, but no scab.

63.—*Fröhlich's Provings upon Rabbits.*

Dr. FRÖHLICH experimented with rabbits, with the tincture, the triturated powder, and with Colocynthin. His experiments are worthy of study, as the gradual poisoning permitted a longer and more careful observation, and they are accompanied by a most conscientious post mortem examination.

1. 1842, Dec. 25. A strong, white rabbit, ten weeks old, received in the morning *ten*, at noon *fifteen*, and in the evening *twenty-five drops of the tincture.* Not the slightest alteration in the creature could be seen, and on the following morning *thirty additional drops* were administered. Nothing was noticed except a little less liveliness in the animal's movements. Towards evening, when it received *two grains* of the finely-powdered pulp, it sat crouched up in a corner; when disturbed and pushed about, it seemed to move with difficulty. It ate with relish, nevertheless, during the whole day, the apples which were thrown

to it, and on the two following days, on which it received no medicine, though it was constantly dull and moved with great lassitude, it continually manifested a strikingly good appetite.

Dec. 29, 30. It had *ten drops of the tincture,* morning and evening of each day. On the 31st, it seemed very sick; was exceedingly feeble; could not, for instance, get over a low threshold an inch high, but remained with the hind legs hanging over it. When pushed forwards, it did not use its feet as usual, but bent up, and went on in a sort of shuffling gallop. *Ten drops of the tincture* were given on the same morning, whereupon it became gradually weaker, and died at about 2 P.M.

Section, twenty hours after death. The animal was emaciated; skin easily separated, tender on the hind legs, and coming off in pieces; the subcutaneous and deeper areolar tissue on the hind legs infiltrated with a gelatinous, perfectly transparent mass, so that the course of the tendons and several injected vessels could be distinctly traced. Muscles pale and flaccid. Nothing abnormal in the fore-paws. Lungs small, thickened in bands, pale pink on the edges, flesh red in the middle. Heart pale, relaxed, with the coronary vessels plainly injected; some serum in the pericardium. Stomach filled with a grayish, amorphous substance; mucous coat pale, with dendritic injection of the vessels, easily torn; the mysenteric vessels injected with bright red blood throughout the whole course of the intestine; chyme, here and there in the ilium; the stomach-like enlargement at the commencement of the colon, stuffed with amorphous masses of fæces; in the lower part of the canal, small, soft, formed fæces scattered about. Liver much enlarged; its upper surface, towards the right exterior lobe, marbled with dark and pale red; section of that lobe presenting a granulated appearance throughout, in other places only in spots, the upper surface decidedly tinged; the whole five lobes exhibiting cavities of the size of millet-seeds, filled with a purulent-looking fluid; gall-bladder distended with a similar liquid. Kidneys pale. Bladder empty.

2. A brownish gray rabbit, nine weeks old, had taken daily, for eight days, *five grains* of the first (decimal) trituration of Colocynth with sugar of milk, without manifesting any particular symptoms. 1843, Jan. 13. At 8 A.M., FRÖHLICH gave him, at a single dose, *forty drops of the clear Colocynth tincture.* He became weak half an hour after the dose, and remained motionless in a single spot, with his eyes fixed and staring. Towards noon, he passed a considerable quantity of loose, light brown fæces, and afterwards some whitish fluid. He squatted sadly in one corner the whole afternoon, with hair erect and half-closed eyes, and died at 7 P.M.

Section, twelve hours after death. Emaciation; veins of the thighs filled with dark-colored blood; nothing abnormal in the sciatic nerve or spinal marrow; cerebral vessels injected dark red; brain and lungs normal; right cavities of the heart and veins at the base turgid with venous blood; left cavities empty. Stomach marked with a few injected vessels of a bright red, radiating from the upper curve, and filled full with a firm mass of food, which was covered with a layer of mucus, especially toward the pyloric extremity; inner mucous coat pale, easily torn. Upper part of the intestines entirely empty throughout; commencement of the colon, and its enlargement, adjacent to the ilium, full of air and a pappy mass of fæces; further on, until this enlargement was lost in the cœcum, firm, well-formed fæces. Adhesions in places between the large and small intestines; the whole mass, as well as the mesentery throughout the entire intestinal tract, was marked with bright red injected vessels surrounding the bowels. The lower portion of the intestine marked with a straight vessel, bright red in its upper part, but dark red towards the end; inner surface tinged entirely red only at its extremity. Liver of normal size, color, and consistence, scantily set with whitish, mullet-seed points, permitting a purulent moisture to escape on being opened; gall-bladder distended with thin, brownish bile.

3. A strong rabbit, five months old, had gradually received, in the course of two months, *forty grains* of the first trituration of Colocynth-pulp, and *seven hundred drops of the tincture* (*twenty to fifty drops a day*), without being strikingly affected by it. Having remained four days without any medicine, it received, April 26, 1843, *one*, 27th, *two*, and 29th, *five grains of Colocynthin*, dissolved in a little water. No change was noticed, except a momentary impression and some sluggishness. From April 30 to May 4, no medicine was given and no symptom perceived; on the contrary, the animal, especially the latter part of the time, was lively, and had an excellent appetite. On the 5th of May, at 4 P.M., *seven grains of Colocynthin* were given with a little water, and the next morning it was found dead.

Section. The animal was not emaciated; on the contrary, pretty copious deposits of fat were found beneath the skin and in the intermuscular tissue; brain, normal; lungs, pale rose color, thickened in bands; heart, dusky red; right cavities and great veins filled with pitch-black coagulated blood, left cavities filled with blood of the same color, but thin and fluid. Œsophagus pale red; stomach distended with gray aliment; injected vessels of a dark color on the anterior and posterior parietes, proceeding from the smaller curvature; mucous membrane on the smaller curvature, especially towards and about the pylorus, flesh red, gradually diminishing in intensity towards the great curvature, and exhibiting, when examined through a lens, red points collected in spots; membrane firm. Small intestine full of a yellowish chyme; mucous lining pale red; mesenteric vessels bright red and injected, embracing the whole extent of the intestine; colon filled with fetid, pappy fæces; mesocolic vessels distended, dark red, especially remarkable in the great veins accompanying the rectum to its termination. The mucous lining of the colon not altered; spleen normal; liver presenting a single protuberant, suppurating point; kidneys, sciatic nerve, and spinal marrow normal.

4. 1843, July 26. Dr. FRÖHLICH administered to a strong doe-rabbit, five months old, *five grains of Colocynthin* in some water; the

dose was repeated the next day, after which the animal became dull, but continued to eat with appetite. On the 28th and 29th, she received *seven grains* each time, and began to seem very ill on the last day. On the 30th, she had, during the day, several thin stools; in the evening, notwithstanding she still fed, she seemed extremely feeble, and died during the night.

Section, about ten hours after death. No emaciation; brain, heart, and lungs healthy; liver of normal consistence, but strewed with cysts from the size of a millet-seed to that of a pea, filled with a serous fluid and distinguished by snow-white, hardish points, not rising above the surface, but a little depressed; the cysts themselves covered with injected bloodvessels. Similar phenomena in the intestines. Stomach eroded in one place to the external membrane; the mucous lining reddened, easily separated, and thickly set with brownish black points; vivid reddening of the mucous lining of the small intestines; mesenteric vessels congested; uterus dark red at its fundus and containing a small fœtus (like a *Proteus anguinus,* but without a trace of an eye,) together with the placenta and membranes.

CHAPTER X.

Homœopathic Cures with Colocynth.

Colocynth has achieved its most brilliant therapeutic triumphs in the province of the *Neuroses.* Neuralgic and hyperæsthesic affections of the *trigeminus,* the *solar plexus,* the *lumbar and femoral nerves,* and their ramifications are those which have been chiefly excited, and therefore cured, by its agency. Such are by far the greater part of the cases recorded in our literature, as having been cured by Colocynth, and even the few hyperæmic and inflammatory difficulties that have disappeared under its administration, are rather to be considered as having yielded to the predominant influence of the affection of the nerves.

1. *Neuralgic and Hyperæsthesic Affections of the Trigeminus.*

1. A young woman, 24 years of age, of scrofulous constitution, fair complexion, and not fully developed growth, became, all at once, subject to attacks of unusually violent, pressive, tearing headache. While it lasted, she could not lie down, but stood bent double, and gave vent to screams and tears. When it subsided she had paroxysms of suffocation; the chest felt constricted, she clenched her hands, and gasped for breath.* She then became composed, spoke, and remained

* The symptoms of the respiration are plainly due to a reflex influence from the brain, and especially from the *medulla oblongata,* the common origin of the *trigeminus and vagus,* upon the peripheric pulmonary branches of the *vagus.* If, however, any one should prefer to consider the foregoing case as a spinal neurosis of the cerebral system, we have no special objection to offer. "The *external headaches,* apparently seated in the integuments and *galea aponeurotica,* which so frequently accompany affections of the cervical portion of the spine, are easily explained, as the occipital and auricular nerves, distributed

quiet for half an hour, or even several hours, when the attack would return. Dr. SCHINDLER, to whom the patient applied, after she had suffered from this affection for 4 weeks, first had recourse to Belladonna, without any result. A dose of Colocynth (how much?) having been administered, the paroxysms became less frequent, but so much the more intense. It was necessary to recur to its use six times (at what intervals?) before the complaint quite gave way.—THORER's *Prac. Beiträge*, Band ii. 10.)

2. Dr. SCHÜLER gives the following interesting case of cure by Colocynth (*Prac. Mitth. der Corresp. Gesellsch. Hom. Aerzte*, 1827, s. 39, *et seq.*) It is one of encephalalgia, complicated with ophthalmia, the latter having come on after the headache had lasted a long time with scarcely any intermission. Dr. Schüler found the left eye quite blind from the previous allopathic treatment, and the other, though still useful, the seat of burning, cutting pain. The patient also complained of congestion in the head, and of a copious acrid discharge from both eyes. *Two drops of tincture of Colocynth, every 3 hours, removed the headache completely within 24 hours, and had a sensible effect in diminishing the pain in the eye. Under a continuance of the Colocynth, the sight of the eye was preserved, and the patient completely restored in eight days.*

Our opinion, subject to correction, on this case is, that the headache arose from cerebral congestion, and was the primary affection; and that the ophthalmia was secondary to it, and produced by the sympathetic affection of the nerves supplying the eye, derived from the *trigeminus*, and the twigs of the *sympathetic* in connection with it. *Colocynth cannot cure a primary ophthalmia, because it cannot give rise to one.*

3. A boy, 13 years of age, had complained for four days of violent stitches in the forehead and eyes, from without inwards. The pain continued day and night, only diminishing for a few moments to return with increased severity. He became feverish, with bitter taste in the mouth, total loss of appetite, and constipation. *Six hours after a dose of Colocynth 30, the pain had disappeared; next day the patient quitted his bed.*—(ATTOMYR's *Briefe über Hom.* I., 4.) We regard the complaint as a hyperæsthesia of the *supra-orbital* and *ophthalmic branches of the fifth.*

4. A hemicrania in a woman turned 50, occupying the left side, returning periodically at 5 in the afternoon, and which had lasted several years, was, after fruitless treatment by allopathic means, somewhat alleviated by *Asarum*, and disappeared entirely and permanently under a few days' use of Colocynth.—(ATTOMYR, *Archiv f. Hom.* H. xi. 2, 144.

5. A violent face-ache, (prosopalgia, neuralgia of the trigeminus,*)

to these parts, arise from the superior cervical nerves, and send branches as far as the forehead." (HIRSCH, *Spinal-Neurosen.* Königsb. 1843. s. 206.—*Watzke.*

* The sensitive fibres of the 5th nerve are the seat of prosopalgiæ. The *facial* nerve is purely motor (*Constatt. Handb. d. Med. Klinik. Erl.* 1843. iii., 218). We have put the above cases of encephalopathia and hemicrania under the head of Neuralgiæ of the fifth, from a conviction, which our experiments have induced, that it is in these cases it is the affected organ.—*Ed. Oest. Zeit.*

which had lasted 3 days, speedily yielded to a single dose of Colocynth. —(GASPARI, *Annal. d. Hom. Klinik*, iii., 411.) The patient was a robust man, 40 years of age. The pains were sticking, tensive, and tearing, extending over the whole left side of the face, appearing periodically, aggravated by warmth, motion, and touch, and allowed the sufferer no respite, either by day or by night. The left side of the face was hot and red. Also thumping pain in the head, as if the left half were being torn from the right; toothache on the same side; general heat, thirst; pulse full and hard. No cause could be assigned for the affection. Colocynth (dose not specified) was given in the evening; the patient slept comfortably the ensuing night, and awoke next morning quite well. On the complaint returning a year afterwards, Colocynth again afforded equally speedy relief.

2. *Neuralgiæ of the Cœliac Plexus and its Branches.*

6. Dr. SCHRÖN removed in a sexagenarian, a violent burning pain in the scrobiculus, with complete intolerance of pressure, vomiting of all the ingesta, small rapid pulse, and restless tossing about in bed with Colocynth, one drop of the 30th, repeated after 16 hours. Arsenic had been tried without benefit.—(*Allg. Hom. Zeit.* V., 149.)

7. A woman, 50 years of age, had complained for a fortnight of constant disgust at all food, without desire to vomit; cutting pains in the abdomen, which often intermitted, and as often returned, and on the left side of the abdomen a feeling as of a hank twisting round. Also sleeplessness, heat, violent thirst, bitter taste, copious eructations, loss of appetite, constipation, frequent calls to make water, with scanty emission. *Colocynth* 10 removed the pain. The bitter taste remained, as well as the disgust and anorexia, but yielded to *bryonia* and *ipecacuanha*.—(*Annal. d. Hom. Kl.* ii., 264.)

8. An anonymous writer (H.) relates a case of a pregnant female, who was perfectly cured in a few hours by Colocynth 30, of a violent sticking burning pain in the left side of the abdomen. He looks upon the affection as an extremely acute inflammation, but whether in the psoas, kidneys, or spleen, he cannot tell! Ruoff, in his Repertory even calls it peritonitis! It was nothing more than nervous irritation—circumscribed hyperæsthesia of the cœliac plexus. At all events the honor of the rapid cure belongs to Colocynth.—(*Allg. Hom. Zeit.* iv., 66.)

9. One cannot conclude from Dr. KRAMER's account (*Hygea*, i. 30), nor is it in itself likely, that *Colocynth* contributed towards the cure of an affection of the abdomen, of five years' standing, in a duchess, who, since her last confinement but one had suffered from almost daily recurring sticking pains in the right side of the lower abdomen, extending to the kidneys and back. There were also hæmorrhoids, frequent and ineffectual efforts to go to stool, constipation, flatulence, distension of the abdomen, swelling and painfulness of the lower limbs, cold hands and feet, disposition irritable and depressed. *Sulph.*, *nux*, *coloc.*, *phosph.*, *nux*, and again *phosph.*, restored the patient to health in 3 months. In our opinion *Nux-vomica* was the specific remedy in this case.

10. We regard the three cases which Dr. Schron (*Hygea*, ix. 503) gives, as acute catarrh of the bladder, occurring in young women of thirty, and which he cured *rapidly with Colocynth*, as hyperæsthesiæ of some branches of the *renal, hypogastric, mesenteric plexus* of the sympathetic, distributed to the urethra, the bladder, and the rectum. The catarrh was a secondary symptom. The following were the circumstances: At first, cutting pain in the umbilical region, extending towards the ovaries; then desire to pass water, with emission of a small quantity of cloudy, mucous urine, which soon deposited a mucous sediment. Next came on pains like labor-pains, in the direction of the ureters, extending to the upper part of the thighs. Then burning in the urethra; the urine could not be retained more than an hour. There was scarce any intermission of the cutting pain about the fundus of the bladder. The stools were increased in frequency, and attended with cutting pains and a kind of tenesmus. Little appetite; fever towards evening.

11. We may here notice two interesting cases given by Dr. Y. (*Hom. Bekehrungsepisteln*, 1837, 43, 44.)

The first was a neuralgia of the *internal spermatic plexus*, with sympathetic affection of the *cœliac plexus*, the *vagus*, and the femoral nerves, with which it is connected directly or indirectly.

A young woman, 25 years of age, of choleric temperament, had suffered *since her 7th year* from pains which, proceeding from the region of the left ovary, extended partly (burning and cutting) towards the umbilicus, and partly as a painful drawing through the whole right foot. During the day the pain would not abate for more than an hour at a time, being worst in the forenoon, and being aggravated by motion, but at night it was frequently scarcely felt at all. When at the worst, the patient rolled about in bed in spasmodic contortions; the head became burning hot, the rest of the body icy cold; the neck and chest swelled; the breathing became labored, and consciousness was lost. At length all the symptoms abated simultaneously with vomiting of a bitter, watery mucus. After such an attack, the pain was much less violent for several weeks.

A few doses of *Nux-vomica* and *Colocynth* sufficed to deliver the sufferer from this complaint, which had lasted so long.*

12. The second case, singularly enough styled by Y. "*Sterno-cœlialgia*," we consider as a neuralgia of the *plexus phrenicus* and *plexus gastricus magnus*, caused by spinal irritation.

A widow, 44 years of age, had been ill for years. Without assignable cause, a constrictive pain was felt in the region of the left false ribs, at first every four weeks, afterwards every day after dinner. It lasted a quarter of half an hour at a time, with ceaseless, forcible yawning, weight in the chest, and profuse sweat, disappeared at night and in the forenoon,

* We omit the long description of the accompanying (sympathetic) symptoms which probably led Dr. Y. to the selection of *bryonia*, and subsequently, after a violent relapse, of *pulsatilla*, as having little to do with the cure by the *Colocynth.*—*Watzke.*

but gradually increased in frequency and severity, and was accompanied with turning and cutting in the abdomen. Almost all the medical lights in the town had plied for four years powders, electuaries, mixtures, clysters, blisters, and plasters, but all to no purpose. Y. found the patient in the following wretched condition: complete loss of appetite—for the last two years she has taken nothing but broth; a constant bitter taste and much mucus in the mouth; a stool generally only once in four days; catamenia very irregular. The pain has become so intense that it never entirely subsides either by day or night; and the violent attacks occur almost every half hour. The patient then bends herself double, kneels in the bed, stretches herself out again convulsively, and twists round and round in an agony of tears and groans, &c. If the pain leaves the side and belly, the chest is seized with a horrible constriction; the patient is seized with unutterable anxiety, and feels as if she was dying. The limbs are cold; the pulse small and irregular; and the whole body drips with a cold sweat; also almost constant sleeplessness, extraordinary weakness and lassitude, great emaciation, despairing frame of mind.

Under the repeated use of *colocynth* 3, *bryonia* 3, and *arsenicum* 30, complete recovery ensued in two months; and after two years she continued to enjoy uninterrupted and robust health, without the slightest trace of her former malady. (It seems to us that the remedies which were employed besides the Colocynth, could have scarce any if at all contributed to the cure.)

13. Dr. Most of Rostock communicates the following case (*Allg. Med. Zeit.*, May, 1834):

An aged single woman had suffered for a fortnight from periodical pains in the abdomen, headache, nausea, and violent pulsation in the region of the spleen. The pulsation began towards evening, and continued three or four hours. Under the use of effervescing powders the abdominal pain had disappeared in a week; not so, however, the periodical headache and pulsation in the belly, which (though the radial pulse was unaffected) was perceptible not only to the touch, but to the sight. In some of these paroxysms the agony rose to distraction. When they passed off, the patient felt quite well. The *Tinct. Valer. Ammon.* employed for fourteen days, alleviated the difficulties, but the beating continued unabated. Constipation also occurring, Most suspected the existence of *infarcta* (*!*) and prescribed *Tart. tart.*, rhubarb, and flowers of sulphur, ordered the patient to drink tea made from valerian and senna, and had the balsam of sulphur rubbed into the side. When he saw the patient again after eight weeks, she was freed from her whole complaint; but not from the medicines mentioned above, but from a household simple—*Colocynth-brandy.* Having drunk this four times, she passed, amid violent pains in the belly, and diarrhœa, seven lumbrici, the expulsion of which was followed by complete recovery.

Does not the periodical type of this affection, with the complete intermissions, distinctly point out its nervous character? Was the abdominal pulsation—arising from increased innervation, directed on the splenic arteries—the necessary result of the irritation from the worms? May we not rather suppose, that the whole complaint, including the worms, was the product of an abnormal influence of the *cœliac plexus* on the digestive apparatus? Was not the headache to be regarded as a reflex action on the central termination of the sympathetic system? Why did not the parasites yield to the laxatives, e. g. the rhubarb, previously employed? In vermicular affections what is it that determines the choice of the anthelmintic? Are we mistaken in saying, that, in the case related above, the headache, the abdominal pulsation, and the lumbrici would have been proof against *Cina*, and *Sabadilla*, and *Spigelia* too?*

By far the most frequent use that has been made of Colocynth, has been for the cure of colics. Indeed it has been employed too indiscriminately in this way, and has become to the adherents of the specific method, what opium is in the old school. NENNING (*Annal. d. Hom. Klinik*, ii. 256) gives several cases.

14. A servant-maid had been tortured with a violent colic for ten days. The pain lasted day and night; she cried out, bent double, and rolled about in her bed. Every imaginable domestic remedy had been tried in vain, and the patient's death was expected from hour to hour. *One drop of the 24th dil. of Colocynth produced almost instantaneous relief.* A drop of the 30th dil. had as prompt an effect in a similar colic occurring in a boy of 13.

15. A cabinetmaker, 50 years of age, undersized, of choleric temperament, was seized with colic, without known cause. It began at ten in the morning, and continued till midnight, with more or less intermissions. He was hot and thirsty, vomited repeatedly all ingesta, and had not a stool oftener than once in five or six days. A single dose of Colocynth 24 removed the complaint, which had lasted fourteen days, notwithstanding the use of laxatives and anodynes.

16. An unmarried female, 42 years of age, was seized, after a fall on the ice, with burning in the left side of the abdomen and groin; the pains abated somewhat under the use, during four weeks, of ointments, poultices, and mixtures. She was so unfortunate, however, as to fall a second time, when violent sticking was experienced in paroxysms in the parts which had previously suffered. The attacks came on once an hour, or once in two hours, and lasted a couple of minutes at a time. Allopathic remedies (chiefly drastic purges, which brought on painful

* Cruvelhier states (*Univ. Lex. d. pr. Med. u. Chir. Art. Entozoa*) that he knows of a domestic remedy of great efficacy against these worms, especially in persons past the age of 14. It is Colocynth, so highly prized by the ancients, for this purpose. He administered Colocynth-brandy internally to two adults, and caused, at the same time, an ointment, consisting of powdered Colocynth and lard, in the proportion of a drachm to the ounce, to be rubbed into the hypogastric region. This was followed, in both cases, by the expulsion of these animals in great numbers; and the symptoms complained of,—which, but for their periodicity, *might have been set down to inflammation of the heart or great vessels*,—speedily disappeared. It is a pity that Cruveilhier has not described these cases more minutely. Their resemblance to the case in the text, and to nervous affections, is, however, apparent, even from this imperfect account.—*Watzke.*

and bloody stools) were used without effect for twenty-two days; the pain continually increased in severity. NENNING found the abdomen large and tense; the left side and groin felt sore and bruised when touched, as if something had been torn there; the tongue was dry; appetite small; frequent bitter eructations; frequent desire to urinate, with discharge of abundant pale yellow urine. A single dose of *Colocynth* 30, sufficed to remove the paroxysms of pain. *Arnica* removed the remaining tenderness of the left side.

17. A man, 49 years old, after drinking a quantity of wine—a beverage that never agreed with him—was seized on the following day with constant retching, not relieved by vomiting, and sticking burning pain in the left lumbar region, drawing towards the umbilicus, so violent as to deprive the patient of all rest, whether in or out of bed; he rolled himself like a ball, sometimes all but resting on his head, sometimes kneeling in the bed, but without relief, whatever the position he assumed. Having removed the sickness with *ipecucanaha* 3, NENNING ordered *Colocynth* 24, which effected a complete cure in three days.

18. Its effect was more rapid in the case of a young man, of weakly constitution, who, as he supposed, from catching cold, suffered such excruciating pains in the belly, that he thought he should go wild. He cried out constantly for help; he felt as if his intestines were being cut in pieces. Occasional intermissions were succeeded by more violent paroxysms. This had lasted the whole night. Bitter drops, the *Spiritus Hoffmanni*, and essence of caraway had no effect. NENNING then gave half a drop of tincture of *Colocynth*, and in half an hour all pain was gone.

19. Violent abdominal pain, making the patient bend herself double, with inclination to vomiting and diarrhœa, occurring after catching cold, in a sickly girl, 19 years old, *at the commencement of the monthly period*, was immediately assuaged by a dose of *Colocynth* 30, and disappeared entirely in a few hours.*

Our colleague, Dr. WEINKE, contributes another case of menstrual colic, cured by *Colocynth*.

* After NENNING has communicated cases of this character to the *Annal. der hom. Klinik*, he complains in the *Allg. hom. Zeit.* xv., 119 (notwithstanding he had in the meantime alternated *colocynth* and *chamomile* every half hour, in cases of colic with constipation "*with the best results*") about the uncertainty of homœopathic remedies for colics particularly and especially of *colocynth*. Allopathy, with its purgatives, clysters, frictions, and baths is by far more efficacious in such cases! "Where," he exclaims "can the homœopath find a sure and certain laxative?" It seems to us that the uncertainty can be fairly charged neither upon Homœopathy nor upon *colocynth*, but rather belongs to NENNING's diagnosis, of which we have not derived the highest idea from reading the remarks accompanying the foregoing cases in the *Annalen*. When the colics which accompany a tubercular state of the peritonæum, and the formation of tubercular ulcers in the intestinal mucous membrane, notwithstanding their resemblance to the colics of *colocynth*, still refuse to be cured or relieved by that drug or by any other, this fact will hardly excite wonder in a physician, except perchance, in one, who cannot spy the tuberculosis behind the colic.—*Ed. Oest. Zeit.*

20. Josefa Binder, 33 years of age, of lively temperament, following a sedentary occupation, accustomed to take wine in moderate quantities, had for some months experienced, 2 or 3 days before the catamenia (which were normal in quantity), violent cutting pains below the navel, from which they extended towards the flanks, and the internal genital organs, only ceasing now and then for half-an-hour; they disappeared when she became warm in bed, and were accompanied by cold feet. The stools were pap-like, and occurred once or twice a day, with griping. Drawing the thighs up to the body relieved the abdominal pain. A single drop of *Colocynth* 1, on sugar of milk, removed the pain in the course of an hour, and the menses came on during the night without any further inconvenience.

21. Paroxysms of colic in a lying-in woman most frequently at night; cutting as if with knives in the abdomen, preceded by discharge of flatulence, and accompanied by chills, violent stitches in the region of the right ovary, and tearing in the foot; during an evacuation, griping constriction in the bowels. TH. RUECKERT cured this case speedily with *Colocynth* 12.

22. Our colleague, Dr. BÖHM, cured radically with *Colocynth* 3, attacks of colic, with pressure at the stomach, flatulence, eructations, and mucous diarrhœa, in a man of 54, subject to hæmorrhoids; the colic came on daily, and was brought on by taking food even of the lightest description. The patient had undergone the water treatment of Gräfenberg for three years, with partial amendment. Soon after the first dose of Colocynth, he was seized with a more violent colic than he had ever experienced. Ten months after he had experienced no return.

23. A girl, 11 years old, was suddenly seized, without assignable cause, with the most violent pain in the abdomen, which refused to yield to the purgative and anodyne remedies prescribed at home. The pain increasing every quarter of an hour, Dr. BETHMANN was sent for, and found her in indescribable agony, bent double, rolling about in the bed, howling and whining; abdomen drawn in, sensitive to the slightest pressure; pulse small, scarcely perceptible; skin dry, hands and feet cold. She dared not take more than a few drops of milk and water at once to quench her burning thirst; if she took more, vomiting ensued. Soon after taking adose of *Colocynth* 24, she fell into a calm sleep, and awoke in the morning quite well.

She had previously been liable to slighter attacks of the same nature, but after this remained, so long as Dr. BEHTMANN kept her in view—fully 3 years—quite free from them. (*Annal. d. Hom. Klinik, iii.* 419.)

24. In the 3d number of the 5th vol. of the *Archiv*, page 27, we find a remarkable cure by *Colocynth* of a chronic tympanites, with periodical attacks of colic.

A young woman had been in bad health ever since her last confinement, in which she had had a profuse hæmorrhage. The abdomen was so swelled and tense, that she seemed pregnant. She also suffered from frequent paroxysms of colic, and had lost much in strength. She had been treated unsuccessfully for two years by allopathic means. On the 29th Nov., 1823, Dr. H. of Z., who had previously treated the patient for half a year with mixtures, being called to her in the evening, found her in the following condition: The most violent pains in the whole abdomen, as if the bowels were bruised between stones; she can only lie doubled together; abdomen swelled and tympanitic; countenance pale, sunk, and pinched; frequent retching; fainting fits; unutterable anguish; constipation.

After a dose of one drop of Colocynth 12, ensued a notable aggravation of the pains for some minutes, which, however, soon entirely ceased. The patient fell into a sleep, from which she did not awake till next morning. The tympanites disappeared in a few weeks. H. observed the patient for two years, during which time there was no return of the colic. Doubtless the tympanites was dependent on the neurosis, and of secondary importance.

25. Dr. Hering removed the colic of the West Indies (dry belly-ache), which is dreaded both on account of the violence of its attack, and its tendency to relapse, and to bring on secondary affections (paralysis of the limbs, chronic diarrhœa, &c.), in three or four days, *by the alternate use of globules the size of mustard-seeds, of Colocynth* 30, and of black coffee, without ever leaving any secondary disease.—*Archiv f. Hom.* H. xiii., 3, 69.

Hering says it was from these cures of colic that he was first led to see the necessity of repeating the remedy in alternation with its antidote. We must confess that we have no great opinion of this alternating system, and that the necessity for it is not at all apparent to us from these cases of Hering; *for they furnish no evidence of the efficacy of Colocynth.* The aggravation which sooner or later succeeded the administration of the globule is simply referable to the process of development of the colic, rising and falling periodically, till it reached its acme. Nor do we regard the black coffee as a curative or specific agent, but it masked the abnormal sensations either completely or partially while its effect lasted; in short, it did nothing but make the disease run its course with less torture to the patient. The pain was renewed each time, not from the globule of *Colocynth* having been swallowed, but from the anodyne effect of the coffee having passed away.

26. The following account of a case of an abdominal neurosis, complicated with a prosopalgia, related by Gaspari (*Annal. d. Hom. Klin.* iii. 19, *et seq.*), is interesting in more than one point of view.

A young woman, 24 years of age, fell ill after catching cold, with high fever, sticking in the chest, and headache. Six bleedings and many mixtures freed her in six weeks of this acute attack, but induced a worse and chronic one, on which the resources of art were fruitlessly expended during three years. G. undertook the case in the following state:—Emaciated to a skeleton; skin harsh and clay-colored; formication and restlessness of the whole body; extreme weakness of the limbs; giddiness, making her footing insecure; want of memory; pressive pain in the brow and temples, most tolerable in the recumbent posture, aggravated by sitting up and walking; pale contracted features; watering of the mouth; desire for milk; eructations and risings of a sweetish fluid after eating anything. The eructations continued with anguish, pain and pressure at the scrobiculus, for half an hour or an hour after eating, when the food came up, and she experienced a sense of emptiness and cramp; rumbling, pinching, burning, and sticking in the abdomen. A stool every three or four days, whitish and hard; the catamenia had not appeared for three years, the duration of her complaint.

But little benefit was derived from *aconite* and *calcarea*, during nearly four weeks. There now occurred, apparently from catching cold, violent tearing, burning, and continual sticking in the left half of the face. The pains became worse on contact, and made her cry out. The patient could get no rest, and passed the night without sleep. The symptoms enumerated led Gaspari to *Colocynth*. It and *sepia*, to which he afterwards had recourse, effected a complete cure. The menses returned; and he says, in conclusion, that the patient, who previously could only be regarded as the certain victim of death, has ever since enjoyed uninterrupted good health.

Are we mistaken when we set this complaint down as fundamentally a nervous one? May not the abdominal affection, which undoubtedly made a near approach to organic change, be referred to depraved innervation? What was the relation of the prosopalgia to the neurosis of the abdomen? Did the *peccant matter* from the gastric branch of the vagus spread to the trigeminus? Was the curative action of the *Colocynth* limited, as Gaspari seems to think, to removing the neuralgic pain in the face? or may we not rather suppose it to have played the principal part in the removal of the whole complaint?

27. *Colocynth* has been recommended by many authorities, and much employed in dysentery. Dr. Mosbauer derived great help from it in an epidemic dysentery (*Archiv f. hom. H.*, vi. 3, 18). Mühlenbein also assures us that he cured several cases of diarrhœa and dysentery by its means (*Archiv f. hom. Heil*, vi. 3, 78). Tincture of *Colocynth* employed by Rau (*Ueber den Werth des hom. Heilverf.*, 1st *Auf. s.* 99), effected speedy cures (in 2 days) in sporadic dysentery. He found it most useful when it was accompanied by violent colic pains. According to the experience of Pauli (*Hyg.* iii. 139), *Colocynth* is most adapted to those kinds of dysentery in which there is great pain, and scanty stools. Dr. Convers (*Hyg.* iii. 269) found it effectual in an epidemic where there were violent tearing pains in the belly, forcing the patient to bend forwards, incarcerated flatulence, and frequent stools streaked with blood. Rummel also resorted to it with success in a case of dysentery, to remove the pains (*Annal. d. hom. Klin.* iv, 322.) A friend of Leo Wolf, at New York, employed *Colocynth* with such extraordinary success in dysenteries, as, he assures us, not to have lost one single patient in three years (*Kleinert's Repert.*, 1832, ii. 155).* None of these

* Gross's assertion (*Archiv für hom. Heilk.* xv. 1, 97) that *Colocynth* had been of no service in his hands in common dysentery, with violent cutting in the

gentlemen, however, have given us a detailed description of a dysentery cured by *Colocynth.*

We are inclined to think that good effects are to be expected from *Colocynth* in dysentery (speaking generally), only so long as the hyperæsthesia of the intestine, and especially of the rectum,—which, according to Verger, Chauvin, Fink, Paterson, and others, constitutes the cause and essence of the disease,—is still predominant, and is not overcome by the (consecutive) inflammatory process; *i. e.*, so long as the dysentery presents the character of a *neurosis.* Against the inflammation, with its organic products—in short, the fully developed form of dysentery—it will be of much less service.

III. *Neuralgiæ of the Lumbar and Femoral Nerves, and their Branches.*

1. *Lumbago.*

28. A man, 54 years of age, tall and thin, given to drinking, and a sufferer for some years past from dyspeptic and severe hæmorrhoidal complaints, fell ill after exposure to cold, and was treated without success for five weeks by several physicians. Rückert undertook the case on the 15th February, 1817. The following is the account of the patient's state:—

Violent thumping pain in the whole costal region; tension of the integuments from the umbilicus to the thigh. He cannot move from the spot, nor put one foot before the other; when he tries to walk, he feels as if all the tendons were torn and cut to pieces. He cannot even stretch his feet out when he lies down. The easiest posture is sitting bent forward. Frequently he cannot make water, which is often tinged with blood. He has some appetite, and regular bowels; sometimes feverish towards evening. Great irritability and moroseness. Rückert first administered a (superfluous) dose of *aconite* 6, and, after twenty-four hours, of *Colocynth* 12. By the 20th his general state was much improved. After a fresh dose, till the 24th, the pains in the abdomen had quite disappeared; but the patient could not yet walk. He now got a drop of *digitalis-purpurea.* At the end of February he could go about the room without a stick. On the 9th March he was able to go out. Dr. R. now gave him, as a prophylactic (!), another dose of *Colocynth.* From this time forward he enjoyed uninterrupted good health.—(*Annalen d. Hom. Kl.* i. 292.)

Rückert entitles this case "chronic psoïtis?" Ruoff and Kirsch have, in their Repertory, left out the note of interrogation. By many the complaint will be held to be chronic nephritis. But the affection of the kidneys was secondary. The *lumbar plexus,* which supplies the *iliacus internus* and the *psoas,* was plainly the part primarily affected.

bowels, and almost incessant scanty discharges of bloody mucus, and subsequently of organic shreds, amounts simply to the assertion that the drug is not homœopathic to such cases.—*Ed. Oest. Zeit.*

2. *Ischialgia.*

29. The Countess ——, 58 years of age, fair, and remarkably robust, the mother of three children, was attacked, when 22 years of age, with sciatica, in consequence of repeatedly taking cold, and, notwithstanding that she tried every remedy, not excepting the actual cautery, she limped *from that time* so much as to making walking difficult and painful in the highest degree. The last medicine used was cod-liver oil, which she had taken for several weeks by tablespoonfuls. The bashful Countess would not permit an accurate manual examination of the painful hip, but she described the pain in the thigh as pressive, constrictive, on walking sometimes sticking. On attempting to walk, she felt a strong tension extending below the knee, so that she could not place the sole on the ground, but only the toes. The heel remained a full inch from the ground.

Colocynth 18, a drop every eight or ten days, had not, after several weeks, effected the slightest improvement. After *Colocynth* 12, she complained of a burning feeling in the hip-joint, which, after lasting five days, went off, but was not followed by any amelioration of her state. *A second dose of the same dilution again caused this burning sensation;* and this time, when it disappeared, the patient was certain she could perceive a lessening of the pressive constrictive pain in the hip-joint. A dose of *Colocynth* was administered every eighth day with slow improvement. After fourteen weeks, the limping was so far diminished as that the heel remained only about half an inch from the ground. In eleven weeks more, she could walk as well with the affected limb as with the other, except that it sooner became tired during a long walk.*—(*Schwarze, Hom. Heilungen*, 1836, p. 125, *et seq.*)

If this cure was entirely due to the *Colocynth*, of which we have not the slightest doubt, stronger doses of the remedy might have hastened it.

30. A woman, 27 years of age, was seized, after exposure to cold, with tearing pains in the right leg, most severe below the knee and in the calf, extorting screams. Warm drinks, sal-ammoniac, with tartrate of antimony, effected but little change for the better in eight days. The whole thigh was now swollen; the leg lay stretched out, incapable of motion, the foot turned outwards, lengthened by nearly an inch; the right side of the posteriors flaccid. Neither the trochanter nor the groin were painful on pressure; but the least attempt at movement caused excruciating pain. *Ung.-Neapol. Liniment.-volat.*, *Ung.-nervin.*, repeated blisters, mixtures of sal-ammoniac and saltpetre, calomel, sulphuret of gold, guaiac, corrosive sublimate, quinine, and opium, were used in vain. *At the end of the sixth week*, the whole thigh was swollen to double its proper size, and extremely sensitive to the slightest touch. Even the tread of a foot in the room, and approaching her bed, caused pain. The patient felt as if her leg were

* A relapse was cured by SCHWARZE in three weeks with *Arsenic* 18.—*Watzke.*

moved convulsively to and fro. She ate nothing, had grown very thin, had much fever, and passed the night in screaming.

After a single dose of Colocynth, the patient passed a tranquil night, —the first for many weeks; *the pains abated; in a few days she could sit up and allow her limb to be moved. Silicea,* given after twelve days, completed the cure.—(*Thorer's Beiträge*, iv. 9.)

31. LOBETHAL (*Allg. Hom. Z.* xiii. 115) treated a similar case. A strong man, about 30 years old, who was exposed by his occupation to frequent chills, had been attacked, eighteen months before, by coxitis, and since then had been entirely confined to bed. The affected foot was shortened; its muscles shrunken; the pain in the hip constant and intolerable. *Colocynth* 30, every second day, did much good. LOBETHAL supposes this to have been morbus coxarius in the third stage. We take it, notwithstanding the difference in the position of the limb in this and the preceding case, to have been ischialgia. *The morbus coxarius is not within the sphere of action of Colocynth.*

32. *One of the most splendid cures to be found* in homœopathic, and perhaps medical literature, was effected by DR. ÆGIDI, (*Archiv f. Hom.*, H. vii. 109), by means of *Colocynth*, in the following case:—

A young lady, 21 years of age, experienced, in August, 1824, a displacement of the *ossa pubis* from a blow on the symphysis. After a speedy cure, nephritis came on, and the urine was finally discharged mixed with pus. The antiphlogistic treatment employed did not remove, but ameliorated her state; so that, by the end of March, 1825, *there only remained a feeling of numbness and paralysis from the small of the back to the thigh, violent long-continued pains about the symphysis pubis on the slightest touch, distended abdomen, and periodical attacks of colic.**

In January, 1826, she grew much worse from over-exertion. She could now only sit on the right nates. The affected limb was stretched out with the toes turned inwards. From time to time (11 or 12 times a day) she felt, for an hour or two together, *agonizing pain proceeding from the region of the left kidney down the corresponding limb as far as the outer malleolus, with constrictive pains, like those of labor, in the abdomen, forcing screams from the sufferer.* Adjoining the sacro-iliac articulation and the *symphysis pubis*, osseous tumors had formed, which, on being touched, were the seat of burning pain; *abdomen tympanitic, tender to the touch; vesical tenesmus with abundant secretion; urine clear while the pain lasted,* at other times reddish, with a gravelly, whitish flocculent deposit; *bowels irregular, sometimes no action for a long time, sometimes several tough and slimy stools in a day; at times burning pain at the anus during the evacuations, quickly followed by a sensation of weakness and paralysis of the anus;* appetite small; *periodical and violent pain in the chest, and still more*

* If these latter symptoms were accompaniments of the renal affection, we should very much doubt its inflammatory character.—*Ed. Oest. Zeit.*

violent headache on the left side; great depression; proneness to faint; troubled sleep; frightful dreams; alternate shivering and heat; excited state of mind; countenance expressive of suffering; *great disinclination to speaking;* tearful mood; irregular menstruation.

Leeches, hyosciamus, aqua laurocerasi, and opium, were tried without benefit for several weeks. Nor was the result of the first 11 weeks of the homœopathic treatment, during which she got cocculus, sulphur, nux, capsicum, aurum, mercurius-solub., and conium, more favorable.

On the 5th of June, resort was had to the actual cautery. The suppuration which ensued relieved most of the sufferings, but only for a few weeks, when, with a diminution of the discharge, the whole train of symptoms returned in all their severity, and on *the wound beginning to heal up, the patient's state became far worse than before the application of the cautery.* Her general feelings were deteriorated; she was pale and her eyes sunken; a slight cough and daily fever, worse in the evenings, came on. The wound was allowed to cicatrize, and a nourishing diet, quinine, Iceland moss, gentian, and barley-water, &c., were prescribed. In a few weeks the strength recovered, and the fever disappeared, *but the original complaint remained untouched.* Warm baths, sal-ammoniac, chloride of gold, were tried for some weeks, but always without relief.

Under these circumstances, Dr. Ægidi again resorted to Homœopathy. The patient took, on the 8th September, at 9 A.M., one drop of *Colocynth* 6, in a teaspoonful of distilled water.

In the evening the sufferings of the patient increased dreadfully. She could not find ease in any posture, and was wrought up nigh to distraction. *A violent tearing pain shot through the whole brain, and became intolerable when the upper eye-lids were moved; in the right eye-ball pain as from a knife, extending to the root of the nose; empty eructations,* causing palpitations and spasmodic action of the fauces, with constant inclination to vomit; *periodically a dreadful cutting in the abdomen, proceeding from the left renal region, spasmodically drawing the left thigh up to the body, and forcing the patient to bend herself completely forward.*

Rightly ascribing the paroxysm to his having given the medicine in an over-dose, Ægidi gave a spoonful of black coffee now and then, and put a solution of camphor to the nostrils. *In a few hours the pain subsided, the patient fell asleep, slept soundly the whole night, and awoke quite well.* On waking she said a peculiar indescribable feeling of comfortableness pervaded her whole frame. She could bend and stretch the left limb, tread with the left foot, and walk without support.

The next morning she proceeded on foot to visit her physician. She told him she felt perfectly well on waking, and her first attempts at walking in her room proving successful, her overflowing joy would not allow her to remain in the house, and she felt her strength increase with every step she took in the open air. So saying, she raised the sound foot from the ground, and turned round and round on the affected one. *No farther medicine was required;* she daily improved; even the osseous tumors disappeared in a short time, and she henceforth enjoyed perfect health.

33. Our colleague, Dr. Böhm, removed with *Colocynth* 3 an *Ischias postica*, which had attacked a hearty, healthy man, of 40, without assignable cause, with violent pain, extending from the trochanter to the ancle, which had for 12 weeks returned every week, and lasted 20 or 30 hours with extreme intensity. *Rhus-tox.* had been tried without effect. The paroxysm returned once, but in a feeble degree, and went away permanently under a continuance of the *Colocynth.**

We close this chapter with a critical review of a few cases, recorded in our homœopathic literature as Colocynth-cures, but which we consider as

IV. *Doubtful or Rejected Cases.*

34. Dr. Schrön (*Allg. hom. Zeit.* v. 150) gives the case of a woman who was suddenly attacked with incessant vomiting, first of food, then of a greenish fluid, and diarrhœa with rapidly recurring stools, becoming constantly thinner and less colored, and attended by violent sticking, cutting, colic and cramps in the calves; suppression of urine; rapid prostration. *Colocynth* 18, every two and afterwards every three hours, removed the attack in twenty-four hours.

It would be an exceedingly easy thing to fit this case into our Colocynth-schema; we need only regard the cholera, with Pinel, Hildebrandt, Rast, Rathke, and others (See Radius, *Cholerazeitung*, B. 1), as a ganglionic neurosis, an affection of the *Plexus cœliacus*, an erethism of the sympathetic, &c. Besides this, the cholera has been cured with many remedies to which anti-choleric virtues have been ascribed with far less probability. But our provings upon the healthy have brought to light too few symptoms like those of cholera, and Schrön's single relation is too isolated a fact to authorize us to consider his case as anything more than an instance of that disease running a natural but rapid course towards recovery.

35. A plethoric brunette of 30 aborted at four weeks; in consequence of passion, the lochia had ceased for four hours; head hot; scrobiculus and abdomen painful to the touch; delirium alternating with sopor, the eyes half open; constant desire to get out of bed. *Colocynth* 30 towards midnight; relief in three quarters of an hour, and in the morning reëstablishment of the lochia and recovery. Melicher, (Attomyr, *Brief. üb. Hom.* i. 153.)

Ruoff calls this *Puerperal Fever!* To us it appears simply an ar-

* Attomyr (*Archiv*, xi. 2, 118), cured three cases of coxalgia, by means of Colocynth, in a few days, but, alas! does not give us the particulars. Dr. Y. also (*Hom. Bekehrungsep.* 1837, 29) mentions having cured an ischialgia of two years' standing with *nux* and *Colocynth* in a short time, but neither does he give us a description of the disease.—*Watzke.*

terial orgasm, with cerebral congestion, the rapid disappearance of which owed little to the dose of Colocynth.

36. Hoffendahl (*Archiv* xii. 2, 172) had the wonderful good luck to meet three patients, two women and one man, in a single day, suffering from *psoitis*, with such violent pain in the right thigh that they could not walk, and to cure them each within twenty-four hours by a single dose of *Colocynth* 30. These were hardly cases of psoas inflammation, as our good colleague conjectures, but rather transitory attacks of rheumatico-ischialgia.

37. Kopp (*Denkwürd.* iv. 329 *und* 338) cured several cases of paralytic weakness of the legs with *Colocynth*, where there were affection of the head, somnolence, confusion, torpidity of the bowels and disproportionably thin legs—a group of symptoms having direct relation to diminished or depraved nervous influence—*paresis* of the femoral nerves?

Can *Colocynth*, in the extreme limits of its operative sphere, produce, on the one hand, a congestive, hyperæmic and inflammatory condition (especially of the brain and mucous membrane of the ileum and rectum); and on the other hand, cause and cure paresis (especially of the lower limbs)? Satisfactory conclusions on this subject may be deduced from the chapter of experiments on animals.

38. Gross (*Archiv für hom. Heilk.* xii. i. 88) relates the following case, which has caused the repertory-makers to insert erroneously *stiffness in the elbow* as cured by Colocynth. A weaver fell upon his arm from a tree upon an old stump nine years before; the arm continued stiff and sore, and two years afterwards five ulcers appeared, which refused to heal, but in the course of several years became gangrenous and discharged several pieces of bone. The arm was swollen, and a pressing tearing pain tormented the patient, particularly at night. He was finally treated for a year in an allopathic hospital; but as the difficulty seemed constantly to become worse, a council of six physicians and surgeons decided upon amputation, which, however, the patient would not submit to, and left the hospital. Under the use of *arnica* the pains disappeared in a week; *silic.*, *calc.*, and *sulph.* cured the ulcers in the course of several months, and a single dose of *Coloc.* removed the remaining stiffness of the arm in a short time.

We are of opinion that the disappearance of the stiffness was a simple consequence of the healing of the ulcers, and not in the least attributable to the Colocynth.

39. Kramer (*Hygea* 1, 25) gives us a case, but whether *Coloc.* had any and what share of the credit in the cure of an affection in which *nux, acon., ars., carb-an., carb-veg., and phosph.* were employed in addition, cannot be gathered from his account.

The patient had suffered for four years from congestion of the liver (?) piles, constipation, flatulence, inflation of the abdomen, violent periodical pains, drawing through the middle of the chest to the hip. The paroxysms of pain lasted an hour, and were accompanied by asthma, redness of the face, very rapid pulse, and dulness and aching of the head. The whole affection disappeared within six weeks from the use of the above-named remedies. For four years he had used laxative, opening, and purgative remedies, bitter extracts and acids, and mineral waters, in vain.

40. SCHELLHAMMER (*Archiv für hom. Heilk.* xvi. 2, 79) employed *Coloc.*, with *ars.* and *seneg.*, for the cure of dropsy of the chest and abdomen, ensuing after the disappearance of itch from external applications. The previously administered *sulph.*, which had reproduced the itch, doubtless had most to do with the cure, and the employment of the subsequent remedies was superfluous.

41. HECHENBERGER'S *cases* (*Colocynthologie*, 25) *almost all belong in the category of doubtful instances of the efficacy of Colocynth.* We give the concisest possible sketch of them; they do not furnish much information, as the author not only administered other remedies, but even *combined* them with the Colocynth.

42. A lively servant girl, æt. 33, small, irr'table, irregularly menstruating, was seized with a gastric nervous fever, with thickly-coated, clammy tongue, nausea, constipation, inclination to vomit, meteorism, attacks of fainting and delirium. Tincture of Colocynth with *spiritus Hoffmanni*, rinsing the mouth with diluted vinegar, mustard plaster on the small of the back, and subsequently Colocynth in a decoction of arnica, with sulphate of quinine, brought the patient to the stage of convalescence in ten days. We think, however, that the cure depended upon Hoffmann's liquor, arnica and quinine.

43. A *Ptyalismus Suecicus*—frequent pyrosis with cardialgia, frequent vomiting of food, emaciation, &c.—was cured in three weeks, during the employment of a mixture of a decoction of quassia and the tinctures of Colocynth and opium, with evacuation of soft, painless stools, and extraordinary discharge of wind. The patient, a poor, sickly woman, a weaver, had been sick for two months, and during the treatment, left her occupation, was forbidden to eat potatoes, and took moderate exercise with easily digestible food. It seems to us that this case would have got well quicker under the diet and hygienic means without the mixtures, the Colocynth having done little towards it, though the symptoms which attended its use are similar to those produced in our provings upon the healthy.

44. A man of 50, intemperate both in drink and passion, suffering for years from abdominal congestions (?), and annually visited with frequently recurring attacks of asthma, colic, gout in the feet, and the venesections and mixtures consequent thereon, was radically cured by the continued use of *Colocynth.* The disorder in this case is so slightly individualized, that we learn little or nothing from the relation. Doubtless the cure would have been considerably hastened if, instead of deluging the patient with nauseous dandelion-tea, he had given him good spring-water to drink.

45. We learn little more from the next two cases. A tavern-keeper, strong, choleric, and high-tempered, subject to a violent ischialgia which

had resisted all remedies, resorted to the purgatives of a quack as a refuge from the actual cautery, and was cured.

46. A miner, attacked after a bilious fever with a painful swelling of the right thigh and leg, had been fruitlessly treated for a year by doctors and surgeons. When they informed him that the enormous swelling was about to suppurate, he fled for consolation to a cobbler, who, to the astonishment of everybody, cured him rapidly and without any subsequent trouble by a remedy containing a portion of Colocynth tincture.

47. A miller, æt. 36, was suddenly seized after a violent fit of anger with stitches in the side and dreadful pain in the right thigh and hip-joint, so that he could neither stand nor go. HECHENBERGER sent him half a drachm of tincture of Colocynth in half a pound of *decoctio graminis,* to take a tablespoonful every hour. He heard two days afterwards that the patient had entirely recovered, the most unexceptionable case which we find in our colleague's whole book!

48. A woman, æt. 43, of an irritable temperament and jaundiced appearance, mother of thirteen children, had had wandering pains in her limbs for two years. During the preceding winter gastric difficulties had been added, until a *febris cacochymica* and atonic dropsy set in. The respiration was oppressed, feet and hands, face and abdomen much swollen. The author considers the case as a *crisis erronea* of an erysipelas of the face, which had been present some days before the appearance of the dropsy, and had been unobserved. He prescribed a mixture of 10 ounces of decoction of Graswurzel, 10 grains sulphate of quinine, 2 drams of tincture of Colocynth, and 15 grains of unwashed, sudorific antimony, of which the patient was to take a teaspoonful every hour, and to drink wine and water. In a week he heard, *to his astonishment,(!)* that the patient was perfectly cured. What a remarkable ability he has displayed, however, in assigning to each of the components of his formidable mixture, the part which it performed in effecting the cure!!

49. A phlegmatic, cachectic, emaciated proprietor, æt. 39, had been troubled for five years with pain in the stomach, heartburn, constant dull pain under the right ribs, and about the pylorus and navel, and constipation—a stool once in four or five days. The malady was aggravated one or two hours after every meal, and the ingesta were frequently vomited with painful retching. Stools of scybala, with burning pain in the small of the back.

Castor oil and Kirsch-water, tea of Graswurzel, Neapolitan salve, and tincture of opium, *ameliorated the condition somewhat in six weeks* (*!*). Small doses of tincture of Colocynth, disguised first in Castor oil, and subsequently by syrup of buckthorn-berries and Seltzer-water, cured him perfectly in *eleven months,* a daily stool containing black blood having come on. Is it possible that any one can put faith in a cure by Colocynth, that it took *eleven months* to complete?

50. A young woman, æt. 24, of strong build, when menstruation came on, and that irregularly, at 22 years old, had been for two years chloro-

tic, face pale and puffed, suffering from palpitations, asthma, heaviness of the legs, and constipation; for four weeks she took a mixture of Colocynth, Graswurzel, and quassia, for three weeks following malate of iron, and then antimony, after which the menses appeared and became regular. What a wonderful demonstration, a splendid *deductio ad absurdum*, of the mighty, not-sufficiently-to-be-estimated virtues of Colocynth in chlorosis!

CHAPTER XI.

Ancient and Modern Notions on the Nature and Essence of the Active Principle of Colocynth.

The phantasies of the physicians of Arabia and the middle ages taught that Colocynth was composed of fiery and calcined earthy parts, and attributed to it a temperament heating and dry in the second or third degree, and suitable only for cold and sluggish natures. AVICENNA gets in a terrible passion with the celebrated ALCHINDUS, who opposed the popular opinion, and ascribed a cold and moist temperament to the drug. Colocynth at that time thinned and dissolved the thick, tough, glassy mucus of the bowels, dulcified the acidities of the stomach, made patent the veins, shook the nerves, and unlocked the noxious, corrupted humors from their most secret organic cubby-holes. (AVICENNA, ETTMÜLLER, and others.)

The iatro-chemical age next found in Colocynth a sharp, biting, caustic salt, which irritated the sensitive and motor nervous fibres (*fibras nerveas sensibiles et motrices*) of the intestinal mucous membrane, and the excretory ducts connected with it, corroded the vascular terminations, and decomposed the humors in a colliquative, feverish fermentation. (JOAN. MAUR. HOFFMANN, *in Eph. Nat. Cur. Cent.* X. *obs.* 30.)

The moderns hold Colocynth to be a powerful irritant of the ganglionic system, *especially of the pelvic cavity* (?), and of the lower portion of the digestive tube, particularly of the rectum; that it excites the functions of these organs, increases the secretions and excretions of the intestinal canal, and of the kidneys; by sympathy raises the activity of the spinal marrow and its nervous connections; and at times excites, at others depresses, the functions of the brain. These opinions are founded partly on physiological observations and experiments, but too unsatisfactory and imperfect to afford a sufficient foundation for any special indication for the use of Colocynth in disease, and are partly set phrases, which you will find, with but slight variations, applied to its immediate neighbors in the *Materia Medica*, and which give you no insight whatever into any ground for selecting *Colocynth* in a given case, in preference to *scammony*, *hellebore*, *gamboge*, or any other drastic purgative.

Most pharmacologists of the present day, however, do not seem to consider it worth while to seem to know anything *specific* about the peculiar powers of Colocynth. They content themselves with setting it down as "*Purgans acre vehemens,*" or "*Drasticum heroicum,*" and with a few words refer to its former dangerous employment.* This seems to us far better than beclouding and confusing the student with a pretended knowledge, which, after all, is but empty fog.

Among our colleagues, HAUSMANN and GERSTEL have ventured theories of the action of Colocynth.

HAUSMANN considers the essence of the action of Colocynth to be excretory. The whole phenomena, composing both the morbific and the curative process, are only preparatives to this end. On this account, it fixes itself more particularly in the large intestine, which is especially an organ of excretion, and chiefly in the rectum, to the care of which the immediate expulsion of the excreted matters is committed. It is to be observed that the excretions, and of course the preliminaries, are repeated at longer or shorter intervals, which indicates an affection, not of a single tissue of the colon alone, but of the whole structure in its muscular, cellular, and mucous tissues, and with its ganglionic nerves and vessels. Since the separation of the excretions from the matters which are to be retained in the organism is effected by means of the bile, and the bile itself forms a part of the excreta, the biliary organ, the liver, is necessarily affected. The most important excretory organ, next to the rectum, the bladder, with its passages, is of course likewise influenced. The brain is affected in consequence of its connection with the liver. The muscular pains, which are the most prominent symptoms next to the colics, seem to be rather hard to reconcile with this hypothesis; but if LIEBIG's theory of the metamorphosis of tissues and animal motion be correct, that the muscles are undergoing a constant change, corresponding in extent to the amount of force expended, by absorption of the inhaled oxygen, and are therefore as constantly demanding an equivalent for the loss of substance, they are more easily accounted for. For a substance which forces the bowel to an excretion will carry along with it the whole contents of the canal, including the undigested material for that very muscular supply, which is called for by these uneasy muscular pains. According to this view, the constant metamorphosis of the muscular substance is the grand original cause and necessity of every excretion.

We have nothing less to urge in relation to this hypothesis, than

* MOLL (*Handb. der Pharmakologie*, Wien, 1839) places Colocynth among the "*Drastica anti-dyscrasica,*" which, by their antagonistic action upon the organism, produce such an irritation, especially of the vascular system connected with assimilation, that an improvement is brought about in the concoction of the organic materials by a sort of *metasyncrasis*, of which the diarrhœa is but a single symptom. (!) Old PAULUS ÆGINETA was a deal nearer the truth when he laid it down that Colocynth was less a sanguineous than a nervous purgative,—a "*Drasticum alterans,*"—and consequently a remedy exerting a powerful influence over the nervous system, and capable of producing alterations in its functional activity.—*Watzke.*

that it applies with equal force to every purgative and laxative, and gives us no distinctive specific information in regard to Colocynth.

GERSTEL's theory (which, with some modifications, we have no hesitation whatever in adopting)* is not put forward as a theory of the nature and essence of the Colocynth-disease, but as a conjecture concerning its seat, the organs primarily and secondarily affected, and the character, connection, and relations of the symptoms presented.

The physiological and clinical materials already accumulated, justify the opinion that Colocynth exerts a direct specific influence on the sensitive filaments of certain nervous centres and nervous tracts (especially of the *cœliac plexus* and its ramifications, the fifth pair, and the lumbar and femoral nerves), and that its action is confined to, or, at all events, begins from the mucous and fibrous membranes, under the influence of these nerves, and from the neurilemma of the nerves themselves.

This action results in the production of an abnormally exalted sensibility, manifested by neuralgiæ and hyperæsthesiæ, which, on the one hand, give rise to congestion, hyperæmia, and, when repeatedly renewed with violence, even to inflammation, particularly in the brain and the very vascular lining membrane of the small and large intestines; and, on the other, though very rarely, may pass over into paresis of the nerves themselves, especially of the sacral plexus, and the sciatic nerves.

At the same time there appear symptoms of the diffusion of the nervous influence, of reflex action and of sympathy, partly at the proximal extremities of the affected nerves in the brain; partly, though more seldom, and apparently in consequence of the mediate connection with the sympathetic by means of the *plexus gastricus magnus*, in the peripheric ends of the *vagus* in the lungs and heart; and partly in the skin, which is directly or indirectly influenced by the affected nerves. To the first cause we ascribe dulness, pressure, sensitiveness, painfulness, and other symptoms of the head; to the second, pressure, stitches in the chest, constriction, asthma, palpitations, anxiety; to the third, creeping, twitching, sticking, drawing, &c., in the skin.

Besides this, the exalted sensibility (most in the mucous membranes,

* We must be permitted, however, to remark beforehand, that this theory —if indeed it deserve the name—is by no means advanced as the best possible, and as putting a final bar to the zeal and energy of our colleagues. We only claim for ourselves, what we cheerfully grant to every one else, the right of interpreting the phenomena caused by Colocynth in our own way; if any one differ from us, we are content. *In respect to theories, our toleration knows no bounds;* since we know of none, not even our own, that is perfectly satisfactory. If any one demand of our theory that it shall explain to him the how, why, and wherefore of the action of the drug, we can only say that that is beyond the limits of our wisdom. Why Colocynth attacks the nervous system almost exclusively, and leaves the vascular unaffected; why it attacks the *trigeminus*, instead of the *acusticus*, or *opticus*, and why it seizes the sensitive and not the motor divisions of it, we can as little say, as we can why pumpkins bloom yellow instead of black or red.—*Ed. Oest. Zeit.*

but sometimes in the cellular tissue*) is accompanied by increased and often perverted secretion, and imparts acridity to the secretions. Hence burning and biting in the tongue, scraping in the throat, pyrosis, flatulence, tenesmus, diarrhœa, frequent urination, lachrymation, catarrh, and symptoms of a similar kind.

CHAPTER XII.

Indications for Colocynth.—Allied Remedies.—Antidotes.—Size and Repetition of the Dose.

The curative indications are essentially identical with the physiological effects of a remedy. The latter once known, so are the former. The study of the effects which Colocynth develops in the healthy body, affords the best guide to its appropriate use at the bedside. *The usus in morbis can afford no fresh indications*;†—it merely sifts and throws light on the materials furnished by pharmacology; it decides on the greater or less availableness, the value and meaning of the medicinal symptoms, obtained by experiments on the healthy; it is the touchstone of the results of provings, confirming faithful observations, rejecting the product of inexact or superficial experiments, the tissues woven by fancy or by falsehood.‡ The clinical study, therefore, of Colocynth, will have an important influence on its therapeutic employment; it forms a necessary supplement to the curative indications drawn from its physiological effects.

Let us first glance at the indications for Colocynth furnished by our colleagues.

With regard to the disposing causes of diseases which the medicine is fitted to cure, according to Noack and Trinks, Colocynth corresponds especially to sthenic, dry, bilious, melancholic, venous-hæmorrhoidal constitutions, and the cholerico-melancholic temperament. But our experiments on the healthy as well as the published cures by Colocynth, show it to have an absolute power over all constitutions and temperaments. Dislike to speaking, irritability, moroseness, and other symptoms, indicate, it is true, an influence, though perhaps not a direct

* See Weinke's proving, *ante*, p. 334.

† We are not at all disposed to throw stones at a Homœopath here and there, who has become acquainted with, and continues to use, a remedy, such as *badiaga*, *filix-mas*, &c., solely *ex usu in morbis*. We must make a virtue of necessity. We must condemn, however, in the strongest terms, the conduct of those who (like Hahnemann in his later editions) insert in the *materia medica* all the symptoms of a disease which has been cured by a particular remedy. This is opening doors and windows, and inviting error in; this is a process for converting a *pure* into an *impure materia medica.*—*Watzke.*

‡ We remind our readers of the pretended proving of medicines by Fickel, the homœopathic Judas. We know not that there can be found in the whole range of homœopathic literature more than two cures effected by Fickel's lying drugs.—*Watzke.*

one, on the mind and temperament; but they appear as the usual accompaniments of abdominal sufferings, from whatever cause they may have arisen. At all events, a great number of medicines have this in common with Colocynth.

The opinion expressed by HAHNEMANN *with regard to the curative indications to be drawn from exciting causes*, that Colocynth was especially adapted for the effects of anger, indignation, vexation, and brooding over the unjust treatment of oneself or others, among which he enumerates cramp in the calves of the legs, spasmodic colic, sleeplessness, rheumatism in the limbs, &c., we believe to be so far well-grounded that the passions sometimes, especially if acting for a length of time, give rise to morbid phenomena similar to those which Colocynth produces in the healthy; but it is not on this account proved that Colocynth has any direct specific effect on the mind. Neither have our experiments shown any aggravation of the symptoms enumerated to arise from mental impressions, nor have we found in our clinical observations a sufficient number of cases in which Colocynth cured the symptoms mentioned by HAHNEMANN more surely and quickly when they proceeded from mental than when they were due to physical causes.

On what grounds FRANZ proceeds, when he affirms that Colocynth takes precedence even of chamomile, for anger and its effects, we cannot tell. There is more foundation for his opinion that it is peculiarly adapted for women with abundant catamenia. The power Colocynth possesses to promote the flow of the menses, and to bring on menorrhagia, and even abortion, is pròved beyond all doubt.

If Colocynth is more often useful to persons who lead a sedentary life than to others, this is not to be ascribed to any especial susceptibility of such persons to the curative action of Colocynth; it only shows that neglect of exercise is not unfrequently the cause of diseases for which the remedy is found in Colocynth.

Homœopathic indications for Colocynth, *drawn from the symptoms of the diseases it has cured*, such as *rheumatismus acutus*, gouty conditions, paralyses, neuralgias, migraine, gastralgia, ischias, psoitis, sporadic cholera, epidemic dysentery, &c., are the counterparts of those which the Arabians set up for it. The reformed science of healing ought to reject every such indication.*

Among HAHNEMANN's therapeutic hints before the third edition of Colocynth, we find among several unimportant symptoms, such as anxiety, toothache, rumbling in the abdomen, the following: "*Deficiency of religious feeling, eczema of the face, and inguinal hernia.*"

* It seems very probable that the (generally unjust) condemnation pronounced by HAHNEMANN upon all nosological names, was founded upon no other ground than a conviction of the utter worthlessness of such names in reference to therapeutic indications. Unfortunately, he fell out with himself a little subsequently. The scheme of diseases, with which he introduced his antipsoric remedies, is but little better than the indefinite, indistinct, generalizing indications of the old school.—*Watzke.*

Neither our somewhat thorough proving, nor yet HAHNEMANN's, has given any sanction to the charge of impiety against Colocynth, and we greatly fear that HAHNEMANN has introduced that symptom from some one of his patients. As to the facial eruption and inguinal hernia, our homœopathic literature presents but a single feeble analogy.*

HAHNEMANN mentions, as a leading characteristic of Colocynth, its power "*to excite cramp-pain, i. e.* (!) *tonic cramp, with constrictive pressive pain in internal and external parts.*" This definition is objectionable, inasmuch as a theory of the cause of the pain is implied; and is also defective, for Colocynth evidently produces its direct and primary abnormal impression on the sensorial sphere of the nervous system.† The influence it exerts over the motor sphere is almost limited to the involuntary muscles; and in this case also is indirect, and to be ascribed to sympathy.

MELICHER's *puerperal fever*, and RÜCKERT's *psoitis chronica*, we have already dissected in Chapter X. They are both to be stricken out of our repertories, and *lumbago* substituted for the latter. Whether the diagnostic criticisms which we have made in reference to SCHÜLER's *ophthalmia arthritica*, RUOFF's *peritonitis*, SCHRÖN's *sporadic cholera* and *vesical catarrhs*, SCHELLHAMMER's *dropsy of the chest and abdomen*, and GROSS's *stiff arm*, are deserving of regard in any future development of the curative indications of Colocynth, is left to the judgment of our colleagues.

The hypothesis of SCHRÖN and HERING, that Colocynth is indicated for ichthyosis and lepra, rests chiefly on phenomena of doubtful value, which occurred in two patients cured by Colocynth.‡

NOACK and TRINKS' indications for Colocynth are chiefly abridged histories of face-aches, megrims, colics, and diarrhœa, treated exclusively by Colocynth, by GASPARI, ATTOMYR, SCHÜLER, NENNING, HARTMANN, and others. Having given these cases in full in our 10th chapter, we have nothing farther to say of them here. We shall only quote some remarks derived from the posthumous papers of Dr. HARTLAUB, senior. According to these observations, *apparently made upon the sick*, the following symptoms are indications for the employment of Colocynth:

* NENNING (*Allg. hom. Zeit.* vii. 73) mentions a single case in which Colocynth *alleviated the pains* of an epiplocele.—*Watzke.*

† Thus Colocynth affects only the sensitive filaments of the fifth pair (of the first division, especially the *frontal* branch, the whole of the second division, and the *lingual* and *auricular* of the third), while its motor portion, which does not run through the ganglion, and is merely destined for the muscles of mastication, is not in the least affected by it.—*Watzke.*

‡ HERING (*Archiv*, xi., 2, 36) proceeds on the following symptoms of Colocynth:—Shortening of the tendons (?); drawing up of the limbs to the body; tractive pain in the tendons of the thumbs; cramp-like pain in the hands, making it difficult to unfold them; pain as from the psoas being too short; tearing in the soles; pain from the side of the nose up to its root,—a precursory symptom of ulcers in the nose (?); scaling off of the skin of the whole body (?); itching in the ham; buboes in the axillæ (?).—*Watzke.*

1. Intense pain in the forehead (especially in the eyebrows) and in the face (especially pulsation and tearing in the cheek-bone) beginning with itching; worst in the evening and night; inflammation of the eyes, on looking at the sky; pain as if the eyes would fall out of the head.

2. Tearing pain, going from the pit of the stomach deep into the abdomen as though the chest would fall, aggravated by coughing and walking; pain in the small of the back; tenderness of the abdomen to the touch; alternation of cold and heat; on going to stool, violent pain from the abdomen to the small of the back.

3. Spasmodic, inflammatory, and flatulent colic; colic from cold and mental emotions; every evening at six o'clock a single vomiting of bitter matter, preceded by cutting pain in the left hypochondrium, drawing to the abdomen, stomach, and back; anorexia, hard fæces.

4. Diarrhœa, with pressure on the abdomen and tenesmus.

5. Sticking pain, sometimes in one place, sometimes in another, in one of the lower limbs, causing limping.

Finally we introduce the diffuse indications laid down by HECHENBERGER, which are derived less from provings on the healthy than from experiments on the sick, and prove abundantly that he scarce dimly appreciated the character of Colocynth, much less defined it in a clear light. It is indicated, according to him, first in affections appearing in winter or spring as a result of a torpid, necessitous, confined life as a *status pituitosus*, *gastrismus chronicus*, *febris gastrico-pituitosa*, *gastrico-rheumatica*, *atrabilaria et venosa Richteri*, or as the hepatic congestion and portal obstruction of the old diagnostics, or as *ptyalismus suecicus*, and presenting the following symptoms:

Peculiar, vertiginous, dull headache, especially in the morning after a restless, dreamy sleep; earthy, puffed face; yellowish conjunctiva; nauseous taste; smell from the mouth; tongue, white coated; inclination to vomit in the morning after rising; loss of appetite; distressing fullness of the epigastric region; frequent pyrosis with boring, constrictive pains in the stomach; vomiting of the ingesta with a feeling as if the stomach were floated with water, at first periodical, finally more constant; flatulence; dull, deep-seated pain in the hepatic region; irregularity of the bowels; expectoration of mucus, with rattling and oppressed breathing; frequent chills; heaviness of the feet, with wandering pains in the limbs; general debility; emaciation; irritability; melancholy frame of mind; thoughtlessness; torpidity of all the intellectual faculties.

HECHENBERGER considers Colocynth indicated in the second place, in disorders which come on secondarily to previous diseases, in consequence of neglect, frequent exposure to cold, &c.—atonic dropsy, hæmatemesis, hæmorrhoidal colic, menostasia, or which appear as metaschematic or *crises erroneæ*, such as ischialgia, jaundice, gout, hemicraniæ.

Were we required to give an exact and complete view of the indications for Colocynth, we should refer the inquirer to the pharmacological and clinical materials already given, (chapters iv.–ix.) Any abstract of those materials would be defective, and could not save the student the trouble of studying those chapters. Besides this, a theory of the indications cannot be derived from a simple abbreviation; it requires abstraction—a disposing of the facts according to some theoretical view. From its very nature it can be nothing more than the glass through which we view the phenomena. In presenting below to our colleagues, therefore, our generalization from the preceding chapters, we do not imagine ourselves to have found medical treasures which they would not have discovered by their own efforts; no, we merely use our right to see things through our own glass, and are neither weak enough to believe it is the best, nor so deficient in modesty as to insist upon its adoption by others.

The great, clumsy, misshapen monster presented by the indications for Colocynth of the old school, embracing almost all the diseases to which the human frame is subject, (need we refer to our second chapter?) is reduced by the physiological provings, and the critical sifting of the clinical materials before us, to a less pretending, but we trust a well-formed, tolerably healthy, and very promising offspring. Colocynth has, in our hands, instead of a neglected and despised polychrest, become an indispensable oligochrest. Its formerly much-lauded powers against dropsies, epilepsies, apoplexies, paralyses, intermittent fevers, chlorosis, and jaundice have proved either illusory, or at least problematical.* The whole curative sphere of Colocynth in the new system, is almost confined to a few neuralgiæ and hyperæsthesiæ, and of these almost exclusively those which affect the *trigeminus*, the *cœliac plexus*, and the *lumbar and femoral* nerves. And even here its efficacy is limited to a few forms of hemicrania, prosopalgia, cœlialgia, colic, and ischialgia, *depending on peculiar conditions, and appearing under peculiar circumstances.* What these are, will best appear from a careful perusal of chapter viii.; we venture, however, on some conjectural hints.

1. The *hemicraniæ* and *prosopalgiæ* which Colocynth cures, proceed from an exaltation of sensibility, from an excitement dependent on rheumatic, gouty, or gastric irritation, or on congestion of the fifth pair, in all cases on a purely functional derangement of the sensitive filaments.† In organic changes from deeper causes, the efficacy of Colocynth is very doubtful.

Hemicraniæ, arising from thickening of the arachnoid, or hypertrophy of the meninges, tumefaction, and induration of the pacchionian bodies, in erosion or exostosis of the bones of the skull, effusion of serum, or purulent deposits in the brain, will receive no benefit from Colocynth.

* If we did not confine ourselves in establishing our curative indications to physiological and clinical observations, but allowed some play to theory and hypothesis, we should incline to argue favorably of the effects of Colocynth in intermittent fever, regarded by many authors as a pure neurosis of the cœliac plexus; in epilepsy, depending on spinal irritation; in dropsy, where the accumulation is owing to exaggerated nervous influence; and in apoplexy, brought on by neurosis of the ganglionic system, with a reflex action on the brain.

† By this we do not by any means intend to deny to Colocynth all efficacy in complaints in which organic changes have taken place, and plastic effusions have been formed. The latter are frequently consequent on abnormal nervous influence, and disappear with it.—*Watzke.*

Recourse may be had in such cases for cure or alleviation to *calc.*, *caust.*, *sep.*, *sil.*, *sulph.*, and *graph.*

In like manner, Colocynth is of no use in organic and centric prosopalgiæ, from exostosis of the teeth, hypertrophy of the bones of the skull or face, fungous and scirrhous tumors of the membranes of the meninges, cartilaginous or aneurismal malformation of the cerebral veins, &c. More may be effected in such cases by *ars.*, *aur.*, *magnes.*, *calce.*, and *sep.*

The Colocynth-hemicraniæ are generally seated in the course of the frontal nerve, and are accompanied by violent pains in the eye, and alternate with neuralgiæ of the cœliac plexus. Next in efficacy to it are *bry.* and *nux-vom.*, and next to them *puls.*, *bell.*, *phosph.*, *valer.*, *cham.*, *agar.*, *verat.*

In the prosopalgiæ to which Colocynth is suited, there are no twitchings of single muscles of the face and palsied feeling of the affected side. The pains follow the course of the infraorbital nerve, are frequently periodical, and are accompanied by toothache, (*neuralgia infraorbitodentalis.*) Next to Colocynth stand in this connection, *bell.*, *caps.*, and *verbasc.*; and, more remote, *china*, *staph.*, *con.*, *nux-vom.*

2. *The neuralgiæ of the cœliac plexus* and its branches, are particularly likely to be quickly and permanently removed by Colocynth, when they occur as substantive affections, not caused by derangement of stomach, but by cold, vexation, or anger, occurring during the period of evolution, complicated with spinal irritation and neuralgia of the femoral nerves, with hæmorrhoidal difficulties, chronic diarrhœa, or vermicular symptoms.* Next in efficacy come *cham.*, *bell.*, *puls.*; then *valer.*, *cocc.*, *coff.*, *nux.*, *secale*, *ign.*, *stann.*

Colocynth will hardly relieve, far less cure colic from inflammation of the great gut or peritoneum from gall-stones or nephritic calculi, perforating ulcers in the stomach, mesenteric tubercles, tubercular ulcers in the intestines, &c. Some of these set all treatment at defiance; others require *merc.-viv.*, or *corr.*, *bell.*, *bry.*, *canth.*, and *ars.*

3. Of the ischialgiæ those most under the control of Colocynth, are such as are caused by affection of the terminating filaments of the spinal cord, as also those arising from cold, from violent emotions, or remaining after mechanical violence, or connected with gout, suppressed hæmorrhoids, or the processes of involution and evolution, or complicated with

* Colocynth is suited in an especial manner to the affection, first described by ROMBERG, (*Lehrbuch der Nervenkranheiten*, 140,) under the title of "*neuralgia hypogastrica.*" It is a hyperæsthesia of the *hypogastric plexus.* The symptoms are,—pains, as of labor, in the lower belly; pressive pain about the sacrum, with sensation of pressure on the rectum and bladder, and in women on the uterus and vagina. *Pains in the upper part of the thighs are a frequent concomitant.* In girls, in whom it not unfrequently occurs at each menstrual period during the development of puberty, the symptoms resemble greatly those of prolapsus or retroversion of the uterus, but come on in paroxysms, and are not relieved by change of posture. *This affection occurring in the male sex commonly passes under the name of hæmorrhoidal colic.—Watzke.*

affections of various parts of the cœliac plexus. *Cham., rhus, puls.* are cognate remedies.

It is of no value in ischialgiæ, from tumefaction of the bones of the pelvis, carcinoma of the pelvic viscera, change in the substance of the nerves, or *morbus coxarius*, or in those which are due to the localization of a morbid condition diffused through the system. Recourse must be had in such cases to remedies that are homœopathic to the fundamental evil, such as *calc., sil., carb.-veg., merc., ars., hep.-sulph., sulph.*, and others.

In the *morbus-coxarius* itself, Colocynth will be found of little service, and Stapf is greatly mistaken in his surmise, (*Archiv.*, xvi. 1, 93,) that it will be found one of the chief remedies in spontaneous (nervous) lameness. Both the cases which Thorer and Lobethal (*vide* chapter x) think they cured with Colocynth seem to us to have been cases of *ischias.* The changes in the position of the foot and trochanter are quite as remarkable in that disease. (Compare Canstatt *Med. Klin.*, 3, 30.) No remedies but such as we have mentioned above will suffice to arrest the progress of a specific inflammation of the hip-joint.

Related and Antidotal Remedies.—The affinities and antidotal relations of Colocynth, and *vice versa*, may be gathered from the foregoing observations.

Where the formidable symptoms of poisoning by Colocynth make their appearance, the mechanical and chemical resources of medicine must be resorted to, as in other cases of poisoning. In addition to copious draughts of oil, warm milk, or water, wet bandages applied to the abdomen, and the administration of tincture of opium and black coffee, effect the most speedy relief.

We do not know on which grounds Jahr asserts Colocynth to be merely the antidote of *causticum;* and Noack and Trinks, that it counteracts only *causticum* and *mercurius.*

Duration of Action.—The average duration of the action of Colocynth may be set down at from 2 to 6 hours; but when it has produced an intense effect, it frequently extends over several weeks.

Dose and Repetition.—No fixed rules can be laid down as to the size and repetition of the dose. *Judging from our own experiments, and the published cases of cure by Colocynth, we are inclined to think, that the sixth (decimal) dilution or trituration is seldom too large, and the first as seldom too small a dose.*

We are in the habit of repeating the dose of Colocynth every hour, or every 2, 3, or 4 hours in acute, and in as many days in chronic cases.

14.—COCCUS-CACTI.

COCCUS.—Coccus indicus, Coccus Americanus, Grana fici indici, Cochineal, Coccinella or Coccionella, Cochenilla, Cotonella, Conzenilla, Cochenille, Scharlachwurm.

1. *Description and Preparation.*

This hemipterous insect is extensively raised in Mexico for the purposes of commerce. It was employed by the natives, long before the discovery of America, as a means of obtaining an ornamental dye, and it is for this purpose that it is now largely imported from that country. Large plantations of Cactus are there cultivated, upon which the animals are placed, and suffered to grow and propagate, from which three harvests a year are gathered.

The female is the only valuable animal. It has a convex body, flattened below, nearly twice as large as that of the male; apterous, bluish red, covered with a white farina; *antennæ* short, eleven-jointed, filiform, and setaceous; *feet* short. When dried, they are one or two lines long, wrinkled, of an irregular figure, convex on one side, and flat, or somewhat hollow on the other. They are inodorous, have a bitterish, warm taste, tinge the saliva violet-red, and yield a dark-red product. Three varieties are distinguished in commerce, the differences in which are said to be due to differences in the method of curing the insect.

1. *Coccus renigrida.*—Killed in boiling water, of a fine uniform reddish or purplish-black, and destitute of the silvery wool.

2. *Coccus jaspeada.*—Killed in ovens, of a purplish gray, and covered with a silvery powder, appearing under the microscope like fine wool.

3. *Coccus sylvestris,* (*Granilla.*)—Consisting of the sifted powder and fragments of the insect.

The second variety is the most esteemed for coloring purposes; the whitish powder indicating the female: the appearance has been simulated by rolling the other varieties in baryta or talc, a deception at once detected by the microscope.

The first variety is the one used in the provings, as being least likely to be adulterated.

Pelletier and Caventou found the constituents of cochineal to be *carmine,* (the coloring principle,) *peculiar animal matter, fatty matter,* (composed of *stearin, olein,* and an *odorous acid,*) and *phosphate and carbonate of lime, chloride of potassium, phosphate of potash,* and a salt of *potash,* containing an *organic acid.*

Preparation.—After being well washed in warm water, and dried, the cochineal is pulverized and macerated in ten times its weight of alcohol, for a fortnight, when the mother tincture is obtained by filtration.

Or, the powder may be triturated in the usual way with sugar of milk.

2. *Digest of the Symptoms.*

We owe our knowledge of this remedy to the Austrian Society of Provers, in whose Journal the experiments were first published, (Band iv. S. 509,) and where may be found the following

AUTHORITIES.

1. Caspar, 509.
2. A. F., 511.
3. Fröhlich, 512.
4. Mad. Kummer, 516.
5. Gottwald, 518.
6. Huber, 523.
7. Huber, 530.
8. Lach, 540.
9. J. G. M., 545.
10. Marenzeller, 548.
11. Muller, 559.
12. Schweikhofer, 562.
13. Mad. Schweikhofer, 566.
14. Rudiger, 567.
15. Wachtel, 568.
16. Mdlle. Thérèse, 574.
17. Wurmb, 579.
18. Zlatarovich, 582.
19. Rudolph, 588.
20. Eduard, 588.
21. Franz, 589.
22. M. H., 589.
23. Adolphe, 589.
24. Reil, *Viertelj.* i. 194.

☞ The figures refer to the authorities; curative symptoms are preceded by a cypher, (0).

MENTAL AND MORAL.—**Exciting.** 1. Gay mood, (13.) Very gay mood, quite unnatural, (4.) Very great flow of spirits, notwithstanding he had been peevish and irritable the evening before; even the headache and sensation of fullness, which come on in the evening, do not affect his spirits, (11.) An unusual gay mood takes the place of his ill-humor in the evening, (5.) 5. Loquacity, (3.) **Depressing.** Ill-humor, without any reason, during the whole day, (5, 12.) Sadness during the whole day, unattended by any physical suffering, (16.) She is very low spirited, and wearied with the pains in the genitals, (16.) Sombre mood, (9.) 10. Indifferent mood in the afternoon; indisposition to labor, but not from ill-humor; he is rather fatigued, overcome, (8.) Great indisposition to labor; ill-humor, and great moral irritability, (8.) He wakes at 6, A.M., physically well, but morally indisposed, and very irritable, (8.) Great moral irritability, (13.) Anxiety in the evening, (5.)

HEAD.—**Headache in general.** 15. General dull headache, aggravated by shaking his head, during the whole morning, (7.) Congestion of blood to the head; on entering a warm room, he was obliged to go out again, which made him feel better; this occurred three times before noon, (7.) Congestion of blood to the head, with pressive pain in the orbital region, and sensation of inflation of the stomach, soon after the dose, (15.) Painful lancinations through the brain; they last for an hour, and are accompanied by an obstruction of the meatus auditorius, (18.) Confused head, (5, 7, 10, 14.) 20. Confused head, with general depression, (6.) Confusion of the head, which disappears in the open air, (10.) Confusion of the head during the whole day, (3.) Confusion in the morning on waking, as though from a drinking debauch; tongue white, and pasty taste, (7.) Confusion of the head in the morning, with feeling as if the temples were too narrow, (9.) 25. Confusion of the head after breakfast, (5.) Confusion of the head, redness of the face and hands, with swelling of the veins, and throbbings in all the arteries, after dinner, (11.) Confusion of the head in the evening, (5.) Confusion of the head in the evening as if intoxicated, (7.) Confusion of the head on entering a warm room; towards evening it becomes a moderate headache, which disappears in the open air, (3.) 30. Great dullness of the head in the evening, with aching in the vertex, and burning in the skin of the forehead, (18.) Transitory stupefaction, (5.) Stupefaction on waking in the morning, like the effects of drink, (7.) Feeling of fullness in the whole head, (4.) Sensation of swelling of the whole head, accompanied by anxiety, in the evening, (5.) 35. Pressive aching in the brain, particularly in the region of the root of the nose, accompanied by pressure on the internal canthus; it lasts ten minutes, (7.) Pressive headache, like that of indigestion, with general coldness, especially in the back, and eructations of wind, (10.) Pressive headache in the morning on waking, as if after excessive drinking, which disappears after having left the bed, (7.) Pressive headache at breakfast, (8.) Pressive headache in the evening, but slight, (16.) 40. Head feels empty during the day, (5.) Beer gives him the headache in the evening, although he is used to it, (7.) **Frontal.** Dull and digging frontal headache in the evening; it lasts the whole of the next day, (2.) Heat in the forehead, (15.) Confusion in the frontal region, with feeling of weight on waking, (9.) 45. Dull, pressive, frontal headache; the rest of the head is only confused, (4.) Pressive ache in the region of the superciliary arch, dryness of the nasal mucous membrane and of the pharynx; he cannot detach the mucus either by spitting or blowing; increase of the lachrymal secretion, particularly copious in the open air; the tears seem thicker than usual, (15.) Two little pimples on the right side of the forehead, (9.) Violent lancination in the head, to the right of the coronal suture, in the afternoon, (18.) Frontal headache in the left frontal eminence: it leaves there to occupy the parietal and temporal regions, extends to the zygoma, and causes in all these parts a dull, rheumatic, and cutting aching, (11.) 50. Pressive aching in the left frontal region, which sometimes extends into the occiput, (2.) Frontal headache, increased by moving or turning the head, and even when using the arms, (7.) **Parietal.** Dull, digging pain toward the posterior edge of the right parietal bone, coming on in paroxysms, like waves, in the morning in bed, (6.) **Vertex.** Heat in the vertex, (7.) Confusion of the head in the vertex, (12.) 55. Dullness of the head, especially in the vertex, (12.) Great dullness of the head, particularly in the vertex, in the evening when walking, (12.) He wakes with a pressive, burning pain in the vertex, which lasts for an hour, but goes off as he has gone to sleep again for a little while, (18.) **Temporal.** Lancinating pain in the temples in the morning, (4.) Pressure in both temples, (5.) 60. Violent throbbing, pressive pain in both temples at 1 P.M.; it lasts an hour, frequently alternating with heat and redness of the face, and unaffected by either motion or rest, (15.) Weak pressure, extending from the temples to the vertex, and disappearing after bathing the parts in cold water, (8.) Drawing and pressure in the temples, (1.) Pressive pain in the right temporal region, (1.) Dull, lancinating pain in the left temple, disappearing on external pressure, and returning when the pressure is removed, (12.)

Mastoidean region. 65. Pressive pain in the right temporal region soon after rising, extending sometimes into the left ear, and lasting all day, (17.) Bruised pain around the left external ear, extending along the left side of the neck to the left clavicular and thoracic region, (6.) Violent pressive and throbbing pain in the left mastoid process, in the heat of the bed before midnight, increasing and becoming boring from within outwards, (6.) Pressive and tensive pain in the temporal bone, but particularly in the mastoid process, (6.) Pressive and lancinating pain in the bones, in the neighborhood of the left ear, in the evening in bed; the pain becomes digging and congestive, has very short remissions, and extends, when most severe, into the cervical and clavicular region, the left inferior molars, and the left occipital region; it is accompanied by lancinations in the left tragus, and a disagreeable roaring in the left ear, (6.) **Occipital.** 70. Dull, digging pain in the left side of the occiput in the evening, extending toward the ear, (6.) Feeling of coldness in the occiput, as though a cold breeze were blowing upon it, (5.) Feeling as if the occiput, from one mastoid process to the other, were encircled by a burning band, at the same time great moral distress; by degrees the whole scalp became involved, and seemed to him to contract and shorten; formication at the roots of the hairs, which stood on end, (11.) Drawing and slight pressure in the occiput, temples, and right eye, (1.) Feeling of pressure and heat in the occiput in the evening, (7.) 75. Pressive pain in the occiput, accompanied by a feeling of swelling in the scalp; this feeling extends to the left cheek and nasal surface, (1.) **Scalp.** Itching in several places on the scalp in the afternoon, (6.) Lancination, causing him to scratch the scalp at midnight on waking, (6.) Painful elevation on the vertex, of the size of a lentil; it disappeared in the evening, but the place was still sore to the touch, (18.) Formication in the scalp, forcing him to scratch, and followed by a disagreeable sensation in the morning on waking, (8.) 80. Feeling as if the scalp were too tight upon the cranium, with formication at the roots of the hair, (11.) Sensitiveness of the scalp on the vertex, (18.)

EYES.—Trembling of the left lower lid, (6.) Feeling as if a hair had got between the eye and the lid in the morning on waking, forcing him to rub, and followed by a forcing pain in the interior of the left eye, (6.) Feeling as if a foreign body were placed between the eye and the lid, in the evening, (17.) Feeling as if the edges of the lids were swollen, (17.) Slight agglutination of the lids in the morning, (18.) Burning of the lids and of the skin of the right leg, (18.) Slight smarting of the edges of the lids, (18.) Drawing and pressure in the right eye, (1.) 90. Rheumatic pain, extending from the eye into the forehead, in the evening, (7.) Violent throbbing pain, extending from the eye into the squamous portion of the temporal bone and its internal surface, and then into the occiput, lasting more than a quarter of an hour; it feels to him as though a liquid were injected into a diminutive vessel by successive strokes of a piston, (6.) The right conjunctiva very much inflamed, (9.) The inflammation of the conjunctiva returns the next day more violently, (9.) The conjunctival inflammation diminishes on the third day, (9.) 95. Sight weaker than usual, (9.)

EARS.—Rheumatic drawing above and behind the left ear, followed by roaring which lasts a long while, in bed, before midnight, (6.) Pressive and tensive pain in the left mastoid process and clavicular region, accompanied by continual roaring in the left ear, (6.) Drawing pain in the convex part of the concha, aggravated by touch, (6.) Violent itching in the right concha and external meatus, (6.) 100. Lancinations and violent itching in the right tragus, (6.) Itching pruritus, sometimes in the right, sometimes in the left tragus, (6). Itching lancination in the external meatus and right temporal region, (6.) Tickling and itching in the left meatus, frequently repeated in the evening, afterward accompanied by pressure in the concha, (15.) Frequent itching in the left external meatus in the morning in bed. 105. Itching in the right external meatus, inducing him to introduce his finger; it frequently changes to lancination, is accompanied by roaring in the left ear and stinging lancinations in various parts of the skin, even of the prepuce, (6.) Itching and voluptuous titillation in both ears, which seems to extend from the external meatus through the internal ear into the mouth, and only lasting fifteen or twenty seconds, (6.) Intolerable itching in the external meatus in the evening in bed, which can only be quieted by introducing the finger, (6.) Drawing in the right meatus lasting all the evening, (17.) Violent lancination in the interior of the right ear, followed by a dull pain in one of the superior posterior molars, (6.) 110. Violent lancinations in the left ear, (5.) Frequent itching in the left ear, (6.) Drawing pain in the interior of the ear, (6.) Cramp-like, drawing pain in the interior of the right ear, (6.) Drawing from time to time in the left ear, (17.) 115. Simmering, as if from boiling water, in the interior of the left ear, (6.) Roaring in the ears, like a tempest among the trees, in the evening in bed, (6.) Itching and noise in the left ear, in the evening, (6.) Heat and tinkling in the ear, (6.) Crepitation in the left ear during deglutition, (6.) 120. Sharp tinkling in the interior of the left ear, (6.) Painful throbbings in the interior of the left ear, isochronous with the beats of the heart, (6.) Feeling as if the ear were stopped with cracking in the interior, (9.) Feeling as if the ear were stopped, not interfering with the hearing, and accompanied by a tensive and pressive pain in the left mastoid process, extending into the left side of the neck into the clavicular region and the last inferior molar teeth, (6.) Hardness of hearing, as if the ears were stuffed with cotton, (5.) 125. Both ears feel stopped up for a quarter of an hour in the evening, with feeling of pressure and forcing in the meatus, (15). The pain in the ear when at its height extends into the interior of the ear, the left occipital region, the posterior inferior molars, and along the sterno-mastoid into the clavicular sternal region, (6.) The pain in the ear is accompanied by a sensation as though liquid cerumen were about to run out, (6.) The pains in the ear are aggravated when lying on the left ear, and last, with little cessation, during the whole day, (6). The pains which extend into the neighboring part, after the severe aching in the ear, produce a sensation of swelling there, (6.) 130. The itching in the ear appears especially when he enters a warm room from the open air, (6.)

NOSE.—Sensation of a pressive pain at the root of the nose and in the frontal eminences, (9.) Two little pustules, of the size of a millet-seed, on the left ala, (15.) Redness and excoriated feeling in the opening of the nostrils, (4.) Yellow pulverulent matter at the internal edge of the nostrils, (18.) 135. Crusts in the opening of the nostrils, (5.) Dry nasal crust, nose obstructed, stopped, (1.) He is obliged, during the day, to snuff up cold water in consequence of the dryness of the nostrils in order to ease the sensation; he is finally enabled to detach, by blowing, a piece of dry mucus, which relieves him for a time, (9.) Feeling of obstruction in the nasal cavity with aqueous secretion, (4.) Much mucus runs from both nostrils without any other catarrhal symptoms, (10, 18.) 140. Secretion of a very fluid nasal mucus during the day, (5, 9.) Slight coryza during the evening, with lancinating pain in both temples and excoriated feeling in the throat, (4.) Nasal and laryngeal catarrh, aggravated in the morning, (5.) Frequent and violent sneezing in the morning, (10.) The attacks of sneezing return the next day at the same hour, but the burning at the edges of the nostrils is continuous, (11.) 145. Very violent sneezing in the afternoon without apparent cause, in several paroxysms, in consequence of which the edges of the nostrils and the furrows of the alæ burn as if from pepper, (11.) Violent sneezing, leaving a sense of roughness in the throat as if from eating high-seasoned food, (15.) Frequent sneezing, accompanied by a dry cough, (5.) Frequent sneezing in the evening, (17.) Itching in the nostrils, followed by repeated, prolonged, and very violent sneezings, (12.) 150. Frequent sneezings, (5, 18.) Feeling of dryness at the posterior opening of the nares, (6.)

FACE.—Heat of the face in a room without a fire in the morning on waking, (3.) Violent heat in the cheeks for half an hour, (3.) Peculiar pricking heat in the cheeks without redness, (11.) 155. Isolated lancinations, violent and deep, between the tragus and the zygomatic process, (6.) Formication and drawing in the left half of the face and nose, analogous to a prosopalgia having its seat in the *pes anserina*, (suborbital branch,) (11.) Feeling of formication in both zygomatic processes, (15.) Formication beginning over the left cheek-bone, extending above the bridge of the nose on the left cheek, and recurring three times on the same day, (15.) Sensation of fullness in the superior maxilla, as if the teeth were about to be forced or pushed out of their sockets, (2.) 160. Pain in the temporo-maxillary articulation when chewing, with crepitation in the joint when swallowing, (6.) Pain in the right parotid region, followed by pain in the right sublingual gland, with increased secretion of saliva, (6.)

MOUTH.—**Lips.** Little furrows (not cracks) in the lips, which look as if sprinkled with flour, (15.) Oblong, reddish-blue spot on the upper lip, disappearing after twenty-four hours, (15.) Slight sensation of contraction of the skin of the upper lip. **Teeth.** 165. Lancinating itching in the gum of the right superior incisor, in the morning in bed, (6.)

Excoriated pain in the inferior alveoli, which have lost their teeth, (15.) He is waked by an excoriating sore pain in the teeth and left upper and lower gums, with great sensibility to the touch; but no sooner had he changed his position, (he was lying on the left side,) than the pain disappeared; he slept quietly until 5 A.M., when he felt an irresistible desire to make water, (10.) Sudden drawing in the incisors and in the right auditory meatus, in the forenoon, (17.) Sudden drawing in the right inferior incisors, and pressure in the left globe, in the forenoon, (17.) 170. Feeling in a lateral inferior incisor, as if it were seized with cold fingers and drawn up, in the evening, (15.) Odontalgia in paroxysms, in the morning on waking, especially in the incisors and left eye-tooth, with a sensation as if a cold wind were blowing upon it, (7.) The pains in the incisors and upper eye-tooth are aggravated by inspiring cold air and in closing them upon the stem of the pipe, (7.) Dull pain in the last inferior molar, (6.) Drawing in the right molars, at noon, (17.) 175. Dull, slightly digging pain in the right superior molars, in the morning on waking, accompanied by dull headache over the right eye, (6.) Aching in a carious third upper molar, at 6 P.M. Very violent toothache in a carious tooth, (1.) The pain in the third upper molar is aggravated by the touch, and is not eased by cold water, nor by heat, (8.) He resorts to extraction of the third superior molar, (carious,) but the pain continues in the alveolus through the whole day, (8.) 180. Sudden drawing in the teeth and itching on the left arm, (17.) Drawing in the teeth of the left side during the whole day, (17.) Teeth painful when closing them against each other, (7.) Teeth exceedingly sensitive to cold, (11.) Sensitiveness of the teeth to cold air, (17.) 185. Great sensitiveness to the cold water when cleansing the teeth in the morning, (17.) Painful sensibility of the under teeth, and feeling as if they had become elongated, (15.) **Buccal cavity.** Roughness in the buccal cavity, (5.) Roughness of the buccal cavity of the throat, with sensation of a foreign body in the throat, and feeling of strangulation. Sensation of heat in the buccal cavity and throat, (12.) 190. Feeling of dryness in the buccal cavity as far as the pharynx, (3.) Dryness of the buccal cavity, and sensation of smarting on the anterior portion of the tongue, as though he had used pepper, (6.) Great dryness of the buccal cavity in the morning in bed, (6.) The buccal and pharyngeal cavities feel as if covered with velvet, which lasts for several hours, (7.) **Tongue.** Tongue coated white, (4.) 195. Clean tongue, (24.) Lancinating itching on the left side of the point of the tongue, and accumulation of saliva in the mouth, toward noon, (6.) Dry tongue, covered with a yellow fur, on waking, (5.) Great dryness of the tongue and whole buccal cavity, with much thirst and desire for cold water, (6.) The tongue is so dry, that in moving it about, and touching the palate, it makes a noise, (5.) 200. Small vesicle on the tongue, (1.) **Saliva.** Increased salivary secretion, (6, 12, 16.) Increased secretion of saliva, and metallic taste, (12, 13,) Increased salivary secretion and great hunger, which compels him to eat at an unaccustomed hour, (11.) Increased secretion of saliva, with continual desire to spit, and metallic taste in the mouth, (12.) 205. Profuse flow of saliva, with bitter taste, colic, sensibility of the epigastrium and hypogastrium, increased by pressure, (12.) Flow of saliva and sensation of emptiness at the pit of the stomach, (13.) The mouth fills with saliva, the head aches, and is not relieved by the open air, (16.) Flow of saliva, followed by pain in the loins and sacrum, (12.)

THROAT.—**Palate.** Tension and great sensibility of the *velum palati*, (5.) 210. Painful tension of the velum, which forces him to drink often, (5.) Sensation in the velum and upper part of the pharynx, as if he had eaten food strongly seasoned with pepper, (2.) The velum is so irritable, that speaking or cleaning the teeth is sufficient to provoke vomiting, (5.) A pustule of the size of a hemp-seed on the right pillar of the velum, (3.) Slight redness of the velum with an attack of hoarseness and dryness of the lips, without any effect upon deglutition, (15.) 215. The pain in the velum is sensibly aggravated by speaking and swallowing, (7.) **Uvula.** Feeling as if the uvula were elongated, occasioning constant hawking, (12.) Tickling in the uvula, after gargling with cold water, which provokes a cough, (2.) Tickling in the uvula which extends over the velum palati, (2.) **Tonsils.** Swelling of the right tonsil, (9.) 220. The inflammation of the right tonsil increases on the second day, (9.) The sore throat increases; the tonsil is very much swollen and red, the velum dry; constant desire to swallow, occasioned by a foreign body which seems to be seated in the pharynx, (9.) **Eustachian tube.** The pressive pain in the Eustachian tube appears suddenly, an hour before dinner, and disappears while eating warm soup, (2.) Aching in the right Eustachian tube, aggravated by turning the head to the right, and when swallowing, (2.) Lancinations in the palate, and even in the tongue, with dryness causing much thirst, (16.) **Pharynx.** 225. The velum palati and pharynx are slightly reddened, (3.) Scraping feeling in the velum and pharynx every morning on waking, accompanied by hoarseness, fits of coughing and expectoration of mucus, which is quieted by tepid gargles, (11.) Roughness of the throat, (5.) Feeling of roughness in the throat which forces him continually to hawk up mucus, (3.) Roughness of the throat and expectoration of mucus in the morning, (18.) 230. Feeling of roughness in the throat, on getting out of bed in the morning, followed by a paroxysm of coughing, which lasted half an hour, (17.) Feeling of roughness in the throat, and expectoration of a fluid mucus at 6 P. M., (17.) Slight burning at the *isthmus faucium*, (11.) Slight burning feeling in the throat in the evening, (8.) Violent burning in the throat, a little relieved by drinking cold water, (8.) 235. Feeling of heat and burning in the pharynx and buccal cavity, (12.) Pressive burning feeling behind the larynx, as if from a caustic liquid, (7.) He is waked in the morning by a tickling in the throat, obliging him to sit up in bed, and exciting fits of sonorous coughing, not followed by expectoration, although much mucus had accumulated in the throat, (11.) Tickling in the throat, (20.) Tickling in the throat which makes him feel like vomiting, (5.) 240. Excoriated feeling in the throat with no effect upon deglutition, (4.) Excoriated feeling in the throat, (4, 5.) Slight scraping in the throat, (18.) Scraping feeling in the throat in the morning after a quiet night, frequent sneezing and some coughing-fits, like the precurrent stage of a cold or catarrh, (10.) Scraping in the throat, lasting until midday and disappearing after dinner, (5.) 245. Scraping in the throat in the evening, which forces him to hack, with expectoration of a considerable quantity of mucus, (10.) Scraping in the throat, and frequent expectoration of easily-detached mucus, (17.) Scraping, lancination, and constriction of the throat, (16.) Feeling of pressure in the throat, (8.) Aching in the throat in the evening, especially on empty deglutition, (18.) 250. Feeling as of a foreign body behind the larynx, (7.) Redness of the fauces without difficulty in swallowing, (4.) Sensation as of the commencement of inflammation in the throat, (3.) The irritation in the throat which causes coughing, is seated in the pharyngeal mucous membrane, only appears in the morning in bed, and disappears after a warm breakfast, (milk-coffee,) (11.) Dryness of the throat, (5, 9.) 255. Sensation of dryness on the posterior wall of the pharynx, (9.) Dryness of the throat as if filled with dust, (5.) Dryness of the throat occasioning cough, (24.) Dryness of the throat lasting several hours, (17.) Dryness of the pharynx and posterior nerves during the whole day, with feeling of a foreign body in the throat, (9.) 260. Dryness of the throat in the morning, and tension on the right side when swallowing, (7.) Dryness of the throat in the forenoon, accompanied by accumulation of mucus about the uvula, (15.) Great dryness of the throat in the afternoon, (5.) Dryness of the throat in the evening, accompanied by burning in the velum palati, (5.) The dryness of the throat wakes him several times in the night; it is relieved by cold water, (5.) 265. Dryness of the throat with scraping, which compels him to be often swallowing, (8.) Dryness of the mucous membrane of the pharynx and nasal cavity, (5.) Very great accumulation of mucus in the throat, (11.) Great sensitiveness of the pharynx in the morning, (5.) Increased sensibility of the pharynx, so that gargling with cold water is sufficient to provoke cough and vomiting of thick, mucous matters, (5.) 270. Feeling as though there were a hair in the throat which, obliges him to hawk up particles of mucus, (3.) Sensation as though a thread were hanging in the pharynx, (14.) The peppery feeling in the pharynx and velum disappears while gargling with cold water, (2.) The sore throat increased by heat, and especially in bed, (15.) The sore throat lasts eleven days; in five minutes after taking *lachesis*, three globules, 7th dilution, the mucus began to be easily detached; the night's rest was good, and in the morning deglutition was unembarrassed, the redness diminished, and the organs restored to their normal state, (15.) 275. Catarrhal affection of the pharynx and respiratory apparatus, (5.) The roughness of the throat, cough, and sneezing last all day, (5.) Burning in the throat when hawking, (8.) Burning in the throat and lips when smoking, which obliges him to give it up, (5.) Tension in the velum palati during deglutition, unmoved by some glasses of wine, (5.) 280. Frequent desire to swallow in the afternoon, with sensation of a foreign body in the throat, (9.) Dryness of the organs of deglutition in the evening, (5.) He is obliged to moisten the organs of deglutition with cooling drinks, (5.) Difficulty of swallowing in the evening, (3.) Burning pain in the organs of deglutition, produced by the fumes of tobacco in an atmosphere filled with it, (5.) 285. The organs of deglutition are deeper red than ordinary, and deglutition is more painful, (15.) Scraping in the organs of deglutition, and constriction of the throat, (29.) Sensitiveness of the organs of deglutition, day and night, (5.) Sensation of a bit of ice sliding along the organs of deglutition at noon, (15.) It seems to him when swallowing liquids, as though they were detained in their course by a spasmodic constriction, (7.) 290. The foreign body in the throat seems at times to descend into the stomach, at others to rise again; this lasts all day, (7.) Burning heat in the œsophagus.

TASTE AND APPETITE.—**Taste.** Bitter taste, (5.) Bitter taste during the whole day, (8.) Taste so acrid and bitter, especially at the root of the tongue, that it makes him feel like vomiting, (18.) 295. Bitter taste in the mouth, and nausea, produced by a scraping in the throat, after having had a pleasant night, (5.) Bitter, nauseating taste, (5, 6, 12, 22, 14, 24.) Sweetish taste in the mouth, (3.) Continual metallic taste with hunger, even after having eaten, (12.) Metallic taste limited to the tip of the tongue, (12.) 300. Nauseating metallic taste, vomiturition, malaise, and pain in the stomach, (14.) Very disagreeable metallic taste in the evening when smoking and drinking beer, (12.) Pasty, disagreeable, almost metallic taste, (8, 17, 18.) Disagreeable resinous taste at the root of the tongue, at noon, after having drunk a glass of water, (18.) **Appetite.** Loss of appetite, (4, 7, 8.) 305. Appetite diminished without disgust for food, and with a feeling as if the stomach were swollen, (16.) Want of appetite without disgust for food, (8.) Loss of appetite, with confusion in the head, (5.) Loss of appetite and increased thirst at noon, (5.) Little appetite, and tongue covered with a white fur at noon, (7.) 310. Anorexia in the morning, followed by very voracious hunger, (5.) Capricious appetite, (1.) Good appetite at noon, (5, 12, 24.) Voracious appetite at dinner, (7, 22.) He seats himself at table with a voracious appetite, but is very soon satiated, (8, 9.) 315. Very strong appetite, but he has scarcely swallowed a spoonful of soup before it is gone; he eats without relish, but without aversion, (10.) He sits down with a good appetite, but does not eat with much relish, and finds himself rapidly satiated, (11, 17.) Good appetite, and after its gratification, pyrosis, (5.) He gets hungry at unusual hours, and is obliged to eat very often; but this frequent eating does not strengthen, but only weakens him, (11.) He is obliged to eat much and often without being incommoded by this unaccustomed course, (11.) 320. Feeling of hunger even when rising from table, (12.) He eats but little at dinner, in consequence of having a disgust for food, (17.) Repugnance to eating any thing, (7.) Coffee is disagreeable to her, and she has an aversion to water, (16.) Smoking gives him no pleasure, (8.) **Thirst.** 325. Thirst not increased, (24.) Absence of thirst, (4.) Thirst, (5.) Thirst increased, especially in the morning, (1.) Increased thirst after dinner, (9.) 330. Violent thirst after dinner, satisfied by cold water; he feels very cold, (3.) Violent thirst in the evening, and great desire to drink beer, (8.)

STOMACH.—**Eructations.** Eructations of wind, (10.) Eructation and desire to vomit, (19.) Daily attacks in the evening of sonorous eructations, and a pain in the loins exactly corresponding to the seat of the kidneys, (11.) **Nausea.** 335. Very great malaise after dinner, which does not disappear until evening, (12.) Food, although of easy digestion, causes malaise, pressure at the stomach, and frequent eructations, which do not afford relief; it is only after repeated regurgitations, by which a part of the ingesta are discharged, that he feels a little better, (11.) Nausea, with insipid, nauseating taste, (13.) Nausea, eructations, and vomiturition, (18.) Nausea and desire to vomit, (7.) 340. Slight inclination to vomit, disappearing after having drunk some wine, (5.) Constant desire to vomit, (5.) She thinks for some minutes that she shall vomit, after which she feels a great heat in her stomach, which frequently returns for several hours, but never lasts long, (16.) The thought of cochineal is sufficient to provoke nausea and inclination to vomit, (5.) Nausea in the pharynx as if his throat were tickled with a feather, (5.) 345. Nausea and vomiturition, (13.) Something ascends from the hypogastrium towards the stomach, and nauseates him, (16.) Vomiturition, salivation, and metallic taste, (12.) Constant vomiturition, (14.) **Epigastrium.** Sharp prickings in the skin of the epigastric region when uncovering it, (3.) 350. Inflated feeling in the epigastric region, (15.) Inflation of the stomach by the introduction of food, (7.) Inflation of the stomach and regurgitation after rising from bed, (7.) Sensation of heat in the epigastrium and region of the small intestines in the evening, as though these parts were bathed with warm water, but without tension or inflation of the abdomen, and directly connected with the dyspnœa and oppression of the inferior portion of the thorax, (11.) Epigastrium painful to the touch, (7.) 355. Painful sensibility of the epigastrium, especially to external pressure, (13.) Slight, undefinable pain in the epigastrium and left hypochondrium, (1.) Lancinating pain in the epigastrium during inspiration for five or six minutes; it disappears during expiration, at 4 A.M., on waking, (6.) Pressive pain in the epigastrium, (1.) Pressure in the epigastrium, (10.) 360. Burning and pressure in the stomach, (18.) Constriction ascending from the stomach into the œsophagus, (13.) Transitory pain in the stomach, as if cramp were about to set in, (13.) Cramp-pain in the stomach, malaise, and peculiar sensation of cold, which extend the whole length of the stomach and into the buccal cavity, (11.) The cramp in the stomach recurs, but is quieted without having recourse to taking food, (11.) 365. Pain in the stomach and diminution of the pain in the toe, on waking, (7.) Several attacks of pain in the stomach in the course of the day, with a disagreeable feeling of violent hunger, (11.) The pain in the stomach, accompanied by fierce hunger, returns several times, and always lasts for several days, as well as the frequent discharge of urine; it is finally accompanied with drawing pain in the back, (11.) Pain in the stomach, with feeling as if there were a large ball there, (14.) Pain in the stomach, with remarkably good appetite and constipation, (13.) 370. Lancinations and griping in the stomach; this pain leaps like an electric shock to the genital parts, but soon vanishes, (16.) Dull lancinations, first in the fundus of the stomach, then in the region of the cœcum; two dull lancinations, (12.) Weakness and fatigue of the stomach, (16.) Cold feeling in the stomach; it seems to him as if a cool breeze were blowing in his stomach, (12.) Cold feeling in the stomach, with hunger, tenesmus, and pain in the sacro-lumbar region, (12.) 375. Pressive griping in the stomach, lasting all day, and which nothing will relieve, (3.) Feeling as if the overloaded stomach was about to empty itself by vomiting, which, however, does not take place, (7.) Fullness of the stomach, and constriction all day, (7.) Feels all the morning as if she had drunk too much water, (16.) Sensation of a stone in the stomach, and a foreign body in the throat, (7.) 380. Pressure in the stomach, (b. 15.) Pressure in the stomach after a light repast, (7.) Pressure in the stomach during the whole day, as if produced by some undigested food, (6.) Very violent pressure in the stomach, constriction and sensation of a foreign body in the throat, continually inducing him to swallow, (7.) Pressure in the stomach, tearings and lancinations through the whole body, even in the knee, with weariness and impossibility to take his usual walk, (16.) 385. Pressure in the stomach with constriction in the throat, (7.) Feeling as if the pressure in the stomach ascended into the pharynx, (7.) Fullness and pressure in the stomach through the whole day, (7.) Sensation of emptiness in the stomach, (13.) **Pyrosis.** Pyrosis and transitory shocks in the left inferior canine tooth, when walking and smoking, (7.) 390. Pyrosis and regurgitation of an acrid liquid in the evening, (7.) Pyrosis for two hours after dinner, (5.) Pyrosis after having taken a small quantity of wine, (7.) Pyrosis at night, (8.) Pyrosis and painful tension in the throat in the afternoon, (5.)

ABDOMEN.—395. Lancinating itching, prolonged into the integuments of the abdomen, as though from leech-bites, in the afternoon, (6.) Inflation of the abdomen and sensitiveness of the epigastric region, especially to the touch, (12.) Full feeling in the abdomen, as though he had eaten too much; this feeling persists even after having been twice to stool, (7.) **Hypochondrium, right.** Lancinating pain in the right hypochondrium, extending from the edge of the false rib to the right side of the back, aggravated by the pressure of the hand upon the parts, and ameliorated by the discharge of flatulence, (6.) Crackling in the abdomen below the right false ribs, (6.) **Hypochondrium, left.** 400. Pain in the left hypochondrium, as if from incarcerated flatulence, (24.) The pains commence in the left hypochondrium, and extend to the left dorsal and lumbar regions, (24.) He is waked by a burning in the region of the left hypochondrium, which is quieted by the application of the warm hand, and he goes to sleep again, (11.) Burning drawing in the splenic region, which ascends into the thorax, does not last long, but returns several times, (11.) Paroxysms of acute, transitory lancinations in the splenic region, (15.) 405. Lancinations in the spleen, at first acute, then dull, changing into obtuse sensations in the left hypochondrium, (11.)

Rapid lancinations in the left hypochondrium, ascending into the left thorax, (11.) Drawing lancinations, extending from the left hypochondrium along the left hip, and lasting several seconds, (6.) **Umbilical.** Pain around the navel, extending from time to time towards the iliac bones and their symphisis, (1.) •Digging pain around the navel, (2.) 410. Violent colic accompanied by headache, (14.) Borborygmi with pains in the loins and sacrum, (12.) Borborygmi and discharge of copious flatus, (18.) Painless gurgling in the abdomen after dinner, but very disagreeable from its long duration and violence, (18.) The borborygmi ceased after the discharge of flatus, when walking about the room, (11.) 415. The same gurgling during the siesta, which annoys him a great deal, and compels him to abandon his accustomed nap, (11.) Borborygmi again during the whole day, removed by the emission of flatus, (11.) A great deal of flatulence, which sometimes rolls about in the bowels, at others is very easily discharged, (24.) Accumulated flatulency in the abdomen, some hours after dinner, accompanied by heat in the stomach, (16.) Flatulence with great general malaise in the afternoon, (9.) 420. Slight colic with fruitless desire to go to stool in the afternoon, (12.) Violent, but transitory griping colic after dinner, (10.) Almost constant, but mild colic in the afternoon, commencing in the stomach and extending towards the region of the cœcum, remitting from time to time, and then returning, (12.) Moderate colic in the morning on waking, followed by efforts to vomit, with nausea and copious salivation, metallic taste, pain in the stomach, and flatulency, (12.) Colic in the morning, followed by a diarrhœa, which is repeated three times during the day, (5.) 425. Violent colic in the morning on waking, but ceasing after a stool, (12.) Colic around the navel, followed by a soft stool at 11 A.M., and several times in the course of the afternoon, (7.) Colic and diarrhœa, towards noon, (5.) Colic, followed by diarrhœa and chills in the evening, (5.) Cutting colic in the abdomen, (5, 17.) 430. Cuttings around the navel at 4 A.M., soon after waking; she is afraid to move, for fear of aggravating the pain, which lasts a quarter of an hour, (4.) **Hypogastrium.** Colic in the hypogastric region, ameliorated by the emission of flatulence, (6.) Pains in the hypogastrium and sacrum during dinner, (16.) The sensitiveness of the epigastrium extends throughout the abdomen; lancinating drawing and pressive pains especially appear in the groins and vesical regions, which oblige her to keep her bed, (13.) The pains in the abdomen, after having lasted an hour, extend towards the hypogastrium; they are not like the menstrual molimina, but lancinating pains, (16.) 455. Rumbling movement in the hypogastrium, followed by very acute lancinations, as if from needles, extending from the bladder through the urethra, toward the glans; they come on again several times within three minutes, when seated, (3.) Twisting pain deep in the abdomen on the left side of the vertebral column, as if in the kidney and ureter, (24.) **Inguinal.** Agitation and lancinations in the left groin in the morning, (15.) Pruritus, itching, and drawings in the region of the groin and pubes, in the prepuce, glans, dorsum of the foot and toes, (12.)

STOOL.—**Rectum.** Sudden feeling of distension and lancinations in the rectum, on the cessation of which a heat extends through the whole hypogastrium, (16.) 440. Lancinating pain in the rectum, lasting several hours, diminishing from time to time, but always aggravated by walking, (16.) Violent jerking and boring lancinations in the rectum in the afternoon, when seated; they are suddenly transferred to the neck of the bladder, follow the direction of the ureter as far as the kidneys, and vanish, (15.) Usual stool followed by burning in the rectum, (15.) Lancinating pain in the rectum during stool, (16.) **Anus.** Secretion of a fluid in the sulcus and at the anus, which stains the sheets yellow, (18.) 445. Exceedingly violent lancinating thrust from the anus through the urethra at 5 P.M., (17.) Slight formication at the anus, (18.) Pretty severe itching at the anus, (9.) **Stool.** Tenesmus and copious diarrhœa in the evening, (12.) Anal tenesmus after a short walk at noon, (18.) 450. Pressing desire to go to stool soon after having eaten, with tenesmus, slight burning, protrusion of hæmorrhoidal tumors, and discharge of matters enveloped in mucus, (11.) Copious discharge of flatus, (18.) Very irregular stools, sometimes hard, sometimes liquid, sometimes two a day, and sometimes a day without one, (24.) Irregular stools during the whole proving. Stool with tenesmus; fæces like potter's clay, and after the passage a very disagreeable transitory cramp-pain in the rectum, opposite the inferior extremity of the sacrum, (9.) 455. Frequent fruitless desire to go to stool, (12.) Frequent fruitless desire to go to stool, during the day, and when the evacuation comes on, the pains in the loins and sacrum vanish, (12.) Constipation for four days, (8.) The usual 8 o'clock A.M. stool does not take place until 2 P.M., and is then straining and slimy, (9.) Desire to go to stool, followed by an evacuation of hard substances, (13.) 460. Evacuation of a hard ball, followed by a pappy stool, (9.) Hard stool, (7.) Consistent but unsatisfactory stool in the forenoon; very copious evacuation an hour after dinner, (noon,) not fetid, with discharge of much flatus, which relieves him, (8.) Three soft stools during the day, mixed with round, solid matters, (7.) Pressing desire for stool on getting out of bed, followed by a pappy evacuation, and accompanied by much flatus, (6.) 465. Three soft stools, (12.) Two diarrhœic stools, (13.) Very hard stools, (13.) Several copious soft stools, (12.) Two copious stools on waking, (12.) 470. Daily stools, copious and pappy, (3.) Copious evacuation, contrary to his usual habit, (7.)

URINE.—**Bladder.** Alternations of cramps, coldness, and heat in the bladder, (16.) Pain in the bladder during the night, and fruitless desire to urinate, (24.) Excoriated, sore pain in the bladder, (2.) 475. Sensation of fullness and tension in the bladder, without desire to urinate, (5.) Sensation of fullness in the abdomen, especially in the vesical region, (12.) Pressure in the vesical region, with discharge of mucus from the vagina, (13.) She is obliged to make water very often after dinner, which, together with a pressure analogous to that which is experienced at the period, makes her think her bladder is diseased, (16.) Feeling of pressure and fullness in the bladder, extending toward the urethra, with constant desire to urinate, and frequent discharge of normally-colored and slightly acid urine, (3.) 480. Attack of pressure, tenesmus, and cutting pains in the bladder, during which the face becomes red, (24.) The pressure and pain in the bladder continue, even after the evacuation of the urine, (24.) Tenesmus of the cervix-vesicæ, (2.) Strong vesical tenesmus for making water, (24.) The tension in the bladder remains even after the discharge of the urine, (5.) 485. Very violent twisting pain in the neck of the bladder at 1 P.M., lasting a quarter of an hour, and not ameliorated by the discharge of urine or of flatus, (17.) **Urethra.** Burning in the urethra when urinating, (24.) Slight burning in the urethra when urinating at noon, (18.) The burning of the urethra continues, even after having urinated, (16.) The burning in the urethra and the titillation in the meatus cease after the discharge of clear, straw-colored urine; the sensation returns, however, several times in the day before urinating, (8.) 490. The burning in the urethra and swelling of the vulva continue for fifteen days, (16.) Very violent lancinating thrusts in the anterior portion of the urethra and glans, a long time after having urinated, when in bed at night; they force him to groan and cry out, and last a minute and a half, (5.) The pains in the uropoetic organs are more violent, especially the pain in the urethra when urinating; it is burning, and accompanied by a sensation as if a little stone were sliding along the urethra, (10.) Sensation in the anterior part of the urethra, twice before urinating, as if he were pricked with a blunted needle, (8.) Very violent lancinations along the urethra toward the glans, lasting several minutes, after the discharge of a deeper colored urine, (3.) 495. Transitory lancinations in the urethra toward the glans, two hours after having urinated, (3.) Painful drawing in the left side of the urethra, (24.) The meatus is so contracted and constricted that the urine flows very slowly, and as the vulva is excoriated, the burning is very violent, and lasts an hour, (16.) Pruritus in the meatus, (8.) Violent pruritus in the orifice of the urethra, (24.) 500. Pruritus and itching in the meatus, obliging him to rub it constantly, (11.) The titillation at the meatus comes on as yesterday, but the urine is less copious, cloudy, and yellow, (8.) **Urine.** Discharge of pale urine in a stronger jet, (17.) Irresistible desire to urinate; the urine was excreted in very great quantity and in a very powerful jet, (10.) Copious urination in a very powerful stream, three times between 5 and 7 P.M., (17.) 505. The urine, in issuing from the urethra of a female, does not form the usual jet, but runs down over the surrounding parts, (16.) Desire to make water several times during the day, (3, 10.) Frequent desire to urinate in the afternoon, (13.) Frequent desire to urinate, followed by discharge of very copious urine, sometimes with pain in the urethra; frequent emission of a clear and copious urine during the whole day, (3.) 510. Very frequent and copious discharge of pale urine, (17.) Very frequent discharge of urine, almost every hour in the afternoon, (17.) Frequent, but scanty discharge of urine, (3.) Very frequent emission of urine, (3, 8.) He woke twice from a desire to urinate; but the emission is difficult, slow in coming, and takes place with straining, (tenesmus of the bladder or cervix,) (20, 24.) 515. Night much disturbed by frequent discharges of urine, (11.) He is obliged, contrary to his usual custom, to rise and urinate during the night, (11.) Diminution of urine, (17.) The quantity of urine is diminished one half, (24.) Nocturnal excretion of urine diminished, (18.) 520. He commonly makes water eight times a day; the number is reduced to six during the proving, (24.) Exceedingly scanty urination at night, (18.) Violent desire to urinate; the urine excreted exceeds the quantity of fluid ingesta, (10.) Increased urinary excretion, (12.) Very much increased urinary excretion, (11.) 525. Urine at first normal in color; it then becomes citron-yellow, brown, and finally red, (24.) Frequent emission of a highly loaded urine, (15.) Frequent emission of pale. urine, (3.) He is obliged to urinate almost every hour; urine pale, aqueous, and inodorous, (11.) Copious discharge of pale, watery urine, (3.) 530. Frequent emission of a deep-colored urine, (2.) Urine excessively loaded, (15.) The urine becomes cloudy, and, during the last days of the proving, jumentous, (18.) Evacuation of a copious watery urine, of an alkaline smell, almost every hour, (11.) Scanty and infrequent urine, of an ammoniacal odor and very high color, (11.) 535. The quantity of urine is not increased, but it is deeper colored, cloudy, and has a cadaverous odor, (15.) The urine seems thicker and hotter than usual, when passing it at 9 P.M., (3.) Frequent and copious emission of pale urine, which seemed to be thicker than ordinary, like oil, (3.) Increased acidity of the urine, (24.) The urine is so acrid that it burns in passing; she perceives this burning to increase for several days, (16.) 540. The urine contains mucus in the form of filaments, clouds, and flocks, (18.) The urinary sediment is entangled in much mucus, (18.) The urine contains neither albumen, pus, nor blood, (24.) Excretion of urine, which deposits a lateritious sediment, (23.) The urine deposits a reddish sediment, of the color of brick-dust, which adheres to the vessel, (6.)

GENITAL.—**Male.** 545. Pruritus in the prepuce and meatus auditorius internus, (15.) Lancinating itching in the prepuce, (6.) Pruritus and itching on the prepuce and glans, (12.) Dull throbbing in the glans during the whole day, and, from time to time, tickling in the urethra, (15.) Pruritus around the glans, (24.) 550. Sensation of disagreeable heat in the glans and left testicle, (17.) A suppurating pimple on the middle of the penis, (18.) The pimple on the penis discharges a fluid on being squeezed, (18.) Violent pruritus on the scrotum in the morning after having quitted the bed, (9.) Drawings and transitory lancinations in the right testicle, which ascend toward the inguinal ring, (3.) 555. Extraordinary lasciviousness, (3.) Lasciviousness without erection, (5.) Excitement of the venereal appetite, (10, 15, 17, 18.) Very great sexual appetite on getting up, (8, 18.) Excessively violent sexual desire during the day, and voluptuous dreams during the following night, (10.) 560. Venereal appetite excited the first four days, afterward depressed, (11.) Diminished sexual appetite and yet a nocturnal pollution, (12.)

Pollution in the morning, (12, 17.) Moderate erection in the morning, with great lasciviousness, (5.) Great desire to urinate in the morning, with erection and longing for coitus, (5.) 565. Very frequent erections day and night, (24.) Erection and pollution toward morning, (9.) Erections in the morning which last longer than usual, (9.) **Female.** Sensation when walking as though the lips of the vulva were swollen, (16.) Pain in the vulva when going to bed so violent as to make her shed tears; she is obliged to sit up in bed, and goes to sleep in that position, (16.) 570. The swelling of the genital parts increases, but it is less troublesome in walking, because it is displaced toward the anterior part of the vulva, (16.) The excoriated feeling at the vulva is very violent in consequence of a continuous discharge of mucus, (16.) The vulvar tumor increases, becomes hard, and is sensitive to the touch, (16.) Throbbing and burning sensation in the vulvar tumor, and excoriated feeling when walking, (16.) The night is restless, but she is not waked by the vulvar pains, which do not come on until she has made water the next morning, (16.) 575. The tumor of the vulva diminishes, but on the other hand, the urine is discharged with difficulty, slowly and with burning pains, accompanied by lancinating thrusts in the excoriated portion, (16.) The menses appear three days too soon, (as they sometimes do,) but they are more than usually copious, (16.) The menses are three days too early, are more free, and the blood is black and thick, (13.) The menses are seven days too early; the blood very abundant, black, and thick, (13.) She feels a sensation on the fifth day of the catamenia, analagous to that which she sometimes perceives at their commencement; tension and constriction in the hypogastrium and something ascending to the stomach, which makes her think she shall vomit water, (16.) 580. Discharge of a liquid which has not the density of leucorrhœa, (16.) Discharge of mucus from the vagina, preceded by drawing and thrusting pains in the inguinal, vesical, and pubic regions, (15.)

LARYNX.—Rough feeling in the larynx all day; his voice after a long silence is hoarse, but it becomes clearer by talking, (8.) Rough feeling in the larynx when speaking and after having spoken, (3.) Pain and rough feeling in the larynx after a short conversation, (3.) 585. Tickling in the larynx, followed by hacking, (12.) Lancinations in the larynx from time to time, and hoarse voice, (15.) The scraping and dry feeling in the larynx are increased toward evening, and accompanied by hacking cough and hawking, (1.) Scraping in the larynx and trachea, with slight hoarseness in the evening, (23.) Scraping in the larynx causing cough, (23.) 590. Sensation of swelling in the larynx, with difficulty of speaking, (3.) Irritation in the larynx obliging him to cough, (5.) Acute prickings in the larynx, (3.) Scraping in the trachea toward evening, obliging him to cough, by which a copious amount of mucus is brought up in the shape of globules, (10.) Roughness in the trachea provoking a frequent cough, (7.) 595. **Hoarseness.** Hoarseness, (45.) Hoarseness sometimes greater, sometimes less, (1.) Persistent hoarseness,

(18.) Hoarseness all day, (7.) Hoarseness in the morning, (3.) 600. The hoarseness and scraping are never entirely absent, except in bed, where the heat produces a quieting effect, (11.) Hoarseness and scraping in the velum palati toward evening, (15.) The hoarseness and cough remain for several days; the expectoration increases, becomes grumous and grayish, (7.) Hoarse voice in the morning, with mucus in the throat, which obliges him to hawk, bringing up every time a little thick mucus, (8.) Constant hoarseness, with mucous expectoration, (8.) 605. Slight hoarseness and scraping in the throat, in the evening, (15.) Hoarseness and pressure on the chest, (2.) Voice constantly veiled, (8.) Veiled voice, deeper than natural, (3.) Weariness of the vocal organs; she becomes hoarse after a short conversation, and her respiration is a little embarrassed, (18.) 610. Fatigue of the vocal organs from speaking a little too long, (18.) His breath seems hotter to him than usual, with hot feeling in the chest, (7.) Warm breath, (3.) **Cough.** Frequent desire to cough and sneeze during the whole day, (5.) Short cough, (2.) 615. Short, dry cough, (4.) Short cough in the morning, with expectoration of thick mucus, (18.) Infrequent cough during the morning, some isolated coughs, (8.) Cough excited by a tickling in the larynx, which hinders sleep, (5.) He is inclined to cough, from a constant irritation in the trachea and larynx, which renders the velum so sensitive that swallowing food and saliva becomes very troublesome; these symptoms aggravated by beer, (7.) 620. Very violent cough, which, notwithstanding the expectoration of mucus, is constantly excited by a tickling in the neighborhood of the bifurcation of the trachea; the attacks go on increasing, (8.) Feeling of mucus ascending and descending in the trachea, causing tickling and cough, (8.) Fatiguing, painful cough on waking, caused by a tickling in the larynx, (18.) Attack of short cough, produced by a tickling in the larynx, in the forenoon, (18.) Dry cough in the morning, which lasts several minutes, and finally causes a vomiting of mucus, (5.) 625. The cough annoys him all day, and at 3 P. M., an hour after dinner, it is so violent as to vomit him, (8.) The cough is so violent as to cause vomiting, and the expectoration of a great quantity of thick, viscous, and albuminous mucus, (17.) Before he vomits from the violence of the cough, he endeavors in vain to quiet it by drinking a glass of cold water; but after having vomited, a second glass has the effect, (8.) Dry cough at intervals, (23.) Dry cough, (1, 19.) 630. Constant dry cough in the morning, (5.) Violent cough without expectoration, which lasts a long time in the morning, (5.) Alternations of dry and moist cough, (18.) Moist cough, small quantities of mucus are detached, (1.) Frequent cough, with expectoration of mucus, (17, 18.) 635. Frequent cough, with scanty expectoration during the day, (8.) Frequent expectoration of mucus after coughing during the whole day, (17.) The cough in the evening is accompanied by a much more copious expectoration of greenish mucus, tasting like licorice, (7.) Less frequent cough, with easy expectoration of a yellowish-white mucus mingled with saliva, (8.) Cough with expectoration of a yellowish mucus, accompanied by sneezings, (5.) 640. A little greenish-yellow mucus tasting like licorice, is detached by the cough, (7.) Paroxysm of short cough, with expectoration of globular mucus, (15.) Cough, with expectoration of globular mucus, (5.) Periodical attacks of cough and expectoration of mucus in the morning, (8.) Paroxysm of coughing produced by a tickling in the larynx and throat, (24.) 645. Paroxysm of coughing for half an hour, and expectoration of a great quantity of mucus, (15.) Attack of tickling at 7 P. M., producing a five-minute paroxysm of coughing, ending by an expectoration of mucus, (17.) Every attack of coughing is followed by a burning sensation lasting some time, (7.) Frequent hacking and hawking, with increase of thirst, (1.) Slight coughing in the morning, with expectoration of gray and globular mucus, (11.) 650. Cough in the morning, with easy mucous expectoration mixed with viscid filaments, (8.) Cough, which wakes him at 6 A. M., having remissions of a minute; it is at first clear, dry, and barking; subsequently some thick mucus is detached, and the effort of doing this causes desire to vomit, accompanied by an excoriated feeling in the throat and pressive headache, (8.) The cough wakes him at 1 A. M., in consequence of which and the burning, excoriating pain in the lungs, and pressive headache, he cannot go to sleep again; he does not sleep, except from 6 to 7 A. M., (7.) Frequent nocturnal cough, with expectoration, (7.) Dry cough wakes him twice in the night, (8.) 655. The cough is aggravated by the heat of the room, and diminished by staying in an unwarmed room, (17.) The paroxysm of coughing is renewed by the heat of the bed, (8.) He can scarcely speak for coughing in a warm room, (8.) He does not cough in the open air, although the temperature is cold, but the cough comes on as soon as he enters a warm room, (8.) The cough is ameliorated by gargling with cool water and swallowing a portion, which very much diminishes the heat of the throat; the cough afterward returns on drinking warm milk, but less violent, (8.) 660. Cleaning the teeth produces violent coughing, and, in consequence, vomiting of a liquid mucus, (5.) Tobacco-smoke, to which he is accustomed, excites cough, (5.) **Expectoration.** Frequent spitting of mucus, (5.) Copious and easy spitting of mucus in the afternoon, (12.) Great abundance of mucus in the respiratory organs, (10.) 665. Expectoration of a very thick mucus, (18.) Increased, sweetish, thick expectoration, (7.) Easy expectoration of pretty copious mucus, (1.) Frequent and easy expectoration of whitish mucus of the size of a pea, (3.) Expectoration of globular mucus, (18.) 670. After slight efforts of hawking, expectoration of a yellow globular mucus, (10.) Expectoration of a viscid mucus in the morning, (18.) Expectoration of easily detached mucus in the afternoon, (17.) Easy mucous expectoration in the morning, (18.) Expectoration of a great quantity of grayish mucus, (3.) 675. Expectoration of yellow mucus of an acid taste, (12.) Expectoration of a yellowish mucus, inclining to red, and of a bitter-sweet taste, (12.) Expectoration of a nauseating mucus, (12.)

CHEST.—Lancinating itching in the skin in the region of the right nipple, (6.) Lancinating itching in the skin of the pectoralis major and right groin, (6.) 680. Lancinating itching in the skin of the right clavicular region. Drawing pain in the right clavicular region, aggravated when lying on that side, (6.) Several rapid lancinations between the sixth and seventh ribs, first on the right, then on the left side, (12.) Acute stitches in the right half of the chest, when seated in the afternoon, along the sternum, and soon after some coughing with easy expectoration of globular, gelatinous, grayish mucus, (15.) Rapid lancinations in the region of the left nipple in the morning, after waking from a sound sleep; they soon disappear, and never return, (2.) 685. Violent, penetrating pains near the left nipple in the afternoon, and dull lancinations between the shoulders, extending in a radiating way towards the anterior part of the thorax, (15.) He wakes at 4 A.M. with a bruised pain in the left clavicular region, (6.) The bruised pain in the left clavicular region continues aggravated by moving the left arm, and terminates, when lying on the left side, in a strained pain, (6.) Transitory lancinations in the left clavicular region in the forenoon, (15.) Bruised pain in the region of the left clavicle, which seems dislocated during the movement of the head or left arm, or when lying on the left shoulder, (6.) 690. Tensive pain in the upper left side of the chest, near the clavicle, more severe in the daytime; it lasts several days, and is aggravated by moving the left arm, (15.) Acute, penetrating lancinations, followed by ulcerative pain in the upper part of the left chest, repeated for several days, several times a day, (1.) Lancinations in the left half of the chest, brought on or aggravated by fast walking, (15.) Lancinating pain in the left side of the thorax, and in a very circumscribed region, aggravated by walking, but not by a deep inspiration, (3.) Not very painful lancination in the middle of the first left false rib, coming on when walking in the street, and ceasing when sitting still in the room, (3.) 695. Pain in the left side of the thorax, extending toward the sternum, with pressive pain on the chest, (4.) Lancinations and itchings on the edge of the left false rib, deep between the stomach and the hypochondrium, (6.) Lancinating pain, short and very circumscribed, on the edges of the cardiac region, which on pressure resembles that which would be produced by an abscess, (6.) Burning and slight lancinations between the fifth and seventh ribs, first on the left, then on the right side, (12.) Frequently an acute lancination on the left side, between the fifth and seventh ribs, which dis appears on a deep inspiration, and comes on immediately on expiring, (12.) 700. Lancinations in the region of greatest curvature of the last left false rib, coming on when conversing, aggravated by walking and going up stairs, but not at all by a deep inspiration; ameliorated by rest, (4.) Dull pressure in the region of greatest curvature of the fifth and seventh ribs, repeated several times during the day, (15.) Several lancinations at the left vertebro-sternal angle of the last rib on the left side, rapidly repeated, (4.) Excoriated feeling at the apex of the left lung, with sensation of pulsation always alternating, with a contraction in the lower lip, (spasm of the orbiculorris,) (7.) Heat deep in the thorax; occasionally burning, especially in the region of the heart, (7.) 705. Transitory burning under the sternum in the forenoon, (18.) Excoriating and pressive pain below the sternum after the noon lunch, (18.) Painful pressure in the middle of the sternum in the forenoon, from before backward; at the same time an analogous pain between the scapulæ, from behind forwards, lasting but a little while, (15.) Pressure and burning below the xyphoid cartilage for a quarter of an hour, (18.) Sensation of pressure on the middle of the sternum, extending into the two scapulæ, (4.) 710. Sharp prickings in the integuments of the chest, (3.) Throbbings like strong pulsations, sometimes near the heart, at others in the middle of the chest, and again at the apex of the lungs, (7.) The throbbing in the chest becomes infrequent, and is succeeded by oppression and a sensation as if the thoracic cavity were too narrow; this lasts till evening, and is followed by chills and nocturnal perspiration, which relieve it, (7.) Throbbing feeling in the lungs, (7.) The feeling of heat in the chest disappears in a quarter of an hour, and is succeeded by a feeling of tension and pressure, and by pulsations at the apex of the lungs, (7.) 715. Sensation of heat in the lungs when walking, lasting half an hour, and disappearing suddenly, (7.) Sensation of heat during a long walk, in the chest, epigastrium, and thigh, accompanied by formications in the skin of the thigh, (7.) Heat in the interior of the chest, especially in the region of the heart, and in the inferior half of the thoracic cavity, (7.) Excoriated feeling at the apex of the lungs, accompanied by short-lived chills, notwithstanding the high temperature of the air, and followed by moderate headache, increased by walking, (7.) The excoriated pain in the chest is by turns dully lancinating, and seems to be seated in the pleuræ and pericardium; he sometimes feels it in the deep regions of the lungs and heart, and it seems to him that the pulsations of the heart, which accompany it, are stronger, (7.) 720. Excoriated pain in the chest below the clavicles, and very great fatigue of the respiratory passages, (10.) Paroxysms of excoriated pain and oppression in the whole chest, lasting an hour, and returning several times during the day, (15.) The excoriated and burning pain in the chest continues; it is accompanied by cough and hoarseness, (7.) The cough becomes harder in the evening, and very painful from the excoriated and burning pain in the chest, which follows it, (7.) The excoriated pain in the chest diminishes, as the expectoration becomes easier, (7.) 725. The pains in the chest gradually increase; the excoriated pain becomes burning, and frequently changes its position; it, nevertheless, most frequently affects the heart and the apex of the lungs, with necessity for deep respiration and cough, (7.) Feeling of weariness in the lungs, accompanied by lancinations in the middle of the sternum, which disappears after breakfast, consisting of burnt barley-coffee, (3.) Lancinations in the lower part of the thorax, (3.) Several rapid lancinations in the inferior part of the left chest in the morning, when walking in the street; they recur in the evening, (3.) Dull lancinating thrust in the right inferior pulminary lobe at 4 P.M., when breathing deeply, (17.) 730. Transitory painful lancinations in the thoracic cavity, sometimes on the right, sometimes on the left side, with oppression and dryness of the throat, (22.) Pressive and lancinating pain, which seems to be seated in the right inferior lobe of the lungs, when getting out of bed in the morning; it is particularly severe when inspiring deeply, but is not affected by motion; sneezing is impossible on account of the pain, which remains until noon, and then suddenly disappears. Pressing, weak and bruised feeling in the chest, (3.) Violent pressure on the chest in the evening, followed by an ulcerative pain about the heart, (15.) Pressive and cramp-like pain in the middle of the chest, (3.) 735. Pressive and fatigued feeling in the chest, (3.) Transitory rheumatic pain in the tendinous aponeuroses of the two forearms, and subsequently in the legs also, (18.) Pressure in the chest in the evening, accumulation of mucus in the air-passages, and almost unconquerable somnolence, (10.) Sensation of pressure on the chest, and increased sensibility around the left nipple, (2.) Difficulty of breathing in the afternoon, which increases toward evening, accompanied by paroxysms and lancinations in the upper part of the left chest, (15.) 740. Transitory oppression of the chest, followed by great moral exhilaration, (12.) Her breathing is a little more difficult than usual when walking, (16.) Oppressed respiration on getting up, (18.) Difficult respiration, oppression, (18.) Deep inspiration, and yawnings involuntarily performed, when walking, relieve, (7.) **Heart.** 745. Palpitation for several minutes, causing anxiety, (12.) Pulsations of the heart accelerated, irregular, and productive of anxiety, after dinner, (6.) The movements of the heart are irregular, at times very tumultuous, at others very labored, (11.) Tumultuous movement of the heart when lying down after dinner, and isochronous throbbings in the ear; radial pulse, accelerated, tremulous, (11.) Palpitations during the night, like those of the evening, but less, and accompanied by pressive pain in the heart, (10.) 750. He is waked during the night by a violent palpitation, which lasts a quarter of an hour; the back, sacral and coccygeal regions are bathed in sweat, (10.) Very violent palpitations, lasting twenty-five to thirty seconds, during a half sleep at midnight, as if from a terrible fright; they shook the whole body, and returned in gradually decreasing strength, (6.) The throbbings in the thorax are composed of five or six consecutive strokes, intermitting for five or ten minutes, and then reappearing in a different place, (7.) Violent chills and a hacking cough, excited by a rough feeling in the trachea, accompany the palpitations, while writing at 10 A.M., and are attended by confusion in the head, and increased nasal secretion, (7.) Sensation of a very accelerated arterial throbbing on the surface of the heart, recurring several times when walking, (7.) 755. The pulsation in the heart alternates with the prickings in the thigh, and with a feeling in the lower lip, as if it were drawn out, (7.) Throbbing pain in the heart, and from time to time pulsations on the surface of the heart, (7.) Transitory lancinations between the sixth and seventh ribs, first on the left side, then on the right, (12.) Dull lancinations through the heart, with throbbings which he thinks he can hear, but which are not confirmed by placing the hand on the spot, (7.) The pains in the heart and pericardium coincide with a pressive, tensive pain, sometimes in the stump of the left shoulder, sometimes in the joints of the left fingers and coxo-femoral articulation; it is never very severe, but is frequently repeated, and disappears towards evening, (7.) 760. Painfulness in the heart from morning till noon, (7.) The pain in the heart is felt during the day also, (10.) Indefinable pain in the heart, frequently interrupted by a pulsation, (7.) Digging and pressive pain in the region of the heart, appearing in the evening when riding in a carriage, and only ceases when he leaves the vehicle, (10.) Pressure in the cardiac and renal regions, (10.) 765. Feeling of an afflux of blood to the heart, (7.)

BACK.—**Nape.** Pressive pain in the nape, between the second and third cervical vertebræ, in the evening, (9.) Violent tension of the left cervical muscles on waking, disappearing on getting up, (18.) Lancinations in the muscles of the left side of the nape, when turning the head, (1.) Drawing and tearing here and there, especially in the neck, between the shoulders and on the forearms, (18.) 770. Lancinating pain in the muscles of the nape, (1.) **Back.** A very small pimple on the back, which discharges a great deal of thick pus, (18.) Pressure between the scapulæ, descending by degrees towards the sacrum, and becoming permanent in the renal region, accompanied by frequent paroxysms of oppression of the chest for six days, (15.) Lancinations in the region of the left scapula, extending to the olecranon, and aggravated by moving the arm, (4.) Lancinations in the scapulæ for two days, (4.) 775. Weak lancinating pain in both scapulæ several times in the day, (2.) Rheumatic pain in the scapula and sacrum, (5.) Violent rheumatic pain, extending from the right scapula over the anterior and external surface of the humerus, during rest at noon, (6.) **Loins.** Pressive pain in the renal region, extending by degrees to the bladder and its sphincter, accompanied by vesical tenesmus and frequent emissions of deep-colored urine, (2.) 780. The pain in the kidneys, accompanied by increased urinary secretion, lasts six or seven days, (11.) Dull pain in the renal region, (11.) Lancinating and boring pain in the region corresponding to the kidneys, in the evening in bed, lasting several seconds, (6.) Sudden, acute, prolonged lancinations, extending from the left renal region, along the ureters into the bladder, (15.) Pressive pain in the renal region, (15.) 785. Attacks of nephritic colic, but seldom, and not violent, (10.) Slight attacks of nephritic colic, urine very copious, and dull pain in the urethra, (10.) He jumps about, bends himself, and rubs his hypogastrium in order to relieve the spasmodic pain in the kidneys, and obtains some relief after some minutes, with discharge of much flatus, (10.) Excessively violent pain in the renal region seizes him suddenly when sitting quietly in the afternoon; it radiates from the two sides of the kidneys, and differs from the pressive and drawing pain previously felt there, by its spasmodic character and extension, and can only be compared to the pain experienced in the testicle in consequence of a bruise, (10.) The pressive pain in the kidneys is more violent than the preceding evening, and is alternated with the drawing pain, which extends through the ureters into the bladder; the latter is relieved by the discharge of flatulence, (10.) 790. Dull pressure in both kidneys during the whole day, especially in the right, aggravated by movements of the trunk, and by external pressure; it disappears in the evening, (10.) He wakes at 5 A.M., and can go to sleep no more; a drawing pain commences in the right kidney, and extends along the course of the ureters, as far as the bladder; at the same time a single lancinating thrust, and continual pressure in the urethra, in the navicular region, (10.) Slight pains in the sacrolumbar region, (12.) Bruised pain in the sacrolumbar and iliac regions, on waking, (6.) Bruised pain in the sacrolumbar region, in the morning, (6.) 795. Bruised pain in the left lumbar region, (6.) Pains in the lumbar vertebræ in the evening, increasing in intensity at night, (5.) Drawing pains in the sacrolumbar region, (12.) Tension and drawing, extending from the loins toward the rectum, (12.) Tension in the sacrolumbar muscles, (18.) 800. Violent pressure and drawing pain in the sacrolumbar region during the evening, (18.) Pain in the loins and sacrum in the evening, (12.) Two lancinating thrusts, beginning in the lumbar region and ending in the region of the cœcum, (12.) Pain in the loins and sacrum, in the evening, (13.) **Sacrum.** Pain in the sacrum, (5.) 805. Pressure in the sacral region, extending downwards and forwards towards the bladder, and lasting a quarter of an hour, (15.) Pain in the sacrum, lasting all the morning; it intermits for some time, and then reäppears, (18.) Violent pain in the sacrum, and pains in the hypogastrium for several hours in the afternoon, with a transitory feeling as though there were ulcerated spots there, (16.)

UPPER EXTREMITIES.—**Shoulders.** Cold feeling in the skin of the right shoulder, and dorsal surface of the same side, (1.) Weight and pressure in the right shoulder and along the lateral posterior side of the body, (11.) 810. Weight and tension across the shoulders and nape, which seems to be connected with the pains in the region of the spleen, (11.) Tension, drawing and tearing in the right shoulder and axilla, (12.) The pain in the left shoulder prevents his lying on the right side; it is relieved by lying on the affected side, and burying himself well in the bed, (11.) Slight drawing in the left shoulder, changing into weight, and in the evening into painful paralysis, such as is experienced when a part of the body in perspiration is exposed to a very strong breeze, (11.) Drawing and tearing in the right shoulder during the day, extending into the forearm and index, (12.) 815. The pain in the shoulder extends in the evening into the forearm, and becomes at times very violent, (5.) **Arms.** Slight rheumatic pain in the humerocubital joint, (2.) Disagreeable drawing in the right deltoid in the evening, rendering the motions of the arm painful, especially that of raising it. (17.) Lancinating and rheumatic pain in the internal fleshy part of the left humerus, lasting but a little while, (6.) Transitory rheumatic pain in the external side of the right humerus, in the evening in bed, (6.) 820. Painful drawing in the muscles of the right arm, (6.) Drawing rheumatic pain along the anterior surface of the humeral muscles during rest, (6.) **Elbow.** He wakes in the night with a pain in the olecranon and humerocubital articulation, which prevents his going to sleep again, (11.) Violent pressive pain in the neighborhood of the elbow-joint, at noon, (6.) Pain in the muscles in the bend of the elbow, (6.) 825. Lancination as from the bite of a leech in the bend of the left elbow, (6.) Violent lancination in the left olecranon and right patella, (6.) **Forearm.** Transitory tearing in the tendinous aponeuroses of the two forearms, in the forenoon; when it disappears, an analogous one appears in the legs, but soon vanishes, (18.) **Hands.** Painful drawings in the metacarpal bone of the right thumb, in the morning in bed, (6.) Paralytic pain in the joint of the right hand during the morning, (17.) 830. Lancinating itching on the back of the right hand, (6.) **Fingers.** Moving the thumb and compressing cause a very acute pain, (7.) The left thumb is swollen, and its movements embarrassed, (7.) Transitory rheumatic pain in the right little finger, and left great toe, during motion, (7.)

LOWER EXTREMITIES.—**Nates.** Lancinating rheumatic pain along the sciatic nerve, when at rest, descending from the left nates along the posterior and external surface of the thigh, (6.) 835. Sensitiveness of the tuberosity of the ischium to external pressure, and when remaining a long while seated, (1.) **Thighs.** Bruised pain in the thigh behind the great trochanter, appearing in the evening, lasting but a little while, reappearing and disappearing when walking, (9.) Great lassitude and weariness of the lower limbs, especially manifest in the calves, (11.) Itching in the lower limbs, forcing him to scratch, (9.) The bruised pain and painful lassitude of the lower limbs is in connection with the pain in the kidneys, and the increased urinary secretion, (11.) 840. Great weariness of the lower limbs in the afternoon, as long as he remains seated, but which disappears as soon as he goes out, (17.) Great fatigue of the lower limbs, and burning in the soles of the feet, after a short walk, (18.) The pains in the hip-joints and ischiatic tuberosities are very persistent, (1.) Lancinating, rheumatic pain in the hip-joint, particularly violent when rising from his seat, and from sudden motions, (1.) Painfulness of the thighs in the evening, as if after a long walk, (8.) 845. Drawing pain in the upper and external part of the left thigh, (6.) Rheumatic lancination along the internal muscles of the thigh in the heat of the bed, (6.) Sudden drawing along the anterior surface of the thigh above the knee-joint, in the right great toe and left thumb, at 8.30 P.M., (17.) Transitory rheumatic pain on the internal and anterior surface of the right thigh, in the morning in bed, (1.) Painfulness of both thighs along the track of the great vessels and nerves, (1.) 850. Pricking on the anterior surface of the thighs, analogous to the sensation experienced on drawing electric sparks from the body, (7.) The heat in the thorax, especially in the cardiac region and the arterial pulsation on the heart reäppear when the prickings in the thighs cease, (7.) The pricking in the thighs causes the thoracic symptoms to disappear, (7.) Formication on the anterior portion of the thighs in the afternoon, when walking, as if a hot stream were running over the skin; lasts ten minutes. **Knees.** Both knees and toes swollen and hot, after a long walk; the pain is pressive, entirely preventing motion, and though he was otherwise well, confining him to his bed, (7.) 855. Slight rheumatic pain in the knee-joint, (2.) A sudden lancinating and tensive pain in the bend of the left knee, in the afternoon when walking, so that he cannot extend his leg, and for several minutes he can scarcely walk, (15.) Dull lancinations in the poplileal region, extending along the left tendo Achillis, the dorsum of the right foot, then between the shoulders and the upper part of the left chest, where they do not remain more than an instant or two, (15.) Pain in the right patella, during a long walk, especially at its internal edge, increased by pressure and motion; in the evening he cannot move, (7.) Pressive pain in the left patella, (6.) 860. Violent lancinating thrust in the right patella, in the evening, as if from an electric spark, (6.) Violent lancination in the edge of the left patella, as if produced by an electric spark, (6.) **Legs.** Great burning and itching on the left leg, (18.) Itching on the legs, forcing him to scratch, (17.) Itching on the legs and left fingers, in the afternoon, (17.) 865. Attacks of momentary burning in the legs, (18.) Feeling of excoriation on the right tibia, (18.) Access of throbbing lancination in both legs; the pain suddenly disappears, and comes on in the upper part of the left chest, (15.) Lancinating and tearing pains, rather severe in the internal part of the right tibia, at noon, and slight burning at the anus, (18.) Weakness of the legs, in the evening, (15.) 870. Great weariness after a very short walk, and pain in the whole right leg, (18.) Grating pain in the bone of the tibia and olecranon, (18.) A pain in the lower half of the left tibia, which rises and descends, when quietly seated in the morning, (2.) Cramp-like drawing pain in the right calf, (1.) Rheumatic lancination along the muscles of the calf, (6.) 875. Cramp-like drawing in the calf, frequently returning, (1.) The cramp-like pains in the calves, shoulder, foot, and elsewhere, frequently return, and with varying strength, (1.) Itching on the legs above the malleoli, rising as high as the knees, towards noon, and returning in the evening to its first position; it lasts several days, and constantly increases, (9.) Transitory lancinations in the right leg, not far from the ancle, after dinner, (18.) Some pimples around the malleoli, (6.) 880. Violent lancinations in the right internal malleolus, (6.) Several sudden lancinations in the right internal malleolus, in the morning in bed, (6.) He cannot extend his foot without increasing the pain in the tendo Achillis, (8.) Crackling felt when placing the fingers upon the tendo Achillis when extending and flexing the foot, perceived for two days past, (8.) Going up stairs renders the tendo Achillis very painful, (8.) 885. The pain in the tendo Achillis becomes so violent, that he is obliged to keep his room; nothing can be seen, but it is a little sensitive to the touch, (8.) The pain in the tendo Achillis is aggravated by walking on the pavement in the street; he is obliged to limp; the foot is turned outwards, and he is obliged to stop from time to time to ease the pain, (8.) The pain in the tendo Achillis is seated, an inch above its insertion into the calcaneum, and is not accompanied by any perceptible external change of appearance; the tendon can be pulled and squeezed without pain, which is only felt when walking and extending the leg, (8.) Pressive drawing pain in the left tendo Achillis, only when walking or extending the leg, (8.) The pain in the tendo Achillis lasts ten days, (8.) **Feet.** 890. Pain as if from a sprain on the internal surface of the calcaneum, and in and around the ancles, when flexing the foot, (12.) Feeling of swelling in the articular surface of the tarsus, which impedes motion, (7.) Very violent sprained pain on flexing the feet, (12.) The left foot is painful when walking, (7.) Great weariness of the feet, and burning in the soles, after a very short walk, (18.) 895. Little lancinating shocks in the left sole, near the toes, (6.) Violent pain in the soles, when seated, especially in the anterior part, most of the time burning, and progressively diminishing until it disappears, (18.) Pruritus, itching, and drawing in and between the toes, (12.) Cramp in the right toes, (1.) Pressive pain in the great toe during a long walk, which increases to such an extent, that in the evening he cannot put his foot to the ground; he feels cold all over, which lasts some time in bed, (7.) 900. Acute prickings in the evening, sometimes under the nail of the right great toe, sometimes in the ends of the fingers, beneath the nails of the thumb and right index, (6.) Intolerable itching in the crease on the inferior surface of the left great toe, at noon, (6.) Prickings as though caused by fragments of glass, on the inferior surface and point of the left toe, (6.) Cramp in the last three toes of the right foot, when lying down, (1.) Very violent pain, in the forenoon, in a corn of the little right toe, which forces him to limp in walking, (18.)

SKIN. 905. Pimples on the forehead, sternum, and end of the nose, which dry up rapidly in two days, (9.) Two other pimples appear on the right side of the sternum, and one on the point of the nose, besides the two on the forehead of the day before, (9.) Disagreeable itching in different parts of the skin, (3.) Lancinating itching in various parts of the skin, (6.) Lancinating itching in the skin, even in the scalp, in the evening in bed, (6.) 910. Lancinations and very frequent itchings in different parts of the skin, the scalp, the external ears, the right side of the neck and nape, on the edges of the rami of the lower jaw, in the neighborhood of the nipples, on the back, pit of the stomach, in the axillary cavity, and bends of the groin; they disappear on getting out of the warm bed, (6.) Itching on the skin of the back and abdomen, and especially on the extensor side of the limbs, (1.) Acute lancinations in different parts of the body, especially in the glans, integuments of the abdomen, and of the head, (15.) Red spots and itching pimples in various parts of the body, (1.)

SLEEP.—**Yawning.** Desire to yawn and stretch the limbs, (pandiculation.) with tensive pain in the sacrum, (5.) 915. Inclination to yawning and stretching, (4.) **Sleep.** Somnolence during the day, (5.) Somnolence, weariness, and drawing pains in the limbs in the afternoon, (16.) Almost insurmountable drowsiness after dinner; he can scarcely keep himself awake; followed by great depression, (10.) Great drowsiness in the evening, (5.) 920. He goes to bed with his head greatly confused, and a general sensation of great debility, after having eagerly drunk a glass of beer, but cannot go to sleep before midnight, (8.) The feeling of painful paralysis, and the constrictive pain in the scalp, compel him to go to bed earlier than usual, where he experiences increased general heat, during which he goes to sleep, (11.) Excellent sleep during the whole proving, (12.) Quiet sleep, (1.) Quiet sleep in the morning, (5.) 925. Sound, but not refreshing sleep, (18.) Troubled sleep, restless night, (4.) Sleep disturbed by pain, (24.) Sleep disturbed by dreams, (9.) Sleep disturbed by vivid dreams; he wakes at 3 A.M. in a great agitation, with general dry heat; sleep interrupted the rest of the night; in the morning general perspiration, and his pulse descends from a hundred to its normal rate, (17.) 930. Sleep disturbed by dreams, and great dryness, with scraping in the throat, especially on the velum palati, (1.) Sleep disturbed by frequent waking, in consequence of vivid, disagreeable dreams, (17.) Sleep agitated the whole night, in consequence of a disappointment he had met with, (5.) Agitated sleep with sexual excitement, but without a sufficient erection, (5.) Sleep very agitated, full of dreamings; he cannot get to sleep again before 4 A.M., (11.) 935. Very disturbed night, sleeplessness, and feeling as if the whole body were swollen, (5.) Very agitated night; the external heat prevents him from sleeping, (7.) Night somewhat agitated and disturbed by a gurgling in the bowels, which is specially perceived when he lies on his right side, (11.) The first of the night good, but on waking, the mucous membrane of the buccal cavity and pharynx is dry, the tongue stiff and hot; he is in a hurry to drink cold water to moisten these parts, (5.) Sleep disturbed by shocks in a carious tooth, (1.) 940. Sleep interrupted by cough, (7.) He does not go to sleep until midnight; very much disturbed, and the least thing wakes him with a start and palpitation, (6.) Agitated sleep, troubled by a dry cough, (5.) After waking at midnight, it takes him an hour and a half to go to sleep again, (9.) Agitated night, he wakes at 4 A.M., (11.) 945. Drowsiness in the morning, disturbed by shocks in a carious right molar, (1.) Desire to sleep longer in the morning, (5.) Groaning in the night when asleep, (18.) **Dreams.** Numerous dreams, (6.) Dreams of disappointment, (6.) 950. Voluptuous dreams, (5.) Dreams of love-affairs and youthful passion, (3.) Very voluptuous dreams with pollution, a phenomenon extremely rare with him, (15.) Vivid dreams of platonic love, which he remembers, (15.) Vivid dream about syphilitic diseases, (6.) 955. Dreams that he is in company, and is afraid he shall fail in the etiquette and usages of society, (9.) Dreams of a great many people, and of anxiety to place some one in safety, (9.) Dreams of a great many people, palaces, churches, and love-affairs, followed by a weak pollution, (9.) Dreams which he forgets, (1.) Numerous dreams, but he cannot remember them, (9.) **Waking.** 960. Frequent waking in the night, with over-excitement, as if he had drunk very strong coffee, (7.) He wakes very early, and is very drowsy, (1.) Frequent waking in the night, with paralytic feeling in both thighs and in the left shoulder; afterwards pressure and dull lancination in the middle of the arm, with general heat, followed by perspiration, after which he sleeps again, (15.) He is waked at night at 12.30, by a tickling in the larynx, followed by a paroxysm of coughing for ten minutes, with expectoration of a great quantity of thick mucus; he cannot go to sleep under an hour, (17.) He wakes at 4 A.M., without any perceptible cause, and soon afterwards perceives a slight lancination under the left great toe, (6.) 965. She wakes two days in succession at 4 A.M., (4.) He wakes very early, (1, 5.) He wakes earlier in the morning than ordinary, (1, 15.) He wakes early in the morning at 6 A.M., with burning heatlong urethra, and an almost insupportable tickling in the meatus urinarius, (8.) He wakes at 6 A.M., and cannot go to sleep again, (9.) 970. He only sleeps six hours every night during the whole proving, (11.) He wakes in the morning earlier than usual, with a great feeling of malaise, (11.) He wakes at 5 A.M., contrary to his usual habit, remains some time wide awake, and then sleeps again until 7 A.M., (18.) He sleeps well, but is waked early by an oppression of the chest, which disappears after a hot breakfast, but appears agan soon afterwards, and inconveniences him from time to time for several days, (15.) Restless night, and on waking, headache, which is soon dissipated, (16.) 975. Headache, hoarseness, and roughness in the throat, on waking, (7.) His headache is better on waking at 7 A.M., but the affection of the chest continues unabated, (7.) He is waked by colic, followed by a diarrhœa, which relieves the colic, (12.) General depression when he awakes, (4.)

FEVER.—**Coldness.** Paroxysm of universal chilliness, (9.) 980. Frequent chills, (5.) Chills over the whole body, in the evening, (4.) Chills which run along the whole length of the spine, (1.) More or less chilliness during the day, moderately accelerated pulse, (17.) Chilliness between 3 and 5 P.M., cuttings in the hypogastrium, and discharge of much inodorous flatulence, (17.) 985. Chilliness, which lasts several hours after dinner, (17.) Chill after dinner, which descends from the shoulders along the arms, with a sensation as if the skin were about to separate from the flesh; this is repeated several times, but ceases during exercise in the open air, (9.) Chills over the whole body at 8 P.M., especially along the back, with thirst, (7.) Chilliness, accompanied by cough and sneezing, in the evening, (5.) Horripilations, which run over the whole body for half an hour, at 9 P.M.; pulse 100, (17.) 990. Horripilation, with heat in the head before going to bed, lasting for half an hour in bed, followed by general dry heat and sweat, which continues all night, and affords much relief; urine red, more scanty than usual, (7.) Feeling of extraordinary coldness, without chills. Transitory coldness runs over the limbs, followed by pressure at the stomach, (16.) Coldness during the whole day; she does not feel the heat of 25° Reau., (88° Fahr.,) (4.) He wakes in the morning with cold feeling in the feet and upper part of the body, (17.) 995. Increased coldness and thirst in the afternoon, (17.) Coldness with umbilical colic all the afternoon, followed by soft stools, (7.) General coldness in the evening, with lancinations and palpitations of the heart, and excoriated feeling in the middle of the chest, (7.) The ordinary covering is not enough to keep him warm in bed, (7.) **Heat.** Skin hot and dry, at night, (5.) 1000. Feeling of general increased heat in the evening in bed, (7.) Universal heat in the bed, (7.) **Sweat.** No sweat even, at night, (4.) Copious general perspiration in the morning, (7.) Slight moisture on the legs and feet in the morning, (11.) 1005. Sweat on the right leg, (18.) Violent sweat and general debility during a long walk. **Fever.** Slight febrile movement in the evening, (5.) Dry heat in the head, in the evening in bed, red face, and the rest of the body cold; by degrees the dry heat becomes general, lasts until midnight, and is followed by sweat on the upper part of the body only, which lasts until 5 A.M.; sleep disturbed and interrupted by pressive and throbbing headache, and by the pulsations of the heart, (7.) On the morning following the feverish night, the tongue is coated white, dry, as if it were excoriated, and the headache continues, (7.) **Pulse.** 1010. Pulse accelerated, 76 per minute, (4.) Great excitement of the circulation in the morning on waking; the arteries throb so powerfully, that he thinks he can hear them, (7.)

GENERAL.—Sensation of throbbings through the whole body, (7.) Great excitement, which does not cease even in the open air; it seems to him as if the arteries were throbbing more forcibly, with sensation of general heat. This state lasted for an hour after dinner, and disappeared when walking, (7.) Agitation and physical anxiety, (5.) 1015. Agitation and constant shivering, (5.) Great agitation during the whole day, (5.) Inexpressible agitation; notwithstanding the foul weather, he is obliged to seek the open air, when his agitation is quieted, (5.) Very great physical prostration; she cannot remember ever to have felt the like, (4.) General prostration, compelling him to keep his bed, (14.) 1020. Debility of the limbs during the day, head feels empty, and nose obstructed, (5.) Weariness, prostration, and great irritability after a short nap, (10.) Very great fatigue from the atmospheric temperature, which nevertheless is not very high, (18.) Great fatigue after a short walk, and painfulness of the right leg, (18.) Great fatigue and somnolence during the morning, (5.) 1025. Great fatigue and much yawning in the evening, (24.) She is fatigued, prostrated, and indisposed to labor during the whole day, (11.) He feels debilitated and fatigued after leaving the bed in the morning, and he cannot decide to do anything until after he has swallowed his coffee, (11.) Weariness so overpowering, that she is obliged to seat herself several times during a short walk, with headache, (4.) Painful lassitude of the limbs during the day, (5.) 1030. Drawing rheumatic lancinations, as if from splinters imbedded, coming on in the evening in the bed, on the slightest muscular effort; they appear, for example, in the arm from holding a book in the hand, (6.) Lancinating rheumatic pain in different muscles, (1.) Tearing in the long bones, (18.) Alternations of fatigue, and pains in the limbs, (16.) Great facility and lightness of all the voluntary motions, (4.) 1035. Voice hoarse, heat of the body increased, drawing in the leg and calves, great fatigue in the calves, and general feeling in the body as if it were stuffed. On touching any part of the body, at night, it seemed to him enlarged, (5.) Coma vigil at night; it seems to him as if his body had attained the enormous size of a bale of wool, (5.) The temperature of an apartment moderately warm, seems to him on entering it, insufferably hot, (3.) The headache and pains in the chest are assuaged by the movement of the carriage, but the cough remains, (7.) **Characteristics.** 1040. In general, the mucus in the throat, and the flatulency, are the most tenacious attendants among the effects of cochineal, (10.) The duration of the effects of cochineal does not correspond with their intensity, that is to say, even the violent symptoms produced by it do not last any great length of time, (11.) *Lachesis* mitigates the symptoms of cochineal.

JUST PUBLISHED

BY

WM. RADDE, 322 BROADWAY, NEW-YORK.

Guernsey's Homœopathic Domestic Practice. With full descriptions of the dose to each single case. Containing also Chapters on Anatomy, Physiology, Hygiene, and an Abridged Materia Medica. 1854. Third thousand. Bound, $1.50.

☞ Dr. Guernsey's book of Domestic Practice is a reliable and useful work. It is especially adapted to the service of well-educated heads of families.—John F. Gray, M.D.

Hahneman (Dr. Samuel).—The Lesser Writings of, collected and translated by R. E. Dudgeon, M.D. With a Preface and Notes by E. E. Marcy, M.D. With a beautiful steel engraving of Hahnemann, from the statue by Steinhæuser. Bound, one large volume (784 pages.) $3.

☞ This valuable work contains a large number of Essays of great interest to laymen as well as medical men, upon diet, the prevention of diseases, ventilation of dwellings, &c. As many of these papers were written before the discovery of the Homœopathic theory of cure, the reader will be enabled to peruse in this volume the ideas of a gigantic intellect, when directed to subjects of general and practical interest.

"The Lesser Writings MUST BE READ by every student of Homœopathy who wishes to become acquainted with the *Master*-mind."—R. E. Dudgeon, M.D.

Hahnemann (Dr. Samuel).—Materia Medica Pura. Translated by C. J. Hempel, M.D. 4 vols. Bound, $6.

Hahnemann (Dr. Samuel).—The Chronic Diseases, their Specific Nature and Homœopathic Treatment. Translated and edited by C. J. Hempel, M.D. With a Preface by C. Hering, M.D., Philadelphia. 5 vols. Bound, $7.

Hahnemann (Dr. Samuel).—Organon of Homœopathic Medicine. Third American edition, with improvements and additions from the last German edition, and Dr, C. Hering's Introductory Remarks. Bound, $1.

☞ The above four works of Dr. Samuel Hahnemann are, and will for ever be, the greatest treasures of Homœopathy ; they are the most necessary works for Homœopathic Practitioners, and should grace the library of every Homœopathic Physician.

Hartmann (Dr. F).—Acute and Chronic Diseases, and their Homœopathic Treatment. Third German edition, revised and considerably enlarged by the author. Translated, with additions, and adapted to the use of the American profession, by C. J. Hempel, M.D. 4 vols. $5.75.

Hartmann (Dr. F).—Diseases of Children, and their Homœopathic Treatment. Translated, with notes, and prepared for the use of the American and English Profession, by Charles J. Hempel, M.D. 1853. Bound, $2.

Jahr (Dr. G. H. G).—Diseases of the Skin; or, Alphabetical Repertory of the Skin-Symptoms and External Alterations of Substance; together with the morbid phenomena observed in the glandular, osseous, mucous, and circulatory systems, arranged with pathological remarks on the diseases of the skin. Edited by C. J. Hempel, M.D. 1850. Bound, $1.

Jahr's (Dr. G. H. G.) and Possart's New Manual of the Homœopathic Materia Medica, arranged with reference to well-authenticated observations at the sick bed, and accompanied by an Alphabetical Repertory, to facilitate and secure the selection of a suitable remedy in any given case. Fourth edition, enlarged by the Author. Symptomatology and Repertory. Translated and edited by C. J. Hempel, M.D. 1853. Bound, $3.50.

Douglas (Dr. J. S).—Homœopathic Treatment of Intermittent Fevers. 1853. 38 cts.

Humphreys (Prof. Dr. F).—The Cholera and its Homœopathic Treatment. Bound, 38 cts.

www.ingramcontent.com/pod-product-compliance
Lightning Source LLC
LaVergne TN
LVHW011148110826
845150LV00006B/1189

* 9 7 8 1 4 2 5 5 4 6 6 2 5 *